W9-CUF-268

Secretarial
Dental Assistant

Secretarial Dental Assistant

Mary Ann Douglas, CDA

Claire Williamson, Technical Consultant
Angela R. Emmi, Series Editor

COPYRIGHT © 1976
BY DELMAR PUBLISHERS INC.

All rights reserved. No part of this work covered by the copyright hereon
may be reproduced or used in any form or by any means—graphic, electronic,
or mechanical, including photocopying, recording, taping, or information
storage and retrieval systems—without written permission of the publisher.

LIBRARY OF CONGRESS CATALOG CARD NUMBER: 75-19522
ISBN: 0-8273-0349-1

Printed in the United States of America
Published simultaneously in Canada
by Nelson Canada,
A Division of International Thomson Limited

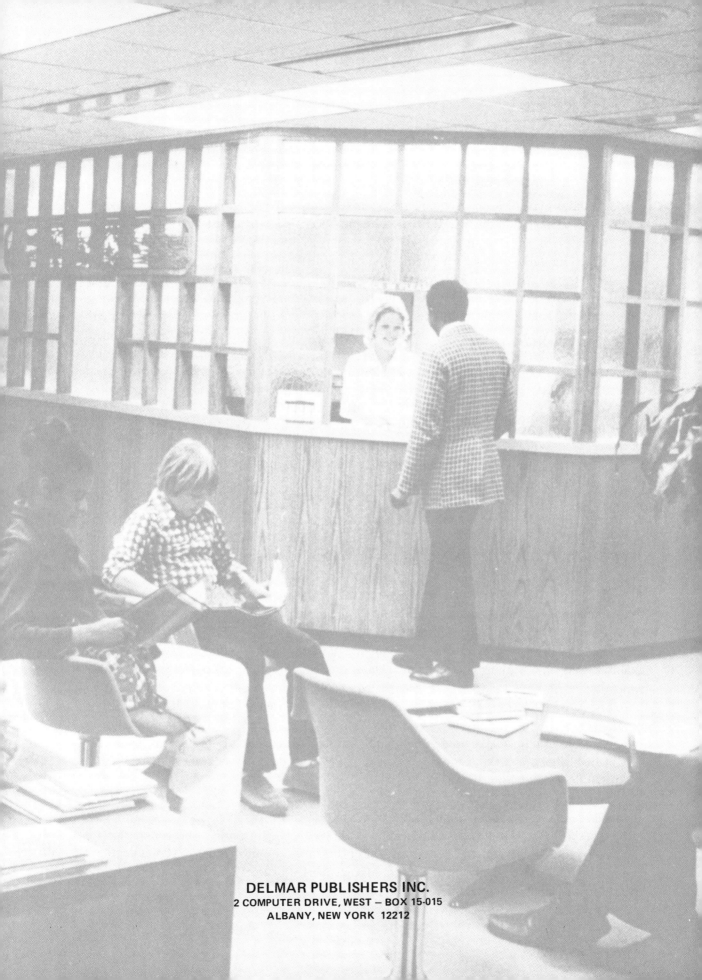

DELMAR PUBLISHERS INC.
2 COMPUTER DRIVE, WEST — BOX 15-015
ALBANY, NEW YORK 12212

Preface

The role of the modern dental assistant involves the performance of a variety of duties in the dental office. Although some dentists employ only one person in the office to assume a complete scope of duties, many dentists employ a chairside assistant and a receptionist-office manager. In any case, it is essential that every dental assistant have a workable knowledge of the secretarial duties performed in the dental office.

At one time, it was possible to walk into the business area of a dental office and find only one dental auxiliary employed sitting at the desk, answering the telephone, making appointments, and greeting the patients. The dentist would be observed in the treatment room working alone. This is no longer the true picture of auxiliary dental personnel.

The modern dental office involves a team approach. The dentist and his chairside assistant utilize two or more treatment areas; the hygienist works in a separate treatment area. A second assistant, called a "roving" assistant, is employed to move among treatment areas, dark room, laboratory, and business office. Sitting at the front desk, a dental assistant is performing various office tasks. This assistant must function as typist, file clerk, receptionist, bookkeeper and office manager. This is the secretarial dental assistant.

The course objective of a dental assisting program is to provide the student with opportunities for learning to function as assistant to the dentist in any routine operative, laboratory, or office procedure. The specific aim of this text is to provide the dental assisting student with information that enables her to perform procedures and practices in dental office management. Many texts have been written on the subject of dental management; however, *SECRETARIAL DENTAL ASSISTANT* places emphasis on the *tasks and the patient* rather than specific items.

Since dental assisting programs recognize the desirability of accreditation status from the American Dental Association, guidelines set up by the Commission on Accreditation of the ADA were used in the preparation of this text.

Unit objectives are presented at the beginning of each chapter so that the student knows exactly what she is expected to learn. Questions and practice sheets, forms and other educational aids serve to teach and test procedures which involve the patient and the staff.

The *SECRETARIAL DENTAL ASSISTANT* may be used in a formal dental assisting program or as a self-instructional text for home study. The only prerequisite is knowledge of typing. A list of terms often used in the dental business office and miscellaneous charts that should enable the student to be more proficient at the front desk of the modern dental office are distributed throughout the text.

The author, Mary Ann Douglas, has years of experience as a secretary, hygienist, chairside dental assistant and as instructor of dental assisting programs. She has served as an officer of both local and state associations of the ADAA. Currently, she is department chairman and instructor of the dental assisting program in a junior college. Her education, experience and active involvement in the advancement of careers in dental assisting contribute to the all-inclusive features of this book.

Contents

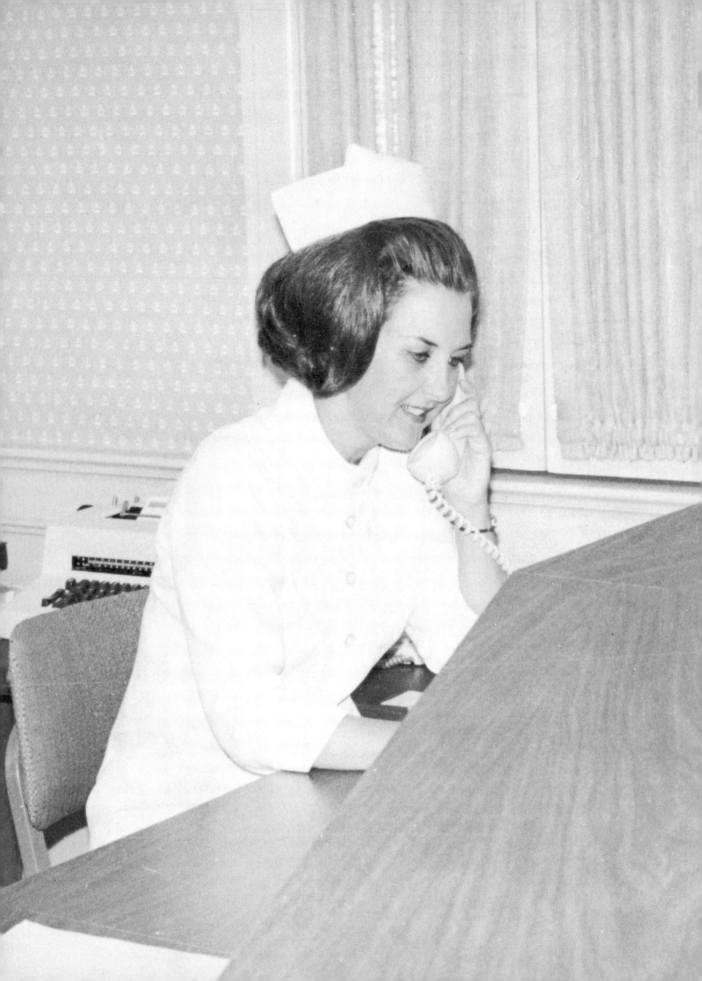

section 1

The Health Team in the Dental Office

Unit 1 Dental Auxiliary Responsibilities

OBJECTIVES

After studying this unit, the student should be able to

- List the duties of a dental hygienist.
- List procedures done by a dental laboratory technician.
- State the duties of a chairside assistant.
- Define the duties of a secretarial dental assistant.

In 1885, Dr. Edmond Kell employed one of the first lady dental assistants in New Orleans, Louisiana. He did not realize that this would be the beginning of a health occupation which would become a tremendously rewarding career. In the United States, dental assisting is one of the most challenging of the health fields.

The first dental assistants could have been called "dental greeters" for their duties implied this title. They greeted the patients, took their wraps, and seated the patients in the dental chair. Today, one or more persons are employed in the modern dental practice to make up the dental health team. In many offices the dental team includes a dentist, a hygienist, one or more chairside assistants, a secretarial dental assistant, and sometimes a dental laboratory technician. If only one dental auxiliary is employed, she acts as a general dental assistant performing varied duties. This includes duties at the front desk, in the treatment area (sometimes called the *operatory*), and in the laboratory. If two assistants are employed, one works at the chair and in the laboratory. The second assistant becomes the receptionist-bookkeeper-office manager. This assistant is often called the secretarial dental assistant. Occasionally where more than two assistants are employed, duties are rotated at different periods between the assistants or definite working assignments are delegated by the dentist.

DENTAL HYGIENIST

The dental hygienist is usually employed specifically to perform *prophylaxis* (cleaning teeth), take radiographs, take impressions for study models, and teach dental health education to the patient. Teaching the patient involves much more than the statement implies. It includes instruction in personal oral hygiene, postoperative measures, and demonstrations to the patient concerning the value of various dental procedures. This is such a broad area that often a dentist will employ a hygienist for the sole purpose of teaching the patient how to care for his teeth. In many offices, the hygienist is also responsible for keeping a recall system. This system is used to call back patients at regular intervals for prophylaxis and examinations. Although the hygienist usually works alone in the treatment area, she is under the supervision of the dentist.

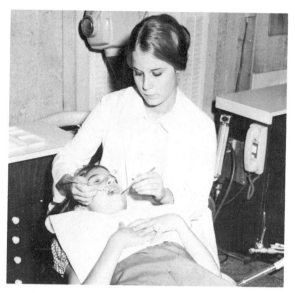

Fig. 1-1 Dental hygienist performing a clinical examination.

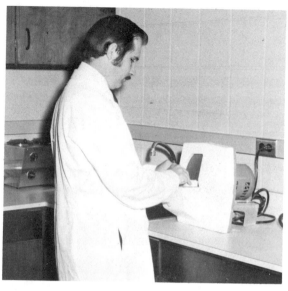

Fig. 1-2 Dental Laboratory Technician trimming a model in a dental laboratory.

It is required that the dental hygienist possess a license in the state in which she resides. The Dental Practice Act of each of the fifty states specifies the requirements. In most states, the hygienist must complete at least two years in an accreditated dental hygiene school before taking the state board examinations. Passing the state boards makes it possible for the hygienist to practice dental hygiene in the state and to use the initials RDH (Registered Dental Hygienist) after her name.

DENTAL LABORATORY TECHNICIAN

The dental laboratory technician is responsible for the laboratory procedures requested by the dentist. The technician performs these procedures after a written work order is prepared by the dentist. These procedures include making dental appliances, casting inlays, crowns and bridges, fabricating (making up) artificial dentures, and many other paraprofessional duties in the laboratory not performed by the dentist. Since about 90% of the dentists in the United States do not have a dental laboratory technician in their office on a fulltime basis, the laboratory work is usually sent to a commercial laboratory.

It is an advantage for the technician to be *certified*. This means that the technician has had a minimum of two years in training and is entitled to use the initials CDT after his or her name. The technician may train as a generalist (one who does all procedures in the laboratory) or as a technician in either full denture, partial denture, ceramics or crown and bridge.

CHAIRSIDE ASSISTANT

The chairside assistant performs most of her duties at the dental chair. They include preparing for the patient, helping in the required dental procedure, dismissing the patient from the dental chair, and sterilizing the equipment and instruments used during the patient's treatment. The procedures at chairside will range from routine examinations to oral surgery. The chairside assistant foresees every need of the dentist and provides him with the materials and instruments needed for each procedure. When four-handed dentistry is used, the assistant will remain seated at the chair

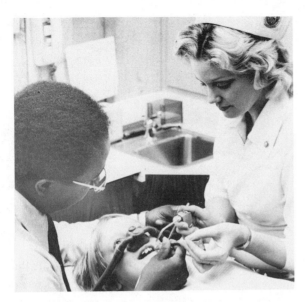

Fig. 1-3 Chairside Dental Assistant and dentist.

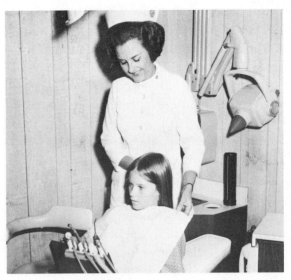

Fig. 1-4 A roving dental assistant preparing a young patient for dental treatment.

during the entire procedure. The seated assistant places instruments in the order they are to be used, keeps the operating field clear during treatment, prepares restorative materials and dental cements, and passes materials and instruments to the dentist.

If a second chairside assistant is employed, she acts as a "roving" assistant. As the name implies, this assistant moves among treatment area, front desk, laboratory, supply area, and dark room. This arrangement makes it possible for the chairside dental assistant to remain seated during the entire procedure being performed. The duties of the "roving" assistant include tasks such as seating the next patient, bringing needed materials to the treatment area, passing messages along, working in the laboratory, and processing X rays. Generally, the "roving" assistant performs any task that frees the seated chairside assistant to remain with the dentist.

It is not required that the chairside assistant be licensed at the present time. However, it is an advantage to both the dentist and the assistant for the chairside assistant to by certified by the American Dental Assistants Association. Eligibility to take the certi-

fication examination offered by the Certifying Board of the American Dental Assistants Association requires graduation from an accredited dental assisting school. Accreditation of a dental assisting school is granted by the Commission on Accreditation of the American Dental Association after it is determined by the Commission that the school meets required specifications. There are other ways to meet the requirement of graduation from a formal accredited program: (1) a person may enroll in a nationally accredited correspondence program or (2) the person with five years of dental assisting experience may challenge a series of tests given by the nationally accredited correspondence school. The names of accredited programs in dental assisting can be obtained from the American Dental Assistants Association. A dental assistant who is currently certified may use the initials CDA after her name and wear the certified emblem on the left side of her cap.

SECRETARIAL DENTAL ASSISTANT

All of the responsibilities delegated to the secretarial dental assistant must be carried out efficiently if a successful dental practice is maintained. The image that is created in the business area by the secretarial dental assistant may be the one thing that determines whether the patient returns or not. Even a hastily written appointment card can create an unpleasant image. The simplest task done in the business area should be performed well.

The secretarial dental assistant is the business manager of the dental office. She is responsible for the smooth operation of the office. Her duties include greeting and dismissal of the patient, making appointments, handling telephone calls, correspondence and records, bookkeeping, maintainance and operation of office machines, and ordering supplies.

Receptionist Responsibilities

Since approximately 90% of all dental patients make their first contact with the office through the secretarial dental assistant, it is important that these duties be performed intelligently, promptly, and tactfully. The dentist does not have time to directly supervise all that goes on at the front desk; he must depend on the secretarial dental assistant to act as a go-between in matters concerning himself and the patient.

Patients, visitors, and salesmen should be greeted promptly and pleasantly. No one likes to go into a reception room (use of the word "waiting room" is discouraged) and wait for someone to decide to greet him. If the new patient has to wait unnecessarily before he is greeted, he may wish he had gone elsewhere. Most people like to hear the sound of their name; greet them by name, and if possible, inform the patient when the dentist will see him. For example, "Good morning, Mrs. Jones. Dr. Simmons will see you in about five minutes."

Salesmen and visitors to the office should be greeted with the same courtesy as patients. Remember that wearing a smile when you

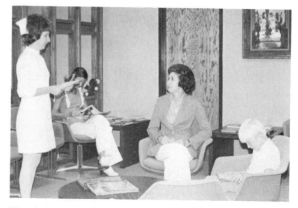

Fig. 1-5 Secretarial dental assistant greets a patient in the dental reception area.

answer the door will help to put the caller at ease. The secretarial dental assistant should converse pleasantly but not excessively with the patient or visitor. As soon as practical, the dentist is informed of the presence of the patient, visitor, or salesman. Since many salesmen are likely to call on the dental office, the person answering the door should know the dentist's policy about seeing salesmen. Usually the dentist will see only about two dental supply salesmen on a regular basis. These salesmen should be recognized and promptly informed of how long they must wait before the dentist can see them. Occasionally a salesman whom the dentist does not wish to see will call. This type of caller should be informed promptly and pleasantly that the dentist is with a patient and will not be able to see him today. Usually this satisfies the caller.

The new patient is requested to fill out a registration form and a personal health record. The forms should be attached to a writing surface such as a clipboard. A sharpened pencil or a ballpoint pen should be attached to the writing surface either by a string or a chain. If the forms are not self-explanatory, it will be necessary for the secretarial dental assistant to help the patient to complete them. It may be necessary to explain to the reluctant patient the importance of the health record. Many laymen do not understand the correlation between the oral cavity and the physical state of the body.

Making Appointments

Similar to handling telephone calls, making appointments should be the responsibility of *one* person in the office. This will minimize confusion. A systematic method of making appointments should be worked out by the dentist and the secretarial dental assistant. Although most patients make appointments by telephone, many appointments are made when the patient is in the office. They may be on a treatment visit to the office or they may drop by just for the purpose of making an appointment.

The appointment book is a vital item in any professional practice. Failure to record appointments properly will result in confusion and increase the possibility of error and poor patient relations.

Dismissing the Patient

After treatment of the patient, the chairside assistant usually brings the patient to the secretarial dental assistant. At this time payment for services just rendered will be accepted unless the patient has already made prior arrangements to be billed at the end of the month. Office policy regarding payment for services will determine which method is to be used. It may be necessary to make an appointment with the patient to return for dental care; if an appointment has already been made, the secretarial dental assistant should confirm the date and time of the appointment. After necessary bookkeeping is completed, the secretarial dental assistant dismisses the patient. This is accomplished by saying something like, "Good-bye, Mrs. Jones. Thank you for visiting our office." Remind the patient of umbrellas, coats, or other accessories that have been placed on the coat rack or in the closet. Remember, a cheerful dismissal leaves the patient with a pleasant image of his visit to the dental office.

Handling Telephone Calls

It is recommended that only one person handle all the incoming calls to the dental office. Only confusion can result if several auxiliary personnel are allowed to answer the telephone. Suggested messages on handling various patient inquiries should be mentioned to the secretarial dental assistant at the beginning of employment to avoid confusion. The office philosophy of the dentist should be reflected in these messages. (This will be covered at length in unit 4). Most outgoing calls are also handled by the secretarial dental assistant. This includes reminding patients of appointments, filling changed appointments, calling delinquent accounts, and making calls of both a business and personal nature for the dentist. In the absence of a hygienist, recalling patients by telephone will be the responsibility of the secretarial dental assistant.

Receiving Incoming Mail

Incoming mail is usually received by the assistant at the front desk, is sorted and placed in its proper place. The dentist should tell the secretarial dental assistant at the beginning of employment how he wants the mail handled. Personal mail should be placed unopened on the dentist's desk where he can easily find it. All other mail should be opened by the assistant and sorted according to several categories; these categories will be discussed in more detail in unit 20.

Incoming mail receives immediate attention. There may be urgent messages from patients regarding treatment or appointments or important announcements from professional individuals or organizations.

Bookkeeping and Other Records

Although some bookkeeping responsibilities are completed at the end of the patient's office visit, most bookkeeping procedures are performed during the course of the working day. Listed below are some specific responsibilities of the bookkeeper.

- Prepare daily work schedule.

- Make changes on work schedule immediately.

- Fill out all records completely, accurately, and neatly.

- Make entries on patient's record card and log book.

- Complete the summary in the log book at the close of each day and each month.

- Reconcile bank statements.

- Handle all financial transactions.

- Complete all county, state, and federal forms.

- Prepare and mail statements to the patient.

- Give estimates to patients when requested by the dentist.

- Maintain cancellation list.

- Fill out insurance, military, and credit card forms.

- Handle incoming and outgoing mail.

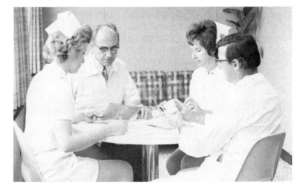

Fig. 1-6 The dental team participating in a staff conference.

Written Communications and Filing Responsibilities

The employee who has the responsibility of handling correspondence and records must understand the importance of filing accurately. A good filing system in the dental office will make it possible for the secretarial dental assistant to locate patient or business records within a matter of seconds.

SUMMARY

The secretarial dental assistant, dental hygienist, laboratory technician, and other dental assistants all work together with the dentist as a team whose goal is to give the very best of dental care to the public.

SUGGESTED ACTIVITIES

- Examine an office manual which is used in a private dental office. List the duties specified for each of the auxiliary personnel.

- Interview a secretarial dental assistant. Ask her to describe her responsibilities. Make a list of the duties she describes during the interview.

REVIEW

A. Indicate what is meant by the following words and abbreviations.

1. R.D.H. _____

2. C.D.T. _____

3. Generalist _____

    4. C.D.A. _____

    5. ADAA _____

    6. Roving assistant _____

B. Briefly answer the following questions.

    1. Name four members of the dental health team. _____

    _____

    2. What members of the dental team are required to possess a license to practice in the dental office? _____

    3. (a) What examination is offered by the American Dental Assistants Association? _____

       (b) What is required of those who wish to take this examination?

       _____

    4. What organization is responsible for accreditation of dental assisting schools? _____

    5. Are dental assistants required to have a license? _____

    6. List two other ways to become eligible for the certification examination, besides graduation from a formal accredited school.

    _____

    _____

C. Briefly answer the following.

    1. The technician may train in one of five areas. Name them.

    _____

    _____

    _____

    2. List four specific duties performed by the dental hygienist.

       a. _____

       b. _____

       c. _____

       d. _____

    3. List five duties usually performed by the chairside assistant.

       a. _____

       b. _____

       c. _____

       d. _____

       e. _____

D. Select the appropriate number from Column I to identify the dental auxiliary who performs the duties listed in Column II.

Column I

1. Secretarial Dental Assistant
2. Dental Hygienist
3. Chairside Assistant
4. Roving Assistant
5. Laboratory Technician

Column II

_____ Performs prophylaxis
_____ Makes artificial dentures
_____ Passes materials and/or instruments to the dentist
_____ Relays messages to chairside
_____ Greets patients and visitors upon arrival
_____ Handles all financial transactions
_____ Teaches dental health education
_____ Keeps operating field clear and dry during treatment.

E. Select the *best* answer.

1. Receptionist duties should be performed intelligently, promptly, and tactfully because

   a. this will guarantee a raise in salary periodically.
   b. 90% of the patients make their first contact with the office through the secretarial dental assistant.
   c. patients will not pay their bills if the receptionist's duties are not fulfilled.

2. When greeting salesmen of dental supplies and equipment, the secretarial dental assistant should

   a. inform all salesmen that the dentist is too busy to see them.
   b. insist that the dentist see all of the salesmen.
   c. inform the salesman promptly if the dentist can or cannot see him and state the approximate waiting time.

3. It is suggested that only one person be allowed to answer the telephone because

   a. confusion may result if several people are given this responsibility.
   b. only the chairside assistant would know how to answer the patient's questions.
   c. the dentist is paying the telephone bill and should handle all incoming calls.

Unit 2 The Office Environment

OBJECTIVES

After studying this unit, the student should be able to:

- Describe appropriate appearance for a secretarial dental assistant.
- Name the environmental factors that may affect reactions of dental patients.
- Prepare a task list to use in maintaining the reception area, business office, and private office.

The impression that a patient has of a dental office is often related to the auxiliary personnel. Since the patient's first contact with the office is usually with the secretarial dental assistant, it is important that this assistant project a good image. This unit discusses the attitude and appearance of the secretarial assistant, and the general decor of the office.

Many patients identify more quickly with the secretarial dental assistant than with the dentist. This assistant acts as a link between the dentist and the patient; therefore, a pleasing personality is extremely important. A cheerful smile on the face of the assistant greeting the patient will help to relieve any anxiety. A soft spoken, "Good morning, Mrs. Jones," will help to make the patient feel secure. Try to always call the patient by name if possible. If the name is not known, greet the patient with, "Good morning. May I help you please." He will give the reason for the visit and usually the name. If the name is not given, it will be necessary to ask. "May I please have your name," is an informal and acceptable inquiry.

The secretarial dental assistant should converse pleasantly and briefly with the patient. A good guide to follow is to talk about the patient rather than oneself. Keeping up with events of the community by reading the local newspaper will help the assistant to converse with the patient. The patient's particular interests may be written in an inconspicuous place on his or her record. Checking this note before the patient's next visit will help the assistant to show and develop a sincere interest in the patient.

APPEARANCE OF THE SECRETARIAL DENTAL ASSISTANT

The dentist decides whether the secretarial dental assistant will wear a uniform or street clothes to work. If she is certified, the dental assistant may want to wear the approved ADAA uniform for clinics as shown in figure 2-1.

Wearing white clothing demands cleanliness. A freshly laundered uniform should be worn daily. Shoes should be cleaned with saddle soap, allowed to dry, and polished daily with white polish. A piece of cheesecloth slightly soaked with alcohol will remove ugly black marks from both leather and vinyl shoes. Extra shoestrings may be purchased very inexpensively. It is wise to just discard soiled shoestrings and replace with new ones. If street hose are worn instead of white hose, they should be natural in color.

Soft fragrances are permissible but effort should be taken to avoid those which may be offensive to others. Makeup should be worn sparingly. Heavy eye makeup is for night-

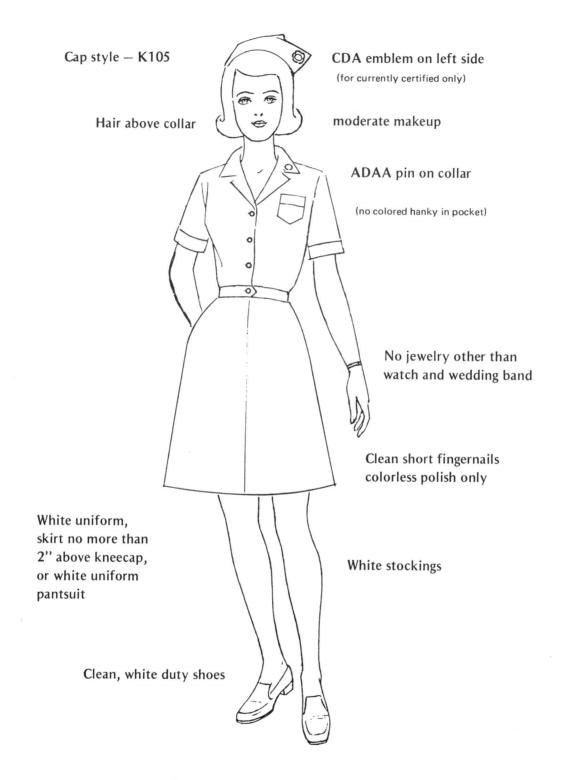

Cap style — K105

CDA emblem on left side
(for currently certified only)

Hair above collar

moderate makeup

ADAA pin on collar

(no colored hanky in pocket)

No jewelry other than
watch and wedding band

Clean short fingernails
colorless polish only

White uniform,
skirt no more than
2" above kneecap,
or white uniform
pantsuit

White stockings

Clean, white duty shoes

Fig. 2-1 Approved ADAA Uniform for Clinics
(Courtesy of *The Dental Assistant,* Journal of the American Dental Assistant Association)

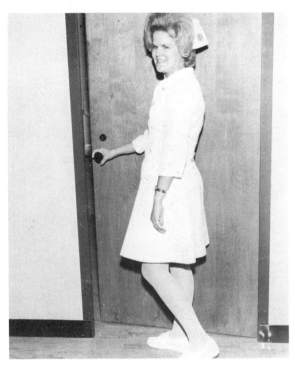

Fig. 2-2 This assistant presents an attractive appearance in her attitude and dress uniform.

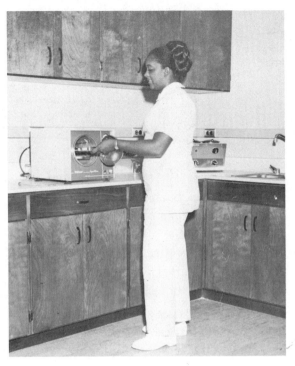

Fig. 2-3 A pantsuit uniform can be comfortable and attractive.

time wear and should not be worn with a uniform. Fingernails should be kept well manicured, relatively short, and polished only with a clear or natural polish, if any.

Hair must be worn in an attractive and easy-to-keep style. Elaborate hair styles are not correct for a professional office. Preferably, the hair should be above the collar. If the hair is longer than the collar, it can be arranged neatly in one of the many upsweep styles; this hair style for long hair is more professional looking. If the secretarial dental assistant must work at chairside, it is necessary to wear the hair in a style above the collar for safety and sanitary reasons.

Jewelry should be kept to a minimum. Only a watch and wedding band is worn with the uniform. Bracelets, necklaces, and dangling earrings are not appropriate or safe; since they cannot be cleaned properly, they may harbor or attract bacteria. Some materials used in the dental office (like mercury) may damage jewelry. Dangling jewelry may present

a problem by catching on equipment or instruments. If the ears are pierced, a small pearl or diamond stud earring may be permissible.

The decision of whether to smoke or not at the front desk is up to the dentist. If the secretarial dental assistant must smoke, this may be done in the employee's lounge. Smoking may be offensive to the non-smoker; it should not be done as, among other things, the stale odor remains on the clothing. More importantly, it is a health hazard to the person who does not smoke as well as to the smoker.

Chewing gum is unattractive and annoying. It has no place in the dental office.

If street clothes are worn, they should be tasteful and modest in design. Many dental offices are now permitting auxiliary personnel to wear pantsuits. If this is permitted, they should be trim pantsuits and not just separate pants and loose shirts. It is desirable that the person wearing a pantsuit, wear one that matches in color, design, and material.

A suggested uniform for a certified dental assistant includes (1) the ADAA pin on the collar, (2) cap K 105 Style with the CDA emblem on the left side, (3) white stockings without runs, (4) clean, white duty shoes kept in good repair, and (5) white uniform with the skirt no more than 2 inches above the knee, or a white uniform pantsuit.

APPEARANCE OF THE OFFICE

Before discussing the decor of the office, it is important that a general knowledge of the basic design of the office be presented. The modern dental office includes several areas which will be discussed as to good taste in appearance and orderliness:

Reception Area	Treatment Area
Business Office	Laboratory
Private Office	Darkroom

Other areas that may be separate rooms or combined with one of the above are:

Recovery Room
Sterilization Room
Consultation Room
Employee Lounge
Patient Education Room

The impression that is created in the reception and business area of a dental office is very important to the success of a dental practice. If the patient finds a pleasant atmosphere, he may refer others to the office. The patient will not be likely to refer a friend to a professional office if the facilities are unpleasant and poorly kept. Many patients discuss the atmosphere of a dental office more than the dental treatment. This is one reason why it is essential that the dental assistant be aware of the things that help to make a pleasant atmosphere.

THE OFFICE ENVIRONMENT

Research has shown that there are four environmental factors that have a psychologi-

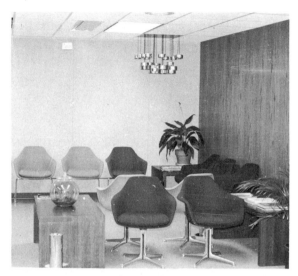

Fig. 2-4 A dental reception area.

cal effect on people: color, lighting, noise, and temperature. Usually these points have been considered before the secretarial dental assistant is employed. However, there are usually opportunities for improving the appearance of any office as the dentist often relies on the staff for redecorating or suggesting improvements.

Color is one of the first things to consider when redecorating the office. Colors have different effects on people. As a general rule, pink, yellow, and orange are considered cheerful colors. Green and blue are more restful. Strong colors (such as red) may cause slight headaches; dull colors like gray tend to make people drowsy. From this information, it is safe to assume that the basic colors for a dental office should be off-white, green, tan, yellow, etc. Lighter colors should be selected for areas where close work is done. Treatment rooms and the business office fall into this category; the color of the walls and ceiling in the reception room may be different.

Since color does affect behavior by influencing the mental attitude, unhurried time should be spent in the color selections. Sometimes, it is possible to reduce fatigue and the electric bills by changing the colors of the walls.

Music

Music has the ability of raising the pain threshold. It has the power of diverting the patient's attention and placing him in a relaxed mood. For this reason, the selection of the type of music is important. Fast and loud music tends to create an increase in tension. It may make the patient and the dental staff feel a little "on edge." Soft, soothing music is relaxing and can raise the *pain threshold,* thereby resulting in feeling less pain.

Office music is usually taped, piped, or played from an AM-FM radio. However, the type of music unit is not nearly as important as the musical selections.

Reception Room

The reception room is considered as the "front window" of the dental office. It should be tastefully arranged and have a pleasant atmosphere in addition to being clean and neat. If the area is dull, dirty, and dreary, the dentist may notice a gradual decline in the number of new patients. Since no one visits a dental office just for pleasure, it is very important that this area maintains a cheerful atmosphere.

There should be plenty of magazines for the patients to read. Outdated magazines should be removed as soon as the new editions arrive. A variety of literature should be available for all ages. Ladies seem to enjoy recipe books with index cards provided for copying favorite recipes. Men usually enjoy the latest edition of the daily paper and sports magazines.

Young children enjoy small storybooks with lots of pictures. Animal stories are very good for the young patient. Older children may enjoy magazines about places and people. Fashion books are suggested for teenage girls and sports editions for teenage boys. Catalogs from mail-order houses seem to appeal to all ages.

A periodic check of the reception room should be made by the secretarial dental assis-

tant as frequently as possible. Magazines and literature are straightened. Litter that is present is placed in waste containers. Ashtrays in the reception room are checked and emptied as soon as possible after a smoker leaves. They should always be emptied and cleaned before leaving the office for the night. Cigarette and cigar butts left in the room overnight will give the air a musty smell. Room deodorizers should always be kept in the office to freshen the air. Since smoking is so offensive to non-smokers, the dentist may wish to place a placard in the office.

FOR THE COMFORT OF
EVERYONE IN THE RECEPTION AREA
PLEASE REFRAIN FROM SMOKING.
Thank you,
THE OFFICE STAFF

Plants should be cared for according to the directions supplied by the florist. Permanent (artificial) arrangements require no care other than cleanliness. Nothing tends to make these arrangements look more artificial than the collection of dust. They should be dusted often and occasionally immersed in a warm, mild soap solution for thorough cleaning.

Business Office

The business office should be comfortable for the secretarial dental assistant and pleasant for the patient. It is here that business transactions take place. The person who is responsible for the reception and bookkeeping duties must have enough room to work efficiently. Many appointments are made here. The secretarial assistant sits in the working area so that she will face the patient. Patients should not be able to stand behind the assistant and peer into the appointment book. Names and dental schedules must be treated confidentially. This reception area should be arranged so that it is possible to write checks following

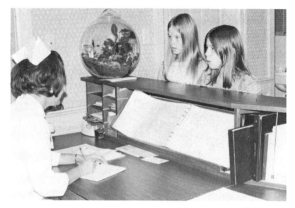

Fig. 2-5 A counter arrangement providing working space and privacy.

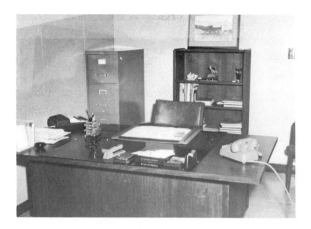

Fig. 2-6 The dentist's private office.

dental treatment. A counter with working space about four feet in height will provide enough room and adequate height for the adult patient.

The business desk must always be neatly arranged. A cluttered desk implies confusion and nonefficient personnel. If treatment plans are to be discussed with the patient in the business area, a comfortable chair should be provided for him or her.

The private office belongs to the dentist. It is an area where the dentist can discuss matters privately with patients, associates, personnel, or visitors. The secretarial dental assistant works in this area only if asked to do so. The dentist will let the office staff know if he wants them to take care of his private office. It is courteous not to disturb the dentist in his office unless it is absolutely necessary.

Both the business and private offices should be kept spotlessly clean at all times. The desks should be given a quick dusting each morning. A can of spray furniture polish is handy for this task.

Operative Areas

The treatment rooms, laboratory, and darkroom are usually maintained by the chairside or roving assistant. General contents of a treatment room include:

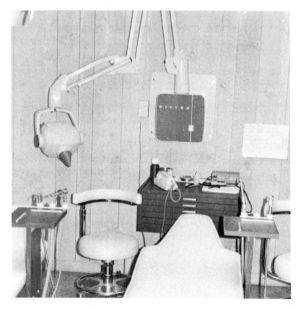

Fig. 2-7 A modern four-handed dentistry operatory. Note that carts and stands have replaced the conventional dental unit.

- A dental chair
- A dental unit
- Waste receptacle
- Cabinets for instruments and supplies
- Sink for the dentist and the assistant
- Operative stools for the dentist and the assistant

The dental laboratory area includes adequate counter space, laboratory equipment

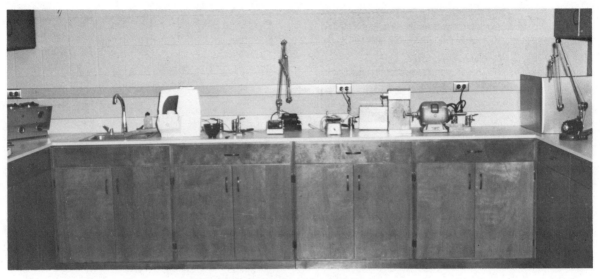

Fig. 2-8 A spacious dental laboratory.

such as model trimmers, lathes, casting equipment, vibrators, vacuum equipment, and various other items.

The darkroom contains the developing tank, a storage area, drying rack or dryer, waste receptacle, and a working space. The optional areas such as a recovery room, sterilization room, etc. will vary according to the needs of the office.

SUMMARY

The impression created by the appearance of the secretarial dental assistant and the general office design contribute greatly to the success of a dental office. Every effort should be made to make the patient have as pleasant a visit as possible. Arrangement and placement of furnishings as well as knowledge of color, lighting, furniture and floor covering all affect the reactions of patients.

SUGGESTED ACTIVITIES

- Prepare a list of "do's and don'ts" for the secretarial dental assistant in reference to personality, conduct, and appearance.

- Visit a dental office and prepare a diagram or sketch of a modern dental office, showing major equipment and furniture.

REVIEW

A. List the items suggested for the official uniform of a certified dental assistant.

1. _____

2. _____

3. _____

4. _____

5. _____

B. Prepare a list of five tasks to be performed daily in maintaining the reception room.

1. _____

2. _____

3. _____

4. _____

5. _____

C. Select the items that are considered as part of good grooming for a secretarial dental assistant.

1. Freshly laundered uniform

2. Dark colored hose

3. Hair style arranged above the collar

4. Diamond watch and dinner ring

5. Manicured nails with a natural polish

6. Clean, white duty shoes

7. Blue eye shadow and dark mascara

D. Select the answer which best completes the statement.

1. Only soft fragrances should be worn by the dental assistant because

a. strong fragrances are too expensive.

b. strong fragrances may be offensive to patients.

c. soft fragrances are reserved for the chairside assistant.

2. The image created in the business-reception area of a dental office is important because

a. patients frequently drop by for a social visit.

b. patients usually refer to the atmosphere of a dental office more than the dental treatment.

c. patients must approve the business-reception area before they will make payments for services.

d. patients are responsible for the success of a dental practice.

3. From the following, select four environmental factors that may affect the dental patient's emotional reaction.

a. color   e. noise

b. period of furniture   f. personality

c. floor covering   g. temperature

d. lighting

4. When selecting colors for the walls of treatment rooms, which color would NOT be recommended.

   a. off-white

   b. mint green

   c. bright orange

   d. light yellow

5. Soft, soothing music in a dental office may

   a. reduce the electric bills.

   b. raise the patient's pain threshold.

   c. make the patient more tense.

   d. make the secretarial dental assistant nervous.

6. The "front window" of a dental office is considered to be the

   a. treatment rooms.

   b. reception area.

   c. business office.

   d. employee's lounge.

7. Ideally, the business office should have counter space available to

   a. aid the patient to view the appointment book for selecting his next appointment.

   b. facilitate payment of fees.

   c. provide women patients a place for checking their makeup.

   d. select a treatment plan for future dental services.

E. Column I lists distinct areas in a dental office. Indicate where the items listed in Column II might be found.

Column I		Column II
1. Treatment Area	2	Model Trimmer
2. Laboratory	4	Developing Tank
3. Darkroom	1	Dental Unit
4. Sterilization Room	2	Lathe
5. Recovery Room	6	Literature about dental health
6. Reception Area	2	Casting Equipment
	6	Unsorted incoming mail
	6	No Smoking sign

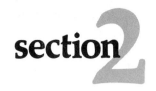

section 2

Telephone Communications

Unit 3 Telephone Techniques

OBJECTIVES

After studying this unit, the student should be able to

- State the items to be kept by the telephone.
- Correctly place a local and a long distance telephone call.
- Explain the five types of long distance telephone calls.

A few years ago, a survey was conducted among 127 dental offices in a city of approximately 125,000 people (Jackson, Mississippi). The purpose of the survey was to determine what course topics should be included in a dental assisting program. The majority of the dentists contacted indicated that proper telephone techniques should be a major topic; some felt that it should be the first procedure taught to a new employee.

The first contact with a dental office for the majority of patients is by way of the telephone. It is important that this first contact leaves the prospective patient with a favorable impression; first impressions are sometimes lasting impressions. To do this, it is necessary for the person answering the phone to:

- be pleasant
- be efficient
- use proper telephone techniques

Proper telephone technique may be the deciding factor that makes a caller become a regular patient. Since the patient cannot see the person answering the phone, the office is judged by the voice that is heard. An effective telephone voice is alert, pleasant, sincere, and expressive. "Please" and "Thank you"

are used frequently; curtly spoken phrases have no place in a dental office. It is of utmost importance to be courteous at all times.

Poor telephone technique can result in losing one who regularly visits the office for dental care, or a prospective patient. Forgetting to deliver an important message or forgetting about the patient who is on *hold* may provoke a patient to call another office. Probably more patients leave a practice because they were rudely treated over the telephone than because they are unhappy with the dental service. Courtesy cannot be overemphasized.

ANSWERING THE TELEPHONE

If at all possible, answer the business telephone after the first ring. Do not let it ring several times to impress the patient that the office is busy. Pick up the phone firmly and quietly. Following are some helpful hints for good telephone etiquette:

- Put the receiver firmly against the ear.
- Put the center of the mouthpiece about an inch from the center of the lips.
- Smile when you pick up the telephone to answer. This will help to convey a pleasant voice.

- Never answer while chewing gum or eating. This will give a mumbled effect to the voice.

- Never answer hurriedly; this makes the patient feel that the office is too busy to be bothered.

- Speak clearly and distinctly into the mouthpiece using a normal tone of voice.

- Speak in a pleasant tone and identify the office. This may be done in one of several ways: "Good morning, Dr. Simmon's office," or "Dr. Simmons's office, Miss Hamilton speaking," or "Dr. Simmon's office, may I help you please?"

It is suggested that all conversations begin with "Good morning" or "Good afternoon." Be sure to change the statement from *morning* to *afternoon* after twelve noon. End all calls by thanking the caller and gently hanging up the receiver. It is polite to let the caller hang up first.

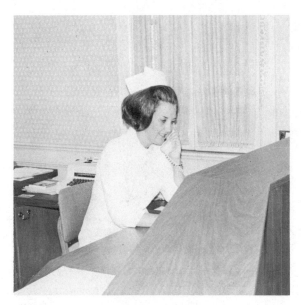

Fig. 3-1 A secretarial dental assistant at the front desk smiling as she talks with a patient.

Use the patient's name when talking, but only if you can pronounce it correctly. Patients enjoy hearing the sound of their own name. When transferring a call to another party in

---

CHECK YOUR PHONE TECHNIQUE

		YES	NO
1.	DID YOU ANSWER PROMPTLY AND PLEASANTLY?	___	___
2.	DID YOU GIVE THE PROPER IDENTIFICATION?	___	___
3.	WERE YOU ATTENTIVE?	___	___
4.	DID YOU DISPLAY PERSONAL INTEREST?	___	___
5.	WERE YOU ALERT FOR OPPORTUNITIES TO BE OF ASSISTANCE?	___	___
6.	DID YOU VOLUNTEER HELPFUL INFORMATION?	___	___
7.	DID YOU GIVE EXPLANATIONS EFFICIENTLY?	___	___
8.	DID YOU TACTFULLY MAKE INQUIRIES?	___	___
9.	DID YOU RECORD THE NECESSARY INFORMATION CAREFULLY?	___	___
10.	DID YOU VERIFY INFORMATION SUCH AS CORRECT SPELLING?	___	___
11.	DID YOU USE THE PROPER TECHNIQUE WHEN IT WAS NECESSARY TO LEAVE THE LINE?	___	___
12.	DID YOU THANK THE PATIENT WHEN CLOSING THE CONVERSATION AND VERIFY INFORMATION?	___	___
13.	WERE YOU CERTAIN THAT THE CONVERSATION HAD BEEN COMPLETED BEFORE REPLACING THE RECEIVER?	___	___

Fig. 3-2 A telephone technique checklist.

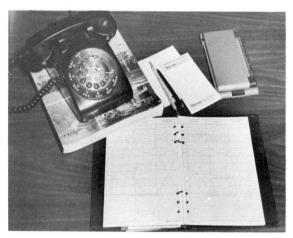

Fig. 3-3 Items needed for handling telephone calls in the dental office.

EMERGENCY NUMBERS	
Fire, Police & Ambulance	911
University Hospital	362-4413
St. John's Hospital	366-9311
Dr. Doe	938-6642
FBI	948-6000
FREQUENTLY CALLED NUMBERS	
Dr. Simmons' home	362-1891
Medical Center	362-4412
Super Drug Co.	354-1789
ABC Dental Supply	354-7896
Black's Dental Lab	453-3478
North's Dental Supply	543-9854
Dr. Dill, Pedodontist	564-9853
Dr. Smithson, Oral Surgeon	432-7649
Dr. Davis, Orthodontist	429-7649

Fig. 3-4 A Sample Telephone List

the dental office, explain to the caller what you are doing. Make sure the patient wants to be transferred. If extension numbers are used, repeat the number to the caller for his future use. Stay with the caller until the transfer is completed.

At times when it is necessary to obtain information away from the telephone, explain why it is necessary to leave. For example: "Mrs. Jones, will you please hold on for a moment? I have to refer to your file." When returning you may say, "Thank you for waiting, Mrs. Jones." This will get the patient's attention again and also show your appreciation. If the delay is going to be longer than one or two minutes, offer to call the patient back. If the patient wants to wait, give an estimate of how long the delay will be.

The following items needed for handling telephone calls in the dental office should be kept close to the telephone:

- Pencil
- Memo pad
- Message pad
- Telephone book
- Appointment book
- List of emergency and frequently called numbers

PLACING A CALL

It is best for callers to place their own calls but, sometimes, a patient may ask the secretarial assistant to make a call. If the dentist asks the secretarial dental assistant to place a call, she should be sure he is free to talk before she dials. When a busy person is called to the phone, it is annoying to hear the secretarial assistants voice instead of that of the dentist or other caller. Allow sufficient time for a person to answer; at least a minute to permit the person to reach the telephone (ten rings equal about one minute in time). This waiting is necessary because situations occur that could cause a slight delay in answering.

When a local call is placed, one must be sure that the number is correct. The telephone directory is consulted whenever there is doubt. If the correct number is not listed, dial the information number for assistance. A list of frequently called numbers should be visible; it may be placed on the desk, on the writing arm of the desk, or neatly arranged on the wall near the telephone.

Emergency numbers such as the fire department, police, ambulance service, medical doctor, Federal Bureau of Investigation, etc. must be included on this list. It should also include dental offices frequently called, dental supply houses, dental laboratories, drugstore, etc.

Suggestions for Proper Dialing

- Look up the number in the directory when in doubt.

- Place the receiver to the ear and listen for the dial tone.

- Dial each digit to the finger rest.

- Release the dial to return at its own speed.

- Hang up if you think you made an error. Listen for the dial tone before dialing again.

- Apologize if you pick up on an extension or party line when someone else is dialing or talking.

Touch-tone telephones require the same accuracy and courtesy. Be careful not to touch the numbers hastily or a mistake will be made.

Types of Long Distance Calls

Station-to-Station calls are made when there is no need to talk to a particular person. In most areas the number can be dialed direct. Charges start as soon as the phone is answered. *Person-to-Person calls* are made when it is necessary or desirable to talk to a particular person. Charges start when the conversation with the requested person begins. Rates are higher for person-to-person calls. *Coin calls* are made from coin-operated telephones; payment for the call is made before talking to the desired party.

Another type of call is the *conference call.* Conference calls are made when it is desirable to talk to more than one person in different places at the same time. The opera-

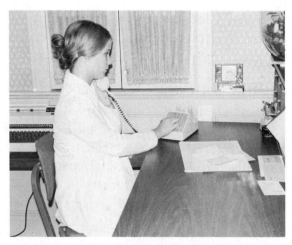

Fig. 3-5 A secretarial dental assistant placing a call to a patient.

tor must be contacted for a conference call. For mobile calls and overseas calls, consult the local telephone directory for instructions.

WATS calls are Wide Area Telecommunications Services. Station-to-Station calls may be made without charge to those who have this service; this may be a state or national service. The digits 800 are part of the WATS number. To determine if a party you wish to contact has a WATS number, dial 1-800-555-1212 for information.

Most areas of the country now have *direct dialing.* This type of service is usually termed as one-plus or zero-plus dialing. To use the *one-plus service,* dial 1 plus the area code (if calling outside the local area code) plus the the telephone number.

To use the *zero-plus service,* dial 0 plus the area code (if outside the local area code) plus the telephone number. The operator will answer after dialing is completed and request information necessary to complete the call. Zero-plus is used for person-to-person calls, collect calls, credit calls, or calls charged to another number. If dialing within the local area code, dial 0 plus the telephone number.

Long distance directory assistance may be obtained by dialing a special series of numbers. To obtain a number within the local area

Section 2 Telephone Communications

code, dial 1-555-1212. To obtain numbers outside the local area code, dial 1-area code-555-1212. When the operator answers, state the city to be called and the name of the person whose number is being requested.

Several pages of dialing information may be found in the front section of the local telephone directory. These pages include information on dialing, charges, area codes, complaints, and general information which may be of interest to the customer; these pages can be easily referred to when a question arises.

One of the many services the telephone company provides to its customers is special public relations personnel that assist the public in working out telephone difficulties. Special equipment, such as a tele-trainer, may be borrowed to teach people how to effectively use the telephone. The tele-trainer consists of two telephones with extra long cords connected to a central unit. One unit is placed in one room; the second unit in an adjoining room. This gives new personnel an opportunity to actually practice placing and receiving calls. This service is excellent for students and new personnel to practice with during training sessions.

SUMMARY

The telephone is a vital instrument in a dental practice. It should be used efficiently in order for a satisfactory relationship to exist between the patient and the dental office. The sound of the voice a caller hears on the telephone conveys the personality of the assistant and the office. An effective telephone voice is alert, pleasant, sincere, and expressive. Proper telephone technique may be the deciding factor that makes a caller become a regular patient.

When placing calls, be sure the number is correct before dialing. There are several ways to place a long distance call: station-to-station, person-to-person, coin calls, conference calls, WATS. Information on dialing, charges, area codes, etc. may be obtained from the local telephone directory. Special equipment, such as the tele-trainer, may be borrowed from the telephone company to teach people how to effectively use the telephone.

SUGGESTED ACTIVITIES

- Prepare a list of frequently called and emergency telephone numbers for your own home and for a local dental office.

- Write a two-page report discussing good telephone techniques; use at least two outside references.

- Make a tape recording of a telephone conversation between yourself and another person. After the playback, list suggested improvements that could be made and discuss them with each other, referring to guidelines in this unit.

- With prior approval of your instructor, contact the public relations department of the telephone company. Ask a representative to come and talk about proper telephone techniques.

REVIEW

A. The majority of dental patients make their first contact with the dental office by using the telephone. It is important that

1. several incoming lines be available for patient use 24 hours a day.

2. the person answering the telephone is pleasant and efficient and uses proper telephone techniques.

3. the dentist always answers the telephone.

4. an automatic answering service be installed for patient convenience.

B. Select two examples of good telephone techniques.

1. Failing to deliver messages.

2. Asking the patient to wait while obtaining information from the file.

3. Transferring a call to the chairside assistant.

4. Keeping the patient on *hold* for an indefinite period of time.

5. Conversing with the patient in a short, curt tone of voice.

6. Asking the patient to allow you to call back after obtaining necessary information.

C. Patients usually leave a dental practice because they

1. are unhappy about fees for services.

2. were rudely treated over the telephone and/or in the office.

3. are dissatisfied with the quality of dental treatment.

4. prefer a more modern office.

D. A dental patient's first reaction, when the secretarial dental assistant speaks hurriedly over the telephone, is likely to be that

1. the office staff is too busy to be bothered with his particular problem.

2. the dentist must have a good practice to have such a busy office.

3. the secretarial dental assistant must really be efficient.

4. the dentist needs to install recording equipment for busy times in the office.

E. Give three examples of how to identify the dental office when answering the phone.

1. _____

2. _____

3. _____

F. State three rules to apply when transferring a call.

1. _____

2. _____

3. _____

G. List the necessary items that should be placed near the telephone.

1. _____
2. _____
3. _____
4. _____
5. _____
6. _____

H. List suggestions that are helpful in dialing a number.

1. _____
2. _____
3. _____
4. _____
5. _____
    _____
6. _____
    _____

I. Match the following.

1. Station-to-Station calls   _____ are made when it is de-
                                               sirable to talk to more
                                               than one person in dif-
                                               ferent places at the same
                                               time.

2. Person-to-Person calls   _____ are made when there is
                                               no need to talk to a par-
                                               ticular person.

3. Coin calls   _____ are wide area telecom-
                                               munications services.

4. Conference calls   _____ are made when it is nec-
                                               essary or desirable to talk
                                               to a particular person.

5. WATS calls   _____ are paid for before talk-
                                               ing to the desired party

J. Types of long distance calls are given below. Select the appropriate number to be dialed.

<u>Calls to be made</u>   <u>Dial</u>

1. Party to be called is out-of-state,
    number unknown.   _____ 1-555-1212

2. Party is within the local area
    code, number unknown   _____ 1-area-code-number

3. Collect call to party outside city
    but with same local area code   _____ 1-phone number (7 digits)

4. Station-to-station call, within
    local area code.   _____ 0-area code-number

5. Call outside the local area code,
    station-to-station.   _____ 1-area code-555-1212

6. Call outside the local area code,
    person-to-person.   _____ 0-number (7 digits)

K. Define the following terms and explain when each would be used.

1. One-plus dialing _____

    _____

2. Zero-plus dialing _____

    _____

3. A tele-trainer _____

    _____

    _____

Unit 4 Communicating with the Patient

OBJECTIVES

After studying this unit, the student should be able to

- Demonstrate the ability to handle incoming telephone calls from patients.
- Correctly place telephone calls to make or change appointments, order supplies, inquire, and collect delinquent accounts.

There are many types of calls the secretarial dental assistant will receive and place during the average working day. It is important that the facts required for each call be obtained and correctly given. The information given must reflect the thinking of the dentist. Since all dentists are different, telephone policies will differ from one office to another. It is desirable for all offices to have a manual with printed statements that reflect the policy and philosophy of the dentist.

INCOMING CALLS

Incoming calls usually fall into one of the following categories:

- New patient making an appointment.
- Regular patient making an appointment.
- Patient changing or cancelling an appointment.
- Patient desiring information related to dental care.
- Patient calling to complain about fees or dental services.
- Private calls to the dentist.
- Personal calls to the office staff.

APPOINTMENT CONTROL

When a patient calls for an appointment, it must first be determined if he is a new or a regular patient. The regular patient may be offended if he is asked, "Are you a new patient?" or, "Have you been here before?" This is especially true if he or she has been a patient for a number of years. A discreet way to determine whether the patient is new or a regular one is to ask, "How is your record listed?" Another way is to repeat the name which was given and ask, "Mrs. Jones, is your record listed as Mrs. Cecil Jones?" Always refer to the established patient as a regular or active patient, never as an "old" patient. Write the name on a memo pad with the letters NP (New Patient) if this is the first visit.

The next fact the secretarial dental assistant needs to know is the reason for the appointment. It will be necessary to ask if the patient does not supply the information. "Is this for your regular checkup?" seems to get more information than, "What is this appointment for?" Many times the dentist prefers that the new patient have a prophylaxis (cleaning) and mouth examination by a dental auxiliary before he starts treatment; the time the appointment is being made provides a good opportunity for explanation of this policy to the patient. Emphasis on the fact that cleaning the teeth includes a thorough preliminary examination because all tooth surfaces are checked helps the new patient understand its value; he becomes more likely to accept it.

Proceed with making the appointment. Facts needed for the new patient include the following:

- Name
- Address
- Telephone numbers (both home and business)
- Nature of treatment
- Age (if the patient is a child)
- Name of the referring party

Obtaining the name of the referring party will tell the office something about the patient. It will also give the office an opportunity to thank the referring party. When all the needed information is obtained, end the conversation with a "Thank you" and repeat the time of the appointment. Repeating the time and date will avoid a misunderstanding of the appointed time. For example, close by saying, "Thank you for calling, Mrs. Jones. We shall see you on *(repeat the day and time of the appointment)."*

When the regular patient calls for an appointment, the nature of the visit should be the first fact obtained. In addition to the name and nature of the visit, secure the telephone number (both home and office). When a time has been established, close the conversation in the same manner as with a new patient.

Many situations arise which make it necessary for a patient to call and change or cancel an appointment. This patient deserves as much consideration as the patient making a new appointment. A changed appointment is rescheduled for a later date; a cancelled appointment is erased on the appointment book and not rescheduled. Office policies will vary concerning changed or cancelled appointments.

INFORMATION REQUESTS

There are many reasons for a patient to call the dental office for information; some of the more common ones will be mentioned.

Calls attempting to determine the fee for dental work may be common. Some people will call several offices hoping to find an office with low fees. These callers might be termed as "dental shoppers." It is very unwise to quote fees over the telephone to anyone. The exact nature of treatment needed can only be established after an examination by the dentist. The caller should be told exactly that. If they do not accept the explanation, give an example. For instance, a fee cannot be quoted for a silver restoration as the restoration may be one of several surfaces and fees vary according to the number of surfaces. An extraction may be a routine extraction or it may require a surgical procedure. Offer to make an appointment for the caller to have a clinical examination at which time an estimate can be given.

Many calls will require technical knowledge of dental procedures. Some questions a secretarial dental assistant may be asked are:

"How long should my filling be sensitive to hot and cold foods?"

"Should I still be having pain from a routine filling yesterday?"

"When should I bring my child in for his first visit to the dentist?"

The secretarial dental assistant and the dentist should discuss the more common problems. Again, an office manual or a specially prepared index file may quickly help answer these problems. Do not attempt to guess at answers just to satisfy patients. The patient's dental and physical health is involved. If unsure, place the patient on *hold* and obtain an answer from the dentist. If the dentist is busy, take the name and telephone number of the caller. Request that the patient wait for a call from the dentist. Record the name, phone number, and the nature of the problem on a message pad for the dentist. Clip the message to the patient's record card and place it in a conspicuous place on the dentist's desk.

A complaint call, whether about services or fees, must be handled courteously. It is

---

EVALUATE YOUR VOICE PERSONALITY

		YES	NO
1.	DID YOU SPEAK DISTINCTLY?	___	___
2.	DID YOU SPEAK DIRECTLY INTO THE MOUTHPIECE?	___	___
3.	DID YOU USE CORRECT GRAMMAR?	___	___
4.	DID YOU USE ANY FORM OF SLANG?	___	___
5.	DID YOU USE PHRASES SUCH AS UH-HUH AND YEAH?	___	___
6.	DID YOU USE POLITE EXPRESSIONS SUCH AS PLEASE?	___	___
7.	DID YOU GIVE THE CALLER A FEELING OR ASSURANCE?	___	___
8.	DID YOU SMILE BEFORE PICKING UP THE TELEPHONE?	___	___
9.	DID YOU REPRESENT THE OFFICE COURTEOUSLY?	___	___
10.	DID YOU MAKE THE PATIENT FEEL YOU CARED?	___	___

Fig. 4-1 A voice personality evaluation

---

possible to be both pleasant and firm at the same time. This type of call will require discipline on the part of the person answering the telephone. Never try to quote information from memory. Tell the patient you would like to refer to their record. Place the patient on *hold* and obtain the correct information from the file. This will also allow a few moments time to review the card and determine what needs to be said to the patient. A pleasant soft voice is the key to successful communication with the complaining patient.

Private calls to the dentist may be from friends, patients, salesmen, or other doctors. It is necessary to establish who is calling by saying, "May I tell Dr. Simmons who is calling please?" If it is a patient, chances are the call may be efficiently handled by the secretarial dental assistant. In fact, most incoming calls can and should be resolved at the front desk. If the patient insists on talking to the dentist, suggest that the dentist return the call (emergency calls are an exception to the rule). When the dentist is busy, tell the caller, "Dr. Simmons is with a patient. May I have him return your call?" Never apologize because he is with a patient. Simply state the fact.

Patients appreciate honesty rather than vague answers; otherwise, they may believe they are being put off. Tell the patient if the dentist is attending an educational seminar, if he is checking on a hospital patient, or if he is out-of-town on business.

There will be times when it is necessary to use discretion in answering. For example, when the dentist is having coffee with the doctor down the hall, the assistant can say, "Dr. Simmons is busy at the moment; may he return your call?" The following phrases should not be used.

- "The doctor is all tied up right now."

- "He is not coming in today."

- "He is having coffee down the hall."

- "He hasn't come in yet." (When it is 11:00 A.M.)

Statements such as these create poor public relations.

When taking messages, be sure to include all of the necessary information. Telephone message pads are convenient for this purpose. The following items should be included on a telephone message pad:

- Name of the calling party

- Time of the call

- Telephone number of the calling party

- Nature of the call

If the caller is a patient, obtain the patient's record and attach it to the telephone message sheet, figure 4-2.

```
┌─────────────────────────────────────────────────────────────────────┐
│  TO _____ Dr. John Simmons _____      │
│  DATE _____ September 17, 1975   TIME _____ 11:35 a.m. _____      │
│                   WHILE YOU WERE OUT                                   │
│  _____ Dr. James B. Fowler _____      │
│  of _____ Medical Arts Building _____      │
│  PHONE _____ 366-1405 _____      │
│  TELEPHONED _____   PLEASE CALL ____ X _____       │
│  CALLED TO SEE YOU _____   WILL CALL AGAIN _____        │
│  WANTED TO SEE YOU _____   RUSH _____        │
│  MESSAGE: _____ Dr. Fowler would like to talk to you _____      │
│  _____ about a patient, Todd Douglas, that you referred __  │
│  _____ to the Fowler office.  Please call Dr. Fowler back _ │
│  _____ before 3:00 p.m. _____       │
│                                        _____ Judy Hutson _____       │
│                                               OPERATOR                 │
└─────────────────────────────────────────────────────────────────────┘
```

Fig. 4-2 Recording a telephone message.

When other doctors call, it is usually a very important call. Try to transfer these calls to the dentist if at all possible. Many times the doctor calling wants to discuss a patient who has been referred. For example, an orthodontist may call in reference to a certain patient. Repeat the calling doctor's name, "Dr. Fowler, let me get John's record and have Dr. Simmons speak with you." This will explain the few seconds delay. It will save time when the doctors talk because the record will be visible.

Personal calls to members of the dental staff should be discouraged unless absolutely necessary. All personnel should recognize that the office phone is a business phone. If friends insist on calling for "visiting" purposes, request that they call back after hours.

OUTGOING CALLS

Outgoing calls are usually made for one of the following purposes.

- Confirm a patient's appointment.

- Remind the patient a checkup is due (Re-call).

- Fill a changed appointment.

- Order supplies.

- Collect delinquent accounts.

- Check on a patient following extensive dental treatment.

Confirming an Appointment

Confirming a patient's appointment serves two purposes; it reminds the patient and tells the office what to expect and what preparations will be necessary. Ask to speak with the person who has the appointment. If the appointment is for a child, ask to speak with a parent. The mother is preferred since she usually brings the child to the office. When the correct party is on the line say, "Mrs. Jones, this is Miss Strickland in Dr. Simmon's office. I am calling to *confirm* your appointment *(tomorrow or today)* at *(state the time)."* Use the word *confirm* instead of *remind.* Patients

---

A RECALL CONVERSATION

Patient:	Hello.
Secretarial Dental Assistant:	Hello. May I please speak to Mrs. Cecil Jones?
Patient:	This is she.
Secretarial Dental Assistant:	Mrs. Jones, this is Miss Hamilton in Dr. Simmon's office. When you last visited our office in January, you asked us to call and remind you when it was time for your regular dental checkup. It is now time for your checkup. Dr. Simmons could see you on Monday. June 17, at 10:00 a.m.
Patient:	Miss Hamilton, I believe June 17, at 10:00 a.m. would be a convenient time for me. Thank you for calling and reminding me.
Secretarial Dental Assistant:	Thank you, Mrs. Jones. We will see you Monday, June 17, at 10:00 a.m. Good-bye.
Patient:	Good-bye Miss Hamilton.

Fig. 4-3 A sample recall conversation.

sometimes are offended at a reminder but not at a confirmation. State the time clearly. Close by saying, "Thank you, Mrs. Jones. We will see you at *(state the time again.)*" Reconfirm the time when closing the conversation. Usually morning appointments are confirmed the day before; afternoon appointments may be confirmed early in the morning of the same day.

Recall

A recall is a systematic method of reminding a patient it is time for a visit to the dental office. Calling the patient for a recall may be the responsibility of either the hygienist or the secretarial dental assistant. In either case, the same guidelines apply. Recall of patients is discussed in Unit 8; only the telephone message will be mentioned in this unit. A suggested recall conversation is shown in figure 4-3.

Determine the best time period for the patient by asking, "Are mornings or afternoons more convenient for you?" This will save valuable time by eliminating the need to suggest numerous appointments the patient

cannot meet. Record this information on the recall record form for future use.

Changed Appointments

Calling to fill an appointment which another patient has changed or cancelled cannot be done without an adequate cancellation list. This list may be kept in a shorthand pad for quick reference. A patient should not be called for an appointment change unless he has requested this service. Many times earlier appointments (other than the time appointed) are desired by the patient. When this situation arises, call the patient, identify the office and say, "We promised to call you if we had a changed appointment so Dr. Simmons could see you earlier. We do have a *changed* appointment today at 3:00 p.m. Could you come in at 3:00 p.m.?" If the patient cannot make the new time, thank the patient and confirm the regularly scheduled appointment. Establish whether he wants to remain on the cancellation list. It is a good practice to always use the word *changed* with patients. The word *cancelled* may make them wonder if the appointment was cancelled because of problems with dental treatment or with the dental staff.

Ordering Supplies

Supplies are often ordered by telephone. The rule to follow when ordering is to know exactly what the dentist wants before picking up the telephone. If a part for a piece of equipment is needed, write the serial number of the equipment, the model number, and the make of the equipment on a memo pad. Dental-supply men should not be expected to remember the equipment that is in each office they serve. State the name of the office calling and an exact description of the item or items needed. If at all possible, ask for the items by brand names if the dentist prefers a specific brand.

Delinquent Accounts

Many times it is necessary to attempt to collect delinquent accounts by telephone. Again, being firm but pleasant is the key. Be very sure that the correct party is on the telephone before beginning the conversation. Identify the office and proceed with one of the following statements.

- "We are calling in regard to your account of *(state the amount)* which is *(state the number of months)* past due."

- "In checking our files, we find your account of *(state the amount)* has not been paid in *(state the number of months)*."

- "We are calling to ask when it would be convenient for you to come to the office so we can discuss your account; it has been overdue for quite some time."

The conversation will vary according to the patient's reply to the opening statement. Thank the patient when closing and state that a note is being made on his record card of his intentions. For example, "Mrs. Jones, I will make a note on your record that you will *(repeat the promise of the patient)*. Let the patient know you will expect exactly what the patient has promised. If collections can be made by use of the telephone, it will save time in writing correspondence and cost of postage.

Follow-up Calls

A thoughtful gesture on the part of the secretarial dental assistant is to call a patient following extensive dental treatment. It is suggested that patients be called the day after routine extractions. Besides showing interest, this call may detect a dental complication. This courtesy also helps to build up the dentist's practice. An example of this type of phone call is, "Mrs. Jones, this is Dr. Simmons' office. We just wanted to call and check on you today. How are you feeling?" This follow-up call makes the patient feel that the dentist and his staff really care about the state of his health.

SUMMARY

Many types of calls will be made and answered by the secretarial dental assistant. Correct, necessary facts must be given for both incoming and outgoing calls. All information given must reflect the thinking of the dentist.

SUGGESTED ACTIVITIES

- Obtain a file box with 3" by 5" or 5" by 8" index cards. Write suggestions for each category of incoming calls received in the dental office. Write suggested telephone messages for each of the six outgoing calls listed in this unit. Maintain the file box for use in future units.

• Call the public relations department of the local telephone company. Request the use of a tele-trainer. Practice receiving and placing telephone calls with another person. Critique each practice call. Make a list of suggested improvements that may be made. Practice the following calls.

Call Mrs. Jack Smith to confirm her appointment on Monday, July 2, at 2:30 p.m. Request that she bring her son, Todd, for an introductory visit to the office when she comes. Determine what other information is needed.

Call Mr. James Fontaine for a recall appointment for his teeth to be checked and cleaned.

Call Mr. William C. Croft from the cancellation list to fill an opening that is available at 4:00 p.m. tomorrow afternoon due to a changed appointment.

Call a dental supply company and order a light bulb (or part) for a dental unit. Obtain information such as model type and serial number from the unit before calling.

Call Ms. Jane Doe about an account of $30.00 which she has neglected paying for the past four months.

Call Miss Beverly Sowell to check on her progress following a surgical extraction performed the previous day.

Assume any information not supplied. If a tele-trainer is not available, write out a conversation for each situation.

REVIEW

A. An office manual with written statements of suggested telephone messages can be helpful because

   1. the new employee may not know how to answer the telephone.

   2. it enables the secretarial dental assistant to convey the office policy and philosophy of the dentist.

   3. the chairside assistant may forget the office policy.

   4. it gives the patient a feeling of assurance.

B. Which of the following statements may offend the regular, established patient? (More than one may be selected)

   1. "Are you a new patient?"

   2. "How is your record listed?"

   3. "Have you been to see the doctor before?"

   4. "Is your record listed, Mrs. Cecil Jones?"

   5. "When was your last visit?"

C. Which is the best statement to use in establishing the nature of the appointment?

1. What is the appointment for, please?
2. Do you need a filling or extraction?
3. Is this for your regular checkup?

D. The best reason for repeating the time and date of the appointment at the close of the telephone conversation is to

1. avoid a misunderstanding by the patient of the appointed time.
2. allow the patient to change the date of the appointment.
3. give the secretarial dental assistant an opportunity to write in the appointment book.
4. draw the conversation to a close on a pleasant note.

E. It is best to refer to a "changed appointment" rather than a "cancelled apppointment" because

1. the patient may not understand the meaning of the word *cancel.*
2. *changed appointment* sounds better than *cancelled appointment.*
3. the patient may wonder if previous appointee was dissatisfied with dental treatment or the office.
4. it is good psychology to use the word *changed.*

F. Dental fees are not usually quoted over the telephone because

1. that would be advertising which is considered unethical.
2. the exact nature of the dental services needed can only be determined after a clinical examination by the dentist.
3. "dental shoppers" should be encouraged to call another office.
4. fees may change every day in the dental practice.

G. One should never answer a patient's dental question with a guess because

1. the dentist may lose the patient because of the answer.
2. the patient can just as easily call another dental office.
3. the patient's dental and physical health is involved.
4. the dentist should have all incoming calls transferred to his private office.

H. Which statement is recommended when answering a complaint call?

1. Place the patient on *hold,* obtain the correct information from the record and proceed with the conversation.
2. Tell the patient you are busy and will return the call later.
3. Tell the patient that the dentist will return the call tomorrow.
4. Be kind and agree with everything the patient has to say.

I. Which of the following statements should *not* be used when telling a caller the dentist is busy?

    1. "The doctor is all tied up right now."
    2. "Dr. Simmons is attending an educational meeting in Atlanta today."
    3. "He is down the hall drinking coffee right now."
    4. "He is not taking any calls this a.m."
    5. "He is at the hospital checking on a patient."
    6. "Dr. Simmons was called out-of-town today on business."

J. List two reasons for confirming a patient's appointment.

    1. _____
    2. _____

K. Define the term *recall*.

    _____
    _____

L. What information should be obtained from a new patient?

    1. _____
    2. _____
    3. _____
    4. _____
    5. _____
    6. _____

M. What information is needed from a regular patient?

    1. _____
    2. _____
    3. _____

N. What four items should be included on the sheets of a telephone message pad?

    1. _____
    2. _____
    3. _____
    4. _____

Unit 5 Telephone Services and Equipment

OBJECTIVES

After studying this unit, the student should be able to

- List the features of a six button key telephone.
- Demonstrate the use of a six button key telephone.
- Explain the use of an 18 Button Call Director®.
- Write messages for an automatic answering service.

The secretarial dental assistant must be familiar with telephone services and the telephone equipment in the dental office. Not knowing how to operate the equipment is frustrating for both the patient and the secretarial dental assistant. There are many different types of telephones that may be installed in a dental office; those that are usually installed will be discussed in this unit.

SIX BUTTON KEY

The six button key is the type of telephone most commonly used in an office with only one dentist, figure 5-1. This type of telephone provides both external and internal communications to the dental office. The average dental office has at least two (usually not more than four) incoming lines to the office. The lines ring at the central phone located on the desk of the secretarial dental assistant. Extensions are usually placed in the treatment areas, in the laboratory, and in the dentist's private office. This phone may be either a regular dial type or a push-button type.

The features of this six button key telephone include multiline, hold, intercom, preset conference, positive visual signal, and an exclusion feature.

The *multiline* feature gives the dental office more than one incoming line. Each

line may serve many telephones. Anyone may talk on any line from any phone within the office. It assures prompt, efficient handling of incoming calls. It saves time and improves patient relations. "Walk to talk" delays are cut down. Everyone has maximum flexibility in making and taking outside calls.

The *hold* feature enables the secretarial dental assistant to leave a call without disconnecting it. This makes it possible to answer or place a second call without being overheard by the party on *hold*. Slow answering is also eliminated.

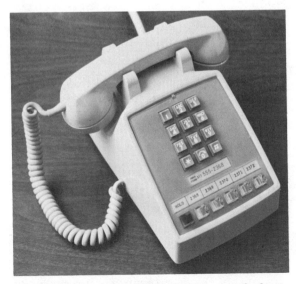

Fig. 5-1 A Six Button Key Touch-tone telephone. The key set features one hold button and five others for calling, signaling or access to other extension.

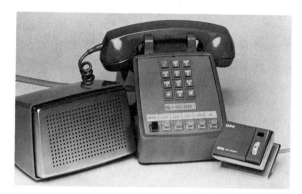

Fig. 5-2 A Speakerphone telephone instrument allowing the secretarial dental assistant or the dentist to talk without holding the receiver.

The *dial intercom* allows all extensions in the dental office to be intercom stations. All the extensions may communicate with each other merely by dialing one or two digits. Additional extensions may be added as the office requires them. The interoffice communications may be improved because internal calls may be made while holding an outside call. This feature allows the secretarial dental assistant to "brief" someone else in the office before transferring an outside call to them.

The *preset conference* feature allows a telephone conference to be made with a fixed group of intercom telephone users. This is done by dialing a code or pushing a button. Many times in the dental office, the secretarial dental assistant needs to consult privately with the chairside dental assistant or the dentist while holding a call on the line. A telephone company representative may be contacted for more detailed information if this service is to be used.

Positive visual signals are small lamps installed to show the status of incoming calls. An unused line shows no light. An incoming call shows a slow flashing light; a line on *hold* shows a rapidly flashing light. A still light indicates the line is in use. These visual signals enable the secretarial dental assistant to glance at the buttons and determine the right line to answer. If more than one light is sig-

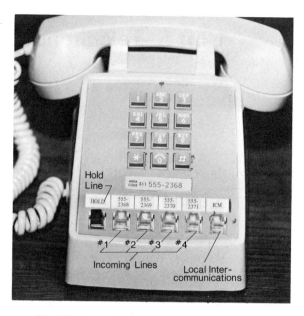

Fig. 5-3 A typical Six Button Key telephone.

naling, the location of the ring, or the tone will help to determine which line is to be answered. This positive visual signal feature avoids confusion and interruption of busy lines.

The *exclusion feature* disconnects all other telephones from a specific line; this may be done automatically or manually. It gives absolute privacy when desired, adds to the communications system.

An optional feature with the six button key telephone is an automatic answering feature sometimes termed "hands-free". This special feature requires an additional piece of equipment such as shown in figure 5-2. This system makes it possible to hear and be heard without lifting the telephone handset. It frees the person to take notes, refer to records or move around while listening and talking. When privacy is desired, the handset is lifted which disconnects the interphone unit. This feature is very useful when making appointments by telephone.

Six buttons are located either below or above the dial or pushbuttons, figure 5-3. From left to right they are:

Button 1 HOLD Button

Button 2 Incoming Line No. 1

Button 3 Incoming Line No. 2

Button 4 Incoming Line No. 3

Button 5 Incoming Line No. 4

Button 6 Local intercommunications button

If the dental office has only two incoming lines, buttons 4 and 5 will be blank. This allows the office to add incoming lines as the need arises.

The HOLD button enables incoming calls to be placed on *hold* for indefinite periods. To place a call on *hold* keep the receiver off the hook and depress the HOLD button for about two seconds. One or more lines may be placed on *hold* during the same time interval. This may be necessary if one line rings while the secretarial dental assistant is talking on another line. If it is necessary to answer an additional line while talking on another, ask the party on the first line to please wait, depress the HOLD button and then answer the second line. Always thank the party for waiting when you have returned.

The local intercommunications button (the last button) allows the secretarial dental assistant to transfer calls to any extension in the dental office. Following is a typical example: Line 1 begins to flash and a bell tone is heard; the secretarial dental assistant (S.D.A.) answers by pressing the button.

S.D.A. Good Morning, Dr. Simmons' office, Miss Eatmon speaking.

Patient Good morning, this is Mrs. Jack Williams. Dr. Simmons asked me to call him today and give him a report on my daughter, Jenny. She was in your office yesterday and had two extractions.

S.D.A. Yes, Mrs. Williams. Dr. Simmons is in his office and can speak with you now. Hold on please.

(The secretarial dental assistant depresses the HOLD button for about two seconds which places line 1 on *hold*. The local button which is the sixth button is depressed and Dr. Simmon's extension number is dialed.)

Dentist Dr. Simmons speaking.

S.D.A. Dr. Simmons, Mrs. Jack Williams is on line 1. You asked her to call today and report on her daughter, Jenny, who had two extractions yesterday.

The dentist depresses line 1 (which is the second button) and speaks with Mrs. Williams. Note that the assistant announced who was calling on *Line 1*. She also gave the dentist a quick review of why the patient was calling. This is very helpful to the dentist. He sees so many patients in a day's time that it is impossible for him to remember every detail about each patient. Help such as this will add to a better relationship between the patient and the dentist.

18 BUTTON CALL DIRECTOR®

A Call Director® is recommended for dental offices or clinics where several dentists are in the same office (The word Call Director® is a registered trademark of the American Telephone and Telegraph Company.) In a clinic setting there may be a number of dentists; one person may be given the responsibility

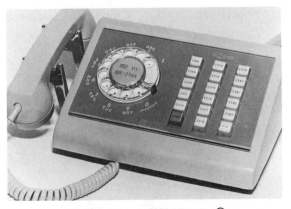

Fig. 5-4 Rotary Call Director®
(Courtesy of American Telephone and Telegraph Company)

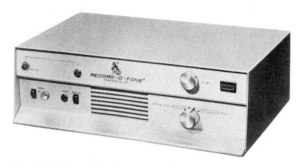

Fig. 5-5 Example of an automatic answering service that may be installed in a dental office.
(Courtesy Record-O-Fone)

of handling all incoming calls. Usually, if there are more than three dentists, one person will probably be employed just to answer the telephone. The individual calls will then be transferred to the proper extension. The 18 or 30 Button Call Director® is usually installed in this type of setting. The number of dentists serviced determine how many buttons will be needed; these machines are usually available with regular rotary dials or with push-buttons.

The operation of the Call Director® is very similar to the six button phone. The main difference is in the number of incoming lines. The six button key telephone has from 1 to 4 incoming lines. The Call Director® may have from 3 to 30 incoming lines.

When a call comes through, one of the incoming lines begins to flash and the tone is heard:

1. The line button is depressed, the handset is lifted, and the operator identifies the clinic.

2. After the caller indicates to whom he wishes to speak and the secretarial dental assistant has asked him to wait, the HOLD button is depressed for about two seconds with the handset still off the hook.

3. The line number will flash rapidly.

4. The Local Intercommunications Button (the last button) is depressed.

5. The digit or digits — of the specific extension of the dentist being called — is dialed.

Contact has been made between the caller and the proper extension when the light of the incoming line stops flashing. The secretarial dental assistant is then free to answer other lines proceeding in the same manner.

AUTOMATIC ANSWERING EQUIPMENT

There are many times — such as before and after regular office hours and during lunch time — that the entire staff is away from the dental office. The staff may also need to attend educational seminars or workshops. Whatever the reason, it is desirable that some method be used to handle incoming calls when the staff is away; patients may need to contact the office at these times. Since it is not practical to employ someone to stay at the office 24 hours a day to answer the telephone, the solution may be an automatic answering service. Automatic answering service companies in the area may be found by consulting the yellow pages of the local telephone directory. The local telephone company may be able to recommend a service that is available. There are many companies, such as Record-O-Fone, that offer automatic answering services. Record-O-Fone is an automatic answer, announce, record, and remote playback system, figure 5-5. The model 100 is suited for the needs of a dental office. This model automatically answers the telephone on the first ring, however; it can be set to answer on any ring. Busy offices may wish to set it for the third or fourth ring. This will answer the needs of an office with a small staff when everyone is busy. During an emergency in the dental office, this service would be very helpful.

The outgoing announcement can be any length up to three minutes. The incoming mes-

An automatic answering service contributes to better patient relations with the dental office. Figure 5-7 shows some examples of recorded phone messages.

SUMMARY

The secretarial dental assistant must be familiar with the telephone equipment in the dental office. Unfamiliarity is frustrating to both the patient and the office staff. The six button key telephone is commonly used in an office with only one dentist. Features of the six button key telephone include:

- Multilines
- HOLD Button
- Intercom
- Preset conference use
- Visual signals
- Exclusion

The 18 or 30 Button Call Director® may be found in offices or clinics where there are several dentists in the same office. The features of the Call Director® are very similar to the six button key telephone; the main difference is that the Call Director® has more incoming lines.

An automatic answering service is suggested for dental offices. When the staff is away from the office, a specially recorded message is heard by the caller explaining the absence of the dental staff; the message of the caller is then recorded. This service contributes to better public relations with the patients.

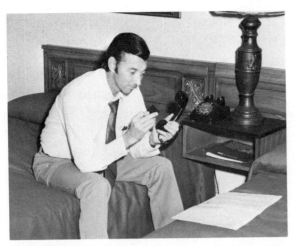

Fig. 5-6 Using a remote signal device to emit a tone into a telephone receiver to receive office messages.

sages are taken immediately following the outgoing announcement. The caller can leave a message before the end of the announcement tape cycle. The unit can be set up so that the time allowed for incoming messages may vary. The remote playback feature makes it possible for the messages to be received without returning to the office. A remote call back signal device is available in pocket size. The dentist and the secretarial dental assistant may each have a signal device to use when away from the office. This signal device has a specially coded double tone signal that is matched *only* to the unit in the particular office; no one else can receive the messages. By emitting the coded double tone into any telephone receiver, the messages may be played back. It is possible to even erase the messages after receiving them or, if preferred, the messages can accumulate for additional review when the staff returns to the office.

"Good afternoon, Dr. Simmons Office. We have installed this answering service in our office for your convenience. We are out of the office but will return at 1:00 p.m. Please leave your name, telephone number, and message at the sound of the buzzer. We will return your call when we return. Please start your message now." (BUZZ) . . .

"Good Morning, Dr. Doe's office. Dr. Doe is in Chicago today attending the Midwest Dental Conference. He will return to the office tomorrow, January 29 at 9:00 a.m. If your call is of an emergency nature, please call 366-1405. Otherwise, please leave your name and number at the sound of the tone. We will return your call approximately at 9:00 a.m., January 29. Thank you." (BUZZ) . . .

Fig. 5-7 Two samples of recorded messages.

SUGGESTED ACTIVITIES

- Make a list of the features available on a six button key telephone.

- Demonstrate the proper method of answering and transferring calls on a six button key telephone.

- Visit a dental clinic using a Call Director®. Request the secretarial dental assistant to demonstrate using the equipment.

- Contact a telephone answering service company; ask a representative to speak and demonstrate automatic answering equipment.

- Prepare index cards for future reference. Write messages to be used with an automatic answering service for the following situations.

    a. During a lunch break
    b. After hours or on holidays.
    c. Staff away attending an educational meeting or convention.

REVIEW

A. Multiple Choice.

1. Failure to know how to use the telephone equipment in a dental office is

    a. frustrating for the caller and the secretarial dental assistant.

    b. a problem that should be kept from the patient.

    c. evidence that the dentist should relieve the assistant of her responsibility to answer the telephone.

    d. a reason for the dentist to take a course in practice management.

2. Identify the type of equipment which is most likely to be used in an office where one dentist is practicing.

    a. 18 Button Call Director®.

    b. 30 Button Call Director®.

    c. Six button key telephone.

    d. Loudspeaker set.

3. The intercom feature on a telephone is useful because

    a. it gives the dental office more than one incoming line.

    b. the secretarial dental assistant may leave a call without disconnecting it.

    c. someone in the dental office may be briefed before a call is transferred to them.

    d. it disconnects all other telephones from a specific line.

4. A "hands free" telephone feature is most useful to the secretarial dental assistant

    a. during the lunch break.

    b. after hours or during holidays.

    c. when making dental appointments.

    d. when the staff is attending an educational meeting.

5. The 18 or 30 Button Call Director® is more likely to be found in

    a. a large 500-bed hospital.

    b. an office where one dentist is practicing.

    c. an office that employes one dental assistant.

    d. an office where there are several dentists.

6. Automatic answering services are suggested for dental offices to

    a. keep the dentist from having to raise his fees.

    b. take the workload off the secretarial dental assistant.

    c. allow patients to leave messages with the office when no office member is available.

    d. be used for income tax deductions.

B. Match Column I with Column II.

Column I	Column II
1. An unused line	_____ shows a rapidly flashing light
2. A line on *hold*	_____ shows a slow flashing light
3. A line in use	_____ shows no light
4. An incoming call	_____ shows a steady light

C. Match the buttons with their functional use on the six button key telephone.

PRESS	FOR
1. Button 1	a. HOLD
2. Button 2	b. Incoming Line #4
3. Button 3	c. Incoming Line #2
4. Button 4	d. Incoming Line #1
5. Button 5	e. Incoming Line #3
6. Button 6	f. Local Intercommunication button

D. Describe the mechanics of answering and transferring a call on a six button key telephone.

E. An automatic answering service is available in the dental office. Write recorded messages for the situations listed; ask for any additional information needed.

a. The dentist is called away from the office due to the death of a close family member.

b. A three-day state dental convention is being attended by all members of the office staff.

c. A serious emergency has arisen in the dental office with a patient. The dentist has requested the secretarial dental assistant and all members of the dental staff to aid him in working with the patient.

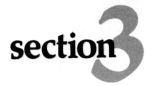

section 3
Appointment Control

Unit 6 Making Appointments

OBJECTIVES

After studying this unit, the student should be able to

- State points to consider when making office appointments.
- Correctly make a dental appointment in an appointment book.
- Prepare a daily schedule to be used in a dental office.

The dental office must have an efficient appointment system as the dental practice revolves around the appointment book. An efficient appointment system makes it possible for the office to run smoothly. Both the patients and the staff suffer when appointments are not planned and recorded accurately. The patient is unhappy if he must wait for long periods of time because of inaccurate scheduling; the dental team is unhappy when there is confused scheduling. Patients make appointments either by telephone or in person. Most appointments made in person are made when the patient is in the office for treatment.

In either case, the same guidelines apply. To avoid confusion, only one person should be delegated the responsibility of making appointments.

PLANNING TIMES FOR APPOINTMENTS

The first step in appointment planning is the selection of an appointment book. The dentist selects a book that will suit the individual needs of the practice. A yearly book that opens to an entire week is commonly used. This gives the secretarial dental assistant a view of the entire week at a glance. The left page of the appointment book is used for making Monday, Tuesday, and Wednesday appointments; the right page is for Thursday, Friday, and Saturday appointments. Each day

Fig. 6-1 Secretarial Dental Assistant making an appointment for a patient.

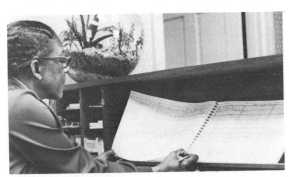

Fig. 6-2 A Secretarial Dental Assistant reviewing an open appointment book.

is marked off in intervals of 15 minutes. The date should be shown at the top and bottom of each day's section. Appointment books with large pages are better because more space is available for writing information about the appointee. Sufficient space needs to be available for the name, telephone numbers, nature of treatment, etc. National and religious holidays should be marked in the appointment book. If the local school holidays and vacation dates are known, they should also be noted.

At the beginning of each week, the dentist should discuss scheduling with the office staff. There may be changes that need to be made because of an unexpected business trip or an upcoming educational meeting or dental convention. These dates need to be marked in the appointment book as early as possible to avoid the necessity of calling patients to change appointment times. Upon receipt of the appointment book, the secretarial dental assistant should begin to mark with an X the times appointments are not to be scheduled such as lunch times and regular afternoons off. All marking in the appointment book *must* be done in pencil. Marking in pen is unsatisfactory because of changes that may have to be made.

As people are generally more alert and function better in the morning, the more difficult dental procedures should be scheduled early in the day. Scheduling long tedious procedures such as crown and bridge preparations late in the day is trying for both the patient and the dentist. Of course, there will be times when the patient cannot make arrangements to come early in the day.

If at all possible, the secretarial dental assistant should try to schedule appointments in such a way that a variety of work is done each day. The dental team would not wish to have all restorations one day and all extractions on another day. Varying the schedule will help to make the working day more enjoyable.

The first appointment for a young child is very important in determining his future as a dental patient. It is not wise to schedule young children too soon after breakfast or during their regular nap times. Midmorning is a good time for these appointments. During the school months, appointments for school children should be scheduled after 3:00 p.m. School age children should not miss school for a routine appointment if a time can be arranged after school. However, there may be times when this is impossible. Explain to the parent that the afternoon appointments are reserved for children who must not miss school. Parents do not like to admit that their children are having difficulty in school and may not be dismissed. This will help to solve some late afternoon scheduling difficulties.

Adult patients who have no preference for an appointment time should be scheduled for the early afternoon hours. This will keep the early morning appointments open for tedious tasks, midmorning appointments reserved for young children, and late afternoon appointments for those who must come late.

Buffer Time

Each day some time should be reserved as a *buffer time;* this time may also be referred to as an "emergency period." Frequently, there are problems and emergencies that arise during the regularly scheduled day; this can create confusion unless a buffer time has been planned. There are three suggested time periods to set aside for the buffer time: 11:30 a.m., 1:00 p.m., or 4:30 p.m. Notice that the suggested times are before or after regular closing times; that is, before or after lunch or near the close of the working day. If the emergency time is not needed, it will give the office extra time to "catch up" on the day's activities.

The buffer time may be used for seeing a patient with a lost restoration. A temporary or treatment restoration may be placed in the tooth until a regular appointment can be scheduled. A patient with a toothache will certainly appreciate being able to receive treatment during the buffer time. Patients with sensitive areas, sutures to be removed, or surgical dressings to be changed may come in during this period. Explain to the patient who is calling that the office reserves the specific time period given to him, for difficulties such as he is having. A buffer time is very helpful in keeping the day running smoothly.

MAKING THE APPOINTMENT

Making the appointment accurately is a must. This includes writing the appointment information neatly and legibly in the correct place. Giving the patient one time while writing another in the appointment book usually results in giving the same appointment to two different patients. This adds much confusion to the office and to poor public relations.

An appointment book, a calendar, a lead pencil, a red-blue pencil, and appointment cards should be available before the secretarial dental assistant attempts to make an appointment. The name of the patient should be printed in *pencil* in the appointment book on the line corresponding to the selected time. Printing is suggested for ease in reading the name of the patient. Spelling must always be correct. If necessary, ask the patient to repeat or spell the name to avoid a misunderstanding. If the name is pronounced differently from the way it is spelled, write how it sounds in parenthesis. If this is the patient's first visit to the office, write the initials NP in red just above the patient's name; it indicates that new-patient forms will need to be completed when the patient arrives. If the patient is a very young child, the age should be written in parenthesis.

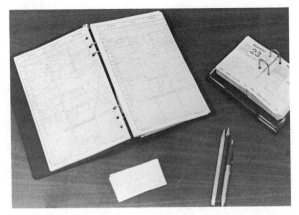

Fig. 6-3 Essential items for making an appointment.

The telephone number where the patient may be reached during office hours should be recorded to the right of the patients name. It is wise to record both the home and business numbers. Denote these numbers by writing (H) by the home number and (B) by the business number. The address of the patient is written if the patient is new to the practice. It may also be written if the address has changed since the last visit.

The nature of the visit should be recorded neatly and legibly just under the patient's name. Abbreviations may be used such as *Ext.* for extraction, *Pro.* for prophylaxis, *Rest.* for restoration, and *Imp.* for impression. If at all possible, record the number of the tooth or teeth involved. If the patient states he is experiencing trouble with both his lower wisdom teeth, write Exam. #17 & 32. (Numbering system will be discussed in detail in the unit on charting.) The nature of the dental visit may require certain preparations by the dental team before the patient arrives. For example, an impression appointment may require heating certain materials. When advance preparation is required, the nature of the visit should be written with red pencil. When the appointment is to deliver an appliance or seat a crown, this is denoted in blue. The blue color signal reminds the assistant to be sure the laboratory prepared the dental case for

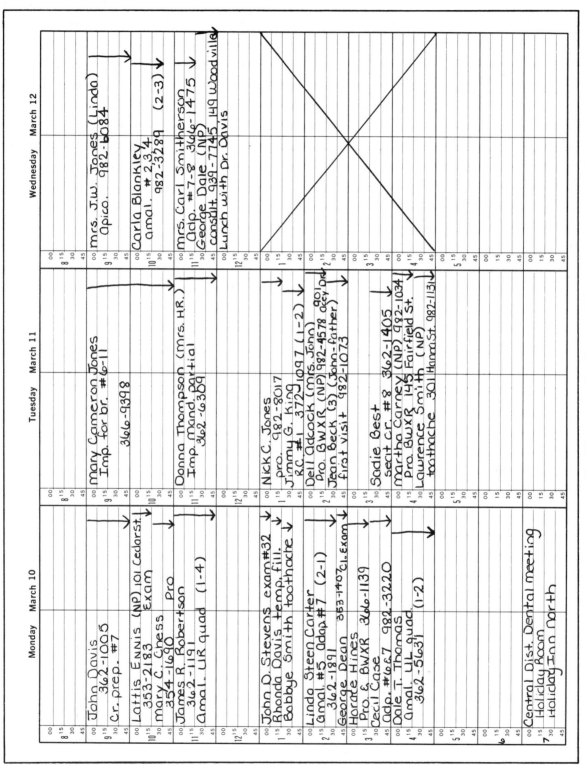

Fig. 6-4 An example of an appointment page.

delivery. The chairside assistant and the secretarial dental assistant may benefit from such reminders.

Many dental procedures require a series of appointments. The number of the sequence should be recorded in the appointment book. A patient may need five appointments in a series, one week apart. The first appointment should show the number 1-4, see third entry in first column of figure 6-4. This indicates that the appointment is the first one in a series of 5. The first number indicates which appointment it is; the second number indicates how many more appointments are to be scheduled. The total of the two numbers indicates the number of appointments necessary. With this system, the dentist can glance at the appointment book and know the exact status of the patient's treatments.

The length of time allotted for the appointment should be indicated by drawing an arrow from the starting time of the appointment to the closing time of the appointment. An arrow is recommended rather than a diagonal slash mark because it is usually neater and more exact. In the event someone else must schedule an appointment, the exact time of the appointments are known. The length of time required for different appointments should be indicated in the office manual of the dental practice. Please refer to figure 6-4 again.

Team Approach

Many offices use the *team approach* in making appointments. Several chairside assistants may be employed in this type of practice. The dentist may desire to appoint patients at the same time for different dental chairs. The same guidelines for planning and making appointments apply in this type of situation. An appointment book is selected that would allow space for scheduling more than one patient at any given time, figure 6-5

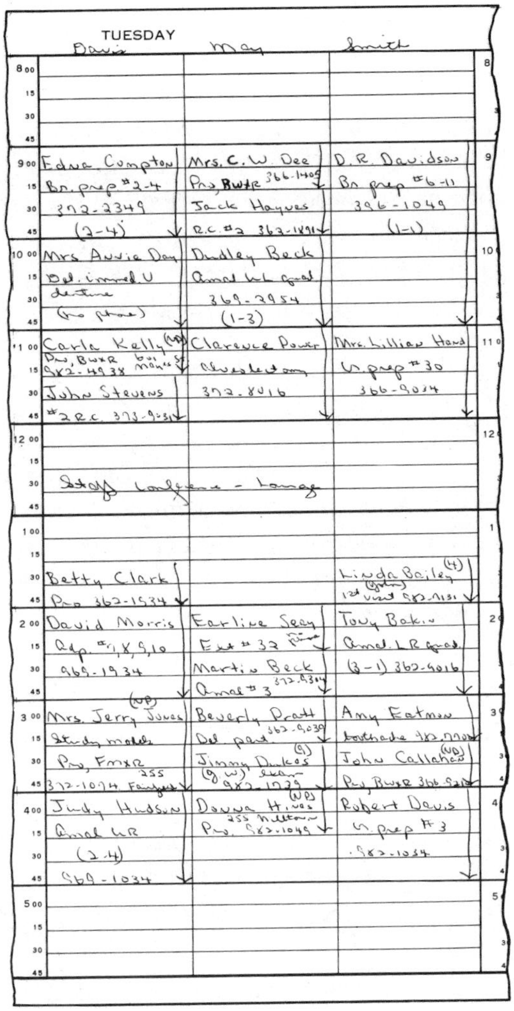

Fig. 6-5 An example of Team-appointment entries for one day.

It is suggested that the name of the chairside assistant assigned to the particular chair be written at the top of the appointed section. Additional time may be needed during weekly staff conferences to effectively plan the appointments. The dentist may decide which type of dental procedure should be assigned to the different chairside assistants.

A message pad should be used to record important information related by the patient concerning the dental appointment. The slip from the pad should be attached to the patient's record card where the dentist can view the message prior to seeing the patient. Any unusual health problem should be recorded in this fashion. If the patient is a referral from another office, the name, address, and telephone number of the referring doctor should be attached to the record card. If confidential information needs to be relayed to the dentist concerning the patient, attach a message slip to the record card states, "Please see me at the front desk prior to treatment."

DAILY SCHEDULE

A daily schedule listing the scheduled appointments should be made for each working day based on the entries already made in the appointment book. It is best to type the daily schedule the afternoon before the appointed day as there may not be time for this task early in the morning. Copies should be made for each treatment area, the laboratory, and the dentist's private office. Printed pads similar to appointment book pages may be secured from dental printing companies. The name of the patient and the nature of the visit should be typed on the daily schedule *exactly* the way it is recorded in the appointment book. Write in red or blue if these colors are used in the appointment book. The age should be written in parenthesis if the patient is a child. The initials NP (new patient) should be written beside the name of the new patient. If the patient has been referred, the name of the referring doctor is written in parenthesis. Length of the appointment is indicated by arrows just as it appears in the appointment book, figure 6-6.

The daily schedule must be placed in a conspicious place in areas where it will be needed. The dentist should be able to glance at the daily schedule and know exactly who is scheduled, the purpose of the appointment and the length of time allotted for the dental treatment.

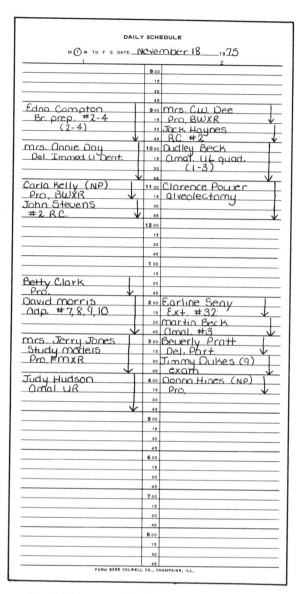

Fig. 6-6 An example of a daily schedule sheet.

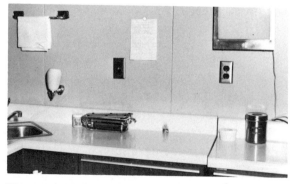

Fig. 6-7 A daily schedule placed on the wall of a dental treatment room easily visible to the dentist.

SUMMARY

Appointment control in planning for and making appointments results in a well-planned working day. The dental practice revolves around the appointment book. Placing one person in charge of the appointment book avoids confusion. The appointment system must be well understood by the secretarial dental assistant. All writing in the appointment book should be neat and legible. Pencil must be used in order to make changes neatly. The name, telephone numbers, and nature of the appointment must be recorded accurately. Each day a buffer time is scheduled to take care of emergencies. A daily schedule list is posted for the dental team to refer to during the working day. The information from the appointment book is transferred to the daily schedule list.

SUGGESTED ACTIVITIES

- Based on what you have learned and using two additional library sources write an essay entitled, "Effective Appointment Planning in a Dental Office."

- With your instructor's approval, ask a dentist to speak to the class about the appointment control as it is handled in his private office.

- Prepare a chart listing steps to use when making an appointment. Use a 5 x 8 unlined index card so that the chart may be used for easy reference by pasting it inside an appointment book or filed in a file box.

- Divide the class into groups of two and role play making appointments.

REVIEW

A. Select the *best* answer.

1. One person should be delegated the responsibility of making dental appointments to

   a. increase the number of patients that can be seen in a day.

   b. avoid confusion.

   c. make the secretarial dental assistant's workload lighter.

   d. provide additional income for the dental office.

2. Appointment books with large pages are preferred in the dental office because

   a. adequate space should be available for writing the name, telephone numbers, nature of treatment, etc.

   b. the book should open to an entire month's schedule.

   c. space should be provided for writing the medical and dental history near the patient's name.

   d. the patient's financial record should be written above the name.

3. Pencil is always used for writing in the appointment book because

   a. using ink pens will be more expensive.

   b. pencil writing looks more professional.

   c. changes may have to be made.

   d. pencil writing is easier to read.

4. Long tedious dental tasks are recommended for early morning hours because

   a. the dental case may need to be prepared for mailing early in the day.

   b. early morning patients are usually better patients.

   c. the afternoon appointments are usually reserved for young children.

   d. scheduling these procedures late in the day is more tiring for both the patient and the dentist.

5. A buffer or emergency time is recommended

   a. before or after lunch or shortly before the office closes for the day.

   b. the first thing every morning.

   c. only on Monday mornings.

   d. from 9:00 a.m. to 10:00 a.m. each weekday.

6. An arrow should be used to indicate the length of time allotted for dental appointments because

   a. it shows the exact length of time allotted.

   b. it can be erased easily.

   c. a diagonal slash mark takes more time to write.

   d. the office manual specifies the time required.

B. Match Column I with Column II according to suggested appointment times.

Column I	Column II
1. Crown and bridge preparations	____ after 3:00 p.m.
2. Very young children	____ middle of the morning
3. School age children	____ early afternoon
4. Adult patients with no preference	____ early morning hours

C. Complete the following.

   1. List five types of dental problems that may be cared for during a buffer or emergency period.

      a. _____

      b. _____

      c. _____

      d. _____

      e. _____

   2. List the desk items needed for scheduling dental appointments.

      a. _____

      b. _____

      c. _____

      d. _____

      e. _____

D. Indicate what the following symbols represent.

   1. NP _____

   2. H followed by a number _____

   3. B followed by a number _____

   4. (3) after a name _____

   5. 1-4 _____

   6. 3-1 _____

   7. Ext. _____

   8. Pro. _____

   9. Rest. _____

   10. Imp. _____

   11. # 17 _____

   12. Appointment written in red _____

   13. Appointment written in blue _____

E.   Complete the daily schedule for Tuesday using information in figure 6-4.

DAILY SCHEDULE

8:00	
15	
30	
45	
9:00	
15	
30	
45	
10:00	
15	
30	
45	
11:00	
15	
30	
45	
12:00	
15	
30	
45	
1:00	
15	
30	
45	
2:00	
15	
30	
45	
3:00	
15	
30	
45	
4:00	
15	
30	
45	
5:00	

Unit 7 The Changed Appointment

OBJECTIVES

After studying this unit, the student should be able to

- Correctly complete an appointment card for a dental patient.
- Write an appropriate message as a written reminder to a dental patient.
- List information needed on a cancellation list.

Although dental appointments are usually changed or cancelled by the dental patient, there may be times when it is necessary for the dental office to request a change. Unexpected illness, death, or personal business may require a sudden change in scheduling. Requesting patients to change appointments should be kept to a minimum. Adequate planning, appointment cards and reminders may keep changed appointments to a minimum. Remember that the word "changed" is suggested rather than "cancelled" when speaking with a patient.

APPOINTMENT CARDS

An appointment card should be given for each appointment made in the office. Patients need a written card to confirm the exact day and time of the appointment or they may forget and come at a different time. The type of appointment card is selected by the dentist. Dental printing or supply companies have several styles from which to choose. Generally, appointment cards which have the days of the week printed for easy checking by the secretarial dental assistant are preferred, figure 7-1. If the days are not printed on the card, the secretarial dental assistant should write the date, the day of the week, and the exact time of the appointment. It is permissible to write the time 15 minutes earlier for the habitual latecomer; if the patient

is usually late, writing the time earlier will help keep the schedule running smoothly. However, the secretarial dental assistant must be very discreet about this.

Writing a duplicate copy for the office may avoid a misunderstanding between the patient and the dental office. A patient may come in and insist that the card (he left at home) stated a different day or hour. Having a duplicate to verify the appointment book may avoid confusion. Appointment cards should be written in ink. Pencil writing is usually not as legible and may become smudged after a few days.

A statement of the office policy regarding changed appointments may be printed on the appointment card: For example:

It is requested that you call our office at least 24 hours in advance when you desire a change in schedule.

Fig. 7-1 Example of an appointment card.

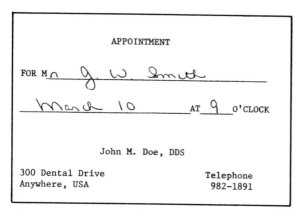

Fig. 7-2 A simple and practical appointment card.

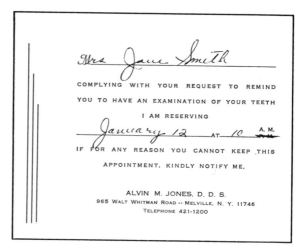

Fig. 7-3 A combination recall and appointment reminder

The office may routinely charge or not charge for broken appointments. Many dentists state that a charge will be made for broken appointments; this is an effective way to emphasize that the patient must notify the office at least 24 or possibly 48 hours in advance. There may always be exceptions to the rule. Many times emergencies or distressful situations arise in which the patient has no control and there may not be time to call the office. Understanding should be shown to these patients.

The name, address, and telephone number of the office should be printed on the appointment card, figure 7-2. The telephone number is more important than the address. Having the telephone number handy will make it easier for the patient to call in advance.

REMINDERS

Patients who live out of the local area or are without telephones should always be sent a notice several days prior to the appointment time. It may be convenient for the dental office to remind the patient by using a postcard. Postcards are usually easier and less expensive to use than letters. Self-adhesive labels may be placed in sheets in a typewriter for quick addressing. This cuts down on time involved in placing individual postcards in the typewriter.

There are numerous printing companies that will print reminder messages for use by the dental office. Space should be available for the secretarial dental assistant to write in the appointment time. The dentist may desire to write his own message and have it printed. If time is available, personal letters may be written to patients.

The written reminder should be mailed so that the patient receives it several days prior to the appointment time and only when a telephone call cannot be made. A five-day notice is suggested. It is easier if the secretarial dental assistant will look ahead *one* week and mail the reminders. This will allow for two-day mail service and still give the patient the reminder five days before the appointment. A five-day notice is usually sufficient since most patients know their personal schedule a week in advance. A combination recall and appointment reminder is shown in figure 7-3.

CANCELLATION LIST

A cancellation list is a written list of patients who wish to come sooner than their appointment time, figure 7-4. Ideally, a patient should not be called unless the secretarial dental assistant has spoken with the patient about

Cancellation List

1. Mrs. Jane Smith 362-8746 Prophy - 30 min.
   Prefers afternoon appts   Appt. June 30, 10.30
2. Mr. D.W. Dudley 947-4638 Two-surface Amal. - 30 min.
   Any time (needs only short notice) Appt. 6-15, 9.00
3. Mrs. C.E. Blankley (for Carla) Ext. UR 1st bi. - 30 min.
   982-4657
   After 3.00 p.m.   Appt. July 1, 2.30
4. Ben Richton (o) 847-3647 (H) 483-4763 Prophy, BWXR-45 min.
   Any Tuesday or Thursday   Appt. June 4, 11.00
5. Mrs. W.O. Ray (Carolyn) 366-3337 Odaptic #7, 8 - 30 min.
   Call only on Wednesdays   Appt. July 3, 8.30
6. Fred O. Klaas 353-5736 Crown Preps #7, 8 (2 hours)
   Any time before 11.00   Appt. July 10, 8.30
7. Mrs. Jerry Jones (Margaret) 356-4836 UR Quad. Amal.
                                                (one hour)
   Prefer Thursday afternoons   Appt. June 19, 4.00
8. Johnny R. Davis 374-6831 Bridge Prep LR (3 hours)
   Monday a.m., Wednesday a.m., or Friday p.m.
   (needs at least two days notice) Appt. June 7, 2.00

Fig. 7-4 A cancellation list to be used for filling changed appointments.

this possibility. Many times the patients will remark when leaving the office, "Call me sooner if you have an opening before my appointment." This name should be added to the cancellation list. When a patient seems distressed about having to wait a long time for an appointment, suggest the cancellation list. Tell the patient the office will try to call him for an earlier appointment by placing his name on the cancellation list. When a cancelled appointment involves a lengthy treatment, it may be necessary to call more than one person to fill the time.

There is usually not room in the appointment book to adequately keep the cancellation list, therefore, a shorthand pad is recommended for this purpose. A shorthand pad is convenient to use and the used pages can be discarded easily. The following information should be recorded on the cancellation list:

- Patient's name.
- Patient's home and business telephone numbers.

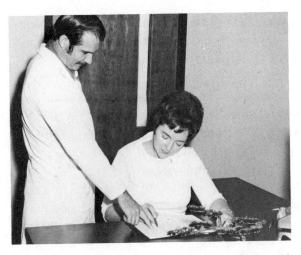

Fig. 7-5 Conference between dentist and secretarial dental assistant.

- Nature of the dental treatment.
- Length of the time needed for the treatment.
- Date of the regularly appointed time.
- The day of the week and time of day most convenient for the patient to come for a changed appointment.
- A notation of whether or not the patient may come on short notice.

Be sure to erase the regularly scheduled time in the appointment book if a patient accepts a changed appointment. Failure to do this will result in time lost from the originally scheduled appointment. Erasing the appointment should be done immediately after talking with the patient. Also, the name should be immediately crossed off the cancellation list; it is embarrassing to call the same patient twice regarding the same appointment. If it is not convenient for the patient to fill a changed appointment, ask if he wishes to remain on the list. Make a notation of his reply on the cancellation list.

If a patient calls to change an appointment only a few hours before the appointment, check with the dentist to see if he desires to have the appointment filled; the dental team may need the time to "catch up." Filling appointments on an hour's notice is more difficult than the appointment changed several hours or days in advance. The office policy concerning changed appointments should be clearly stated in the office manual. In the absence of a manual, the dentist should tell the secretarial dental assistant the policy at the beginning of employment.

When a patient calls to change or cancel an appointment, be as courteous as possible. The reason given for the change may seem unimportant; however, it may be very important to the patient. It is not necessary for the patient to even tell the dental office the reason for the change. Never should the patient be asked the reason. If the patient states he is unhappy with the fees or dental service, suggest that he visit the office for a consultation with the dentist. Try to be understanding of the patient's problem or concern.

BROKEN APPOINTMENTS

When the patient does not come or call the office during the time scheduled for the appointment, it is called a *broken appointment.* Some patients may not come even after they receive a written reminder or a telephone call

from the office. They should be notified in writing that they have missed an appointment. The note should be short and to the point. It suggests that the patient call or write for another appointment. The office manual should include the procedure to follow when a patient habitually breaks appointments; dentists vary in ways to handle the problem.

SUMMARY

Dental appointments may be changed or cancelled by the patient or the dental office. Changes requested by the dental staff should be kept to a minimum. Adequate planning, the use of appointment cards and reminders may avoid many requests for changed appointments. Duplicate copies of appointment cards help avoid misunderstandings about appointments. Patients without telephones should always be sent a reminder notice several days prior to the appointment time. A cancellation list may be maintained for patients who wish to come for treatment sooner than their appointment time. This type of list is very helpful in filling changed appointments. The cancellation list also aids in maintaining an even flow of patients during the day.

SUGGESTED ACTIVITIES

- Compose and write three reminder messages on 5 x 8 index cards suitable for filing.
- Using a shorthand pad, set up a cancellation list for a dental office.

REVIEW

A.   Select the *best* answer.

1. When a patient is habitually late, a suggestion is to

    a. charge for the number of minutes he is late.

    b. make the appointment time 15 minutes earlier on the appointment card than the time shown in the appointment book.

    c. refuse to see the patient when he comes in late.

    d. tell the patient it is fine that he is late because the doctor needs to catch up on his work.

2. Maintaining a duplicate appointment card for the dental office

    a. may increase the productivity of the office.

    b. may keep the daily schedule running smoothly.

    c. may avoid a misunderstanding between the patient and the dental office concerning the appointed time.

    d. may avoid the use of a cancellation list.

3. The telephone number should always be printed on an appointment card because

    a. it will make it easier for the patient to call in advance if a change in scheduling is desired.

    b. the patient may want to give the doctor's number to a friend.

    c. space is not available for both the telephone number and the address.

4. Postcards are preferred for written recalls because they

    a. are less expensive and easier to use.

    b. look more professional.

    c. get better mail service.

    d. lend themselves to detailed messages.

5. If only an hour's notice has been given by a patient, the secretarial dental assistant should check with the dentist before filling appointments that have been changed because the

    a. dental team may be tired of working.

    b. chairside dental assistant may have other plans for the time.

    c. hygienist may need the dentist to check her patients.

    d. dental team may need the time to "catch up" on the day's activities.

6. If a patient states he is cancelling the appointment because he is unhappy about the fee, suggest that he

    a. visit the office and consult with the dentist.

    b. need not call the office again.

    c. forget about it and keep the appointment anyway.

    d. pay for the cancelled appointment.

B. List three suggestions that may aid in keeping changed appointments to a minimum.

    1. _____

    2. _____

    3. _____

C. List the information that should be recorded on a cancellation list.

1. _____
2. _____
3. _____
4. _____
5. _____
6. _____
7. _____

D. Define.

1. A cancellation list.

    _____

    _____

2. A broken appointment.

    _____

    _____

E. Write an appropriate message to send to a patient who has broken an appointment on February 23, at 2:00 p.m. The appointment was scheduled to cover one hour's time.

Unit 8 Recalling Patients

OBJECTIVES

After studying this unit, the student should be able to

- Define and give the reasons for maintaining a dental recall system.
- Describe four specific methods of recall.

A *recall system* is a systematic method of reminding a patient it is time for a visit to the dental office. The visit may be for a routine checkup and prophylaxis or to check on a particular, diagnosed dental condition. In orthodontics, it may be used to check on the progress of a particular appliance. Although there are many reasons for a dental recall, the most common reason is for a regular checkup and examination. The time of the recall depends entirely upon the patient's needs; each patient is different. Some patients need to be recalled for routine examinations and prophylaxis at 3, 6, 12 or 18 months; the dentist will determine the length of time between recalls. A six-month recall is the most common time span.

The new patient should be asked if he would like to be placed on the recall system. In most instances, an explanation of the recall system will be necessary. For example, "Mr. Moore, our office has a recall system that reminds you when it is time for your regular checkup and cleaning. If you would like, we will telephone you in ____ months. You are not obligated. However, most of our patients find the reminder very helpful. Dr. Walker recommended on your chart that you return in ____ months." An explanation such as this may make the future recall conversation easier. When the call is made, it is suggested that the patient be reminded that he agreed to the recall system. If the patient expresses a desire to be reminded, his record should be placed immediately in a desk rack labeled "Charts to be Recalled." As soon as possible, a recall file system should be made up for the patient.

The dentist may assign the task of recalling to either the secretarial dental assistant or the dental hygienist; the same guidelines apply for both. There are different methods of setting up recall systems. The dentist will decide which method is best suited to his practice. The telephone method of recall has been mentioned. Many offices use a postcard or letter for the recall. Four methods of recall will be discussed: the advanced appointment method (at dismissal); the appointment book (telephone recall); the postcard (single file method); the postcard (double file method).

ADVANCED APPOINTMENT METHOD (AT DISMISSAL)

An uncomplicated recall method is to make the appointment in advance. When the

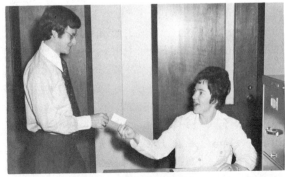

Fig. 8-1 A patient upon dismissal of dental treatment is given an advanced appointment card.

patient is dismissed, he is encouraged to make his next appointment for X number of months in advance. The patient is given an appointment card and reminded that the office will call to confirm the time one week before the appointment. Each day the secretarial dental assistant should look ahead one week and make calls to confirm appointments. If a reminder is to be written, it is important that it be sent at least one week in advance. Some dentists may prefer that the card be sent two weeks in advance.

It is suggested that the dental office have a message printed on postcards by a printing company. Space should be provided for writing in the day, date, and time of the appointment. This card may be filled out and handed to the patient for the address to be written. Afterwards, the card will be filed for mailing at least one or two weeks prior to the appointment time.

APPOINTMENT BOOK (TELEPHONE RECALL)

The appointment book recall is probably one of the simplest of all recall systems. It is recommended for the office that employs one dental assistant to do all the duties. This person would be responsible for the front desk, the treatment area, and the laboratory. The one-girl office needs an effective but simple method of recalling patients.

Most appointment books have at least 12 pages in the back of the book to be used for recalls. The name of the month is printed at the top of each page. If the present month is January, a six-month recall would be scheduled for July. The proper month is turned to in the appointment book and the necessary information is written. The name, telephone numbers, nature of the recall and how the recall is to be made (phone or written) is recorded. If a preferred time is known, this should also be recorded. It will take an entire

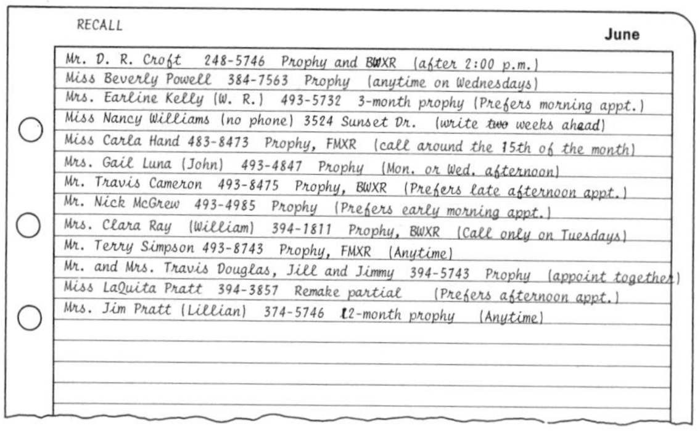

Fig. 8-2 Example of a recall record kept in the daily log. Notice additional information recorded for each patient.

line for each recall patient in order to record the proper information. If more than 25 or 30 patients are to be recalled each month, additional pages will be needed for the appointment book. Space for keeping recall records may also be provided in the daily log. Special pages may be purchased for the daily log recall method, figure 8-2.

Recalls for the month are begun at the beginning of each month. The person in charge may want to set up specific time goals; if forty patients are to be recalled, two calls may be made daily. Spacing the recalls throughout the month will give the office an even flow of recall appointments.

Before dialing the patient's number, his record card should be removed from the files. This is important as information may be needed from the card, or information may need to be recorded on the card following the conversation. With the appointment book open, the call is made. (A sample recall conversation can be found in unit 4, figure 4-3. When the recall is completed, the patient's name is marked through on the recall list. An alternate method is to put an asterisk directly to the left of the patient's name. The date the recall was made should be recorded on the patient's dental treatment card just as a treatment date is to be recorded. The results of the call are noted under the service rendered

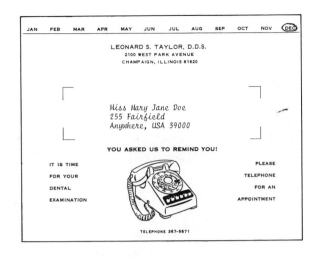

NAME Doe, Mary Jane (Miss)			DATE 6-7-75			AGE 32
ADDRESS 255 Fairfield				PHONE 366-1891		
OCCUPATION Nurse	County Health Dept.		303 Medical Drive			
CHARGE TO Self			ADDRESS Above			
PHYSICIAN Dr. John Smith		306 Medical Drive			CARE NOW? No	
GENERAL HEALTH Good					MEDICATION? No	

REACTION TO: ANESTHETICS Penicillin ANTIBIOTICS
HISTORY OF RHEUM FEVER HT DIS
DIABETES T B
ALLERGIES Pen. ANEMIA
BLEEDING

DATE	TOOTH	SERVICE RENDERED	CHARGE		PAID		BALANCE	
6-7	75	Prophy, BWXR	15	00			15	00
7-1	75	ROC ck.			15	00	–	–
12-2	75	Recalled: Discontinue						
		(Pt. moving to Denver)						

Fig. 8-3 A treatment card showing the proper method to record a discontinued recall.

column. For example, "6-18-75 Recalled: Appointment made for 6-25-75." If the patient desires to discontinue the recall system, the following may be noted: "6-18-75 Recalled: Patient wishes to discontinue recall." If the patient states a reason for discontinuing, note it on the treatment card, figure 8-3.

POSTCARD (SINGLE FILE METHOD)

The postcard method is an effective way of maintaining recall records. When the patient is dismissed, a postcard reminder is written and addressed for X number of months ahead, figure 8-4. The card is filed under the proper month in a file box. During that particular month, several cards are removed daily from the file box and mailed. Mailing all the cards at one time during the month would create confusion as many patients would call the office at the same time of the month. It is best to divide the number of cards among the number of working days in the month. On the day the card is mailed, the patient's record card should be removed from the files and a notation made stating the recall card was mailed.

JAN FEB MAR APR MAY JUN JUL AUG SEP OCT NOV DEC

LEONARD S. TAYLOR, D.D.S.
2100 WEST PARK AVENUE
CHAMPAIGN, ILLINOIS 61820

Miss Mary Jane Doe
255 Fairfield
Anywhere, USA 39000

YOU ASKED US TO REMIND YOU!

IT IS TIME   PLEASE
FOR YOUR   TELEPHONE
DENTAL   FOR AN
EXAMINATION   APPOINTMENT

TELEPHONE 367-6671

Fig. 8-4 A recall reminder written on a postcard.

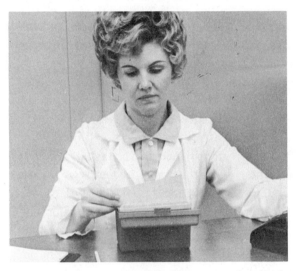

Fig. 8-5 A secretarial dental assistant working with a Single File to recall patients.

Another method is to make the appointment two weeks ahead and mail a notice such as the following:

Dear Mr. Moore:

As you requested, we have reserved a time for you to see Dr. Allen for your regular dental examination. Dr. Allen can see you Thursday, June 19th at 10:00 a.m. If this is not convenient for you, please call our office at 366-1405. Otherwise, we will look forward to seeing you June 19, 1975 at 10:00.

Sincerely,

Ms. Elizabeth James
Secretarial Dental Assistant

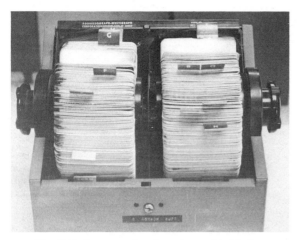

Fig. 8-6 An example of a rotary wheel index.

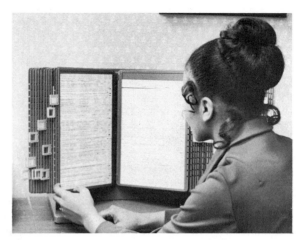

Fig. 8-7 An example of a book index system used in some dental offices.

The monthly file would contain only an index card listing the patient's name, address, nature of recall, and a preferred appointment time. The preferred appointment time is essential information when using this recall method. If a preferred time is known, it may eliminate a number of calls back and forth to the dental office changing the time. When hygienists are assigned to the task of recalling patients, daily time may be reserved on the hygienist's appointment book for work on this recall system. It is essential that the appointment notice be mailed at least two weeks in advance to allow ample time for changes to be made.

POSTCARD (DOUBLE FILE METHOD)

A double file method is recommended for an office when the secretarial dental assistant is assigned to the recall task. It is a double check method of recalling patients. File A is an *alphabetically* arranged file of all the patients in the active recall system. It contains an index card for each patient showing the name, address, telephone numbers, and a notation of the recall month. It is faster and easier to type this information on self-adhesive rolled labels which can then be placed on the index cards. A 5 x 8 file box or a rotary wheel index may be used to file the index cards, figure 8-6

REGISTRATION				
MR. MRS. MISS			S M W D	DATE OF BIRTH
HOME ADDRESS			HOME TEL.	
			SOC. SEC. NO.	
EMPLOYER		ADDRESS		
OCCUPATION		BUS. TEL.		
PREVIOUS ADDRESS		CITY		STATE
PERSON RESPONSIBLE FOR ACCOUNT				
ADDRESS				
REFERRED BY				

RECALL RECORD

DATE OF LAST VISIT	RECALL DUE	NOTIFIED	RESULTS
1-17-74	July	Phone	Appt. made 7-15
7-15-74	January	Phone	Appt. made 1-22
1-22-75	July	Phone	Call again in Aug.

Fig. 8-8 A recall record may also be kept on the reverse of a Registration form.

A book index system could also be used, figure 8-7.

File B contains a 5 x 8 index card for all the patients in the active recall system, filed by the *month* of their recall appointment. Each month individual cards are removed from File B and the recall procedure is carried out.

The double file makes it possible to readily locate the patient's recall time earlier by name (File A) or by month (File B). This method is a little more time-consuming than other methods but it is more efficient.

The four methods explained may need to be modified to suit the needs of the individual dental office. Special recall record cards can be obtained from dental supply companies, figure 8-8. These record cards may make it quicker for the secretarial dental assistant to carry out the recall.

RECALLING CHILDREN

A *pedodontist* is a dentist who has been specially trained in the practice of dentistry for children. Patients in a pedodontist's practice are usually from 3 to 15 years of age; they may be younger or older depending on the individual office or patient. Recall procedures for patients in a pedodontist's practice should follow the same guidelines.

If written reminders are sent to the patients, they should be designed especially for children. The message should be one that the child can understand; if the child is of school age, he should be able to read the message. Address the recall reminder to the child. Children are usually delighted when they receive mail addressed to them.

A good relationship is very important between the dentist and the young patient.

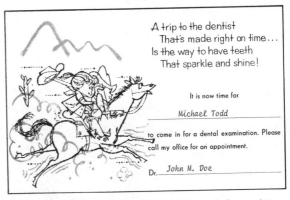

A trip to the dentist
That's made right on time...
Is the way to have teeth
That sparkle and shine!

It is now time for

Michael Todd

to come in for a dental examination. Please call my office for an appointment.

Dr. *John M. Doe*

Fig. 8-9 An example of a recall reminder written especially for a child patient.

Recall cards written especially for and addressed to the child patient may kindle a good relationship, figure 8-9.

SUMMARY

A recall system is a systematic method of reminding a patient it is time for a visit to the dental office. A regular checkup and examination is the most common reason for a dental recall. The patient's individual need will determine how often the recall should be made. The four suggested recall methods are: the advanced appointment method (at dismissal); the appointment book (telephone recall); the postcard (single file method); the postcard (double file method). A pedodontic recall may follow one of the four suggested methods; however, the pedodontic recall should be attractive to the child patient.

SUGGESTED ACTIVITIES

- Select one of the suggested recall methods and write an explanation of how it should be used in a dental office.

- With the approval of the instructor, interview a Registered Dental Hygienist; ask her to explain the recall system used in her practice of dental hygiene. Obtain permission to visit her office and see the system at work. Prepare a report and discuss it with other class members.

- Describe how you would explain a recall system to a new patient by role playing with a class member.

REVIEW

A.   Define.

1.   Recall System.

_____

_____

2.   Pedodontist.

_____

_____

B.   Briefly summarize each of the four suggested recall methods.

1.   Advanced Appointment Method (At Dismissal).

2.   Appointment Book (Telephone Recall).

3.   Postcard (Single File Method).

4.   Postcard (Double File Method).

C.   List the necessary information to be recorded for the Appointment Book (Telephone Recall).

1.   _____

2.   _____

3.   _____

4.   _____

5.   _____

D.   Select the answer which best completes the statement.

1.   The time of a dental recall

a. will depend on the desires of the patient.

b. will be decided by the secretarial dental assistant.

c. is in six months from the last appointment.

d. depends upon the needs of the patient.

2. Usually, the task of recalling patients is a responsibility delegated to

    a. the secretarial dental assistant or the hygienist.

    b. only the dental hygienist.

    c. the chairside dental assistant.

    d. the dentist, as he is the one to determine future treatment.

3. The Appointment Book (Telephone Recall) is recommended for the office that

    a. employs more than five dental assistants.

    b. has more than one dentist.

    c. employes one dental assistant to carry out all the duties.

    d. employs a dental hygienist on a full time basis.

4. Recalls made by telephone should be spaced out during the month to keep

    a. the office busier during the first two weeks of the month.

    b. an even flow of recall appointments during the month.

    c. the dental team alert during the entire month.

    d. the telephone lines open at various times of the month.

5. The patient's card should be removed from the files before dialing a patient for a recall because

    a. additional information may need to be recorded.

    b. the patient may want to discontinue the recall system.

    c. the patient may wish to change his appointment time.

    d. an asterisk may have to be placed to the left of the patient's name.

6. If an advance appointment is made by the secretarial dental assistant for the recall patient, the patient should be reminded

    a. immediately by telephoning the patient.

    b. the day before the appointment.

    c. at least two months in advance.

    d. by mailing a card two weeks prior to the appointed time.

7. Writing a preferred appointment time on the recall record

    a. tells the dentist when he can expect to see the patient.

    b. may eliminate having to change the appointment several times.

    c. is necessary only if the hygienist is working with recalls.

    d. is really unnecessary and time consuming.

8. The double file method makes it possible to

   a. allow anyone in the dental office to work with recalls.

   b. give an estimate of the number of patients for the coming month.

   c. locate the patient's recall status by name or by month.

   d. plan the appointment schedule more effectively.

9. Pedodontic recall reminders are designed

   a. with the parents in mind since they pay the bills.

   b. as economically as possible.

   c. the same as any other recall card in the office.

   d. especially for the child patient.

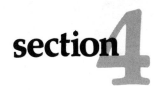

section 4

Patient Records

Unit 9 New Patient Forms

OBJECTIVES

After studying this unit, the student should be able to

- Accurately complete the patient registration form.
- Specify what points must be emphasized to show patients the value of a medical-dental history.
- Complete a medical-dental history.
- Demonstrate how drug allergies are to be shown on the patient's records.

There are two essential record forms that need to be completed by all new patients. The one is a registration form; the other is a medical-dental history. Ample time should be allowed for the new patient to complete these forms when he arrives at the office. Clipboards that have pens or pencils attached with a chain or string should be provided for the patient's ease in filling out the forms. It is very important that the secretarial dental assistant explain the purpose of the forms to the patient. The information provided by the registration form is needed to make up the patient's dental record. For the safety and protection of the patient it is essential for the dentist to know the general medical and dental condition of the patient. The seemingly healthy patient may be more reluctant to fill out the medical-dental history. This reluctant patient may need further explanation of the importance of the health record. The patient should be told that all records are confidential. This may ease the patient's concern about giving personal information.

It is possible to obtain one form that has a registration form on the front and a health history form on the back. Otherwise, two separate forms may be needed. The dentist will select the forms that best suit the dental practice. Many dentists write their own forms and have them printed. This insures the dentist that he has all the information that he desires on each patient.

REGISTRATION FORMS

The registration form is usually a card that asks for all the information needed to complete a dental record, figure 9-3.

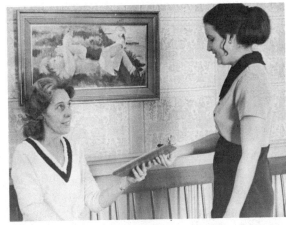

Fig. 9-1 Clipboards simplify the filling out of forms.

67

REGISTRATION SLIP

PLEASE PRINT Date ____________

Name ____________

Address ____________

City ____________ Zip Code ____________

Telephone ____________ Birth Date ____________ Sex ____

☐ Single ☐ Married ☐ Widowed ☐ Divorced

Occupation ____________ Phone ____________

Employed by ____________

Employer's address ____________

Name of Spouse/Parent ____________

Occupation ____________ Phone ____________

Employed by ____________

Employer's address ____________

Referred by ____________

Physician ____________ Soc. Sec. Number ____________

HEALTH QUESTIONS:	Yes	No
Is your general health good?	☐	☐
Are you under a physician's care now?	☐	☐
Have you ever had heart trouble, rheumatic fever, diabetes or infectious hepatitis?	☐	☐
Have you ever had trouble with bleeding after surgery?	☐	☐
Have you ever had an unusual reaction to any drug or local anesthetic?	☐	☐
Is there any other information about your health which should be known?	☐	☐

FORM 3370 COLWELL CO., CHAMPAIGN, ILL.

Fig. 9-2 Example of a registration form with health questions.

REGISTRATION

MR.
MRS.
MISS ____________ S M W D DATE OF BIRTH

HOME ADDRESS ____________ HOME TEL.

SOC. SEC. NO.

EMPLOYER ____________ ADDRESS

OCCUPATION ____________ BUS. TEL.

PREVIOUS ADDRESS ____________ CITY ____________ STATE

PERSON RESPONSIBLE FOR ACCOUNT

ADDRESS

REFERRED BY ____________ PHYSICIAN

DENTAL INSURANCE PROGRAM ____________ LOCAL NO.

PURPOSE OF CALL

PREFERRED DAY FOR APPTS. ____________ TIME ____________ AM PM

REMARKS

FORM 1060 COLWELL CO., CHAMPAIGN, ILL.

Fig. 9-3 Registration form requesting information necessary to complete a new patient's treatment record.

Name of the patient. This should be printed on the form by the secretarial dental assistant before handing it to the patient. For ease in filing, the last name should be printed first, e.g., Sims, Miss Jennifer. When unsure about the full name, ask the patient when he arrives at the office. However, if the appointment was made correctly, the full name will be written on the appointment book. As there may be male patients with the same last name and initials, a man's name should be fully written, e.g., Black, Mr. John David. A married lady's name should be recorded using her husband's name. Her given name should be written in parenthesis after the husband's name, e.g., Moore, Mrs. John Allen (Charlotte). Children's records should record the child's given name with the parent's name in parenthesis. The symbol *P* indicates the name written is the name of the parent, e.g., Douglas, Michael Todd (P-Mr. David L.). In some cases, *G* may be written to show that the name listed is the legal guardian of the child.

Marital status of adult patients. The letters SMWD after the name shows if the patient is single, married, widowed, or divorced. The patient may need an explanation of these initials.

Date of birth. This is an important item. Some patients prefer not to give their age but do not object to writing the date of birth; the age of the patient may then be calculated from the year of birth. If the form asks for the specific age, the date the form is completed must be recorded.

Social security number. This number is needed as dental insurance claims may be made by the patient. Also, many offices use the patient's social security number as the patient number.

Home address and telephone number. This information is necessary in order to send dental statements to the patient. These statements are sent to the home address unless the patient requests otherwise. The street or box number, the name of the city, and the zip code should be recorded.

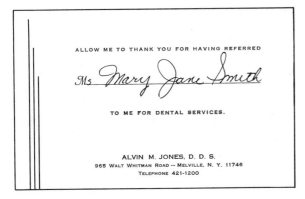

Fig. 9-4 Expressing thanks for a referral.

Name, address, and telephone number of the place of employment. Explain to the patient that the business number would be called only in emergencies. If a patient seems concerned about being called at the office, make a note to always call the home number. Some employees are not free to receive telephone calls at work. This important fact should be noted on the record.

Financial Responsibility. Those responsible for the account should be indicated. In most cases, this will apply to parents of the child patient. However, in an accident case, the name of a company may need to be recorded. The address of the individual or company, if it is different from the home address, is also recorded.

Referral Source. The *Referred By* line is used to record the name of the person who referred the patient to the office. It is courteous to send a note of thanks to the source of the referral. The message may be one such as shown in figure 9-4.

In emergency situations, the referring person may be able to help locate the patient. If the patient should leave the city with an unpaid account which is a considerable amount, a forwarding address may be available from the referring person. The referring person is never held responsible for the account. If a telephone call is made to a referring person because of an overdue account, mention should

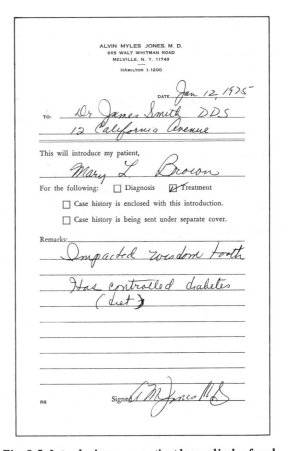

Fig. 9-5 Introducing a new patient by medical referral.

NOT be made of the reason for wishing to contact the patient. Otherwise, the referral source may not make referrals to the office again. When a physician refers a patient, a note of introduction is sometimes written by him, figure 9-5. It may be handcarried or mailed to the dentist. After the patient's visit, a message of thanks, and an evaluation of the dental condition should be written to the referring doctor as soon as possible.

Dental Insurance Program. If dental insurance is carried, the name of the insurance carrier should be recorded. The only information needed for the registration card is the name of the carrier.

Purpose of the call. This should be recorded by the patient; he will usually write what he hopes may be accomplished on this first visit. He may list a procedure that is impossible to perform in one visit. The dentist will explain the treatment and give an explanation of the reasons why the procedure cannot be completed in one visit.

Preferred time and days for appointments. If the patient can only come on Wednesdays, only Wednesdays should be suggested to the patient. Recording this information will save a lot of time when making future appointments. This information should be transferred to the treatment card and the recall system.

Remarks. The patient should record any additional information or important facts that he wants the dental team to know.

Special registration forms can be purchased for the registration of child patients. Usually a combined registration and health history is available, figure 9-6.

MEDICAL-DENTAL HISTORY

Adequate medical-dental histories are very important in the practice of dentistry. It is essential that the dentist know about specific diagnosed medical or dental conditions. For example, a seemingly healthy person may be reluctant to complete the medical history; this patient may be on heavy medication for a heart condition. The injection of certain types of anesthetic solutions would cause a serious emergency, sometimes resulting in death. Explain to the patient the importance and value of a complete medical-dental history. For example, the following explanation could be used:

"Completing the history form is a routine procedure that we ask of all our patients. A complete medical and dental history is very important for us to have before Dr. Fowler can treat you.

Fig. 9-6 Child's registration form to be completed by the parent or guardian.

There are many physical conditions that may be revealed by the condition of the teeth and the tissues in the mouth. Also, certain medications used in dental treatments are not advisable for certain medical conditions. For your protection and safety, we need to have this information."

If a patient refuses to complete the history, consult with the dentist. After an adequate explanation, most patients will cooperate. When they realize that it is for their protection and safety, they are usually more understanding.

Long medical terms should be avoided in the wording of the questions on the medical-dental history. The average dental patient may not understand the questions if technical terms are used. Simply written questions should be asked. The secretarial dental assistant should tell the patient to come to the front desk if help is needed in answering any of the questions.

Certain statements seem to give patients more concern than others. The question, "Are you taking any kind of medication at this time?" bothers many patients. The secretarial dental assistant should realize that this question refers to any and all medications being taken. If the patient is hesitant about listing the medication, reassure him that the record

PATIENT MEDICAL-DENTAL HISTORY

Date _____

Name _____ Residence _____
    Last   First   M. In.   Date of Birth _____

PATIENT MEDICAL HISTORY

Physician _____ Office Phone _____ Home Phone _____

Approximate date of last physical examination _____

		Yes	No
1.	Are you under any medical treatment now?	☐	☐
2.	Have you had any major operations? If so what?	☐	☐
3.	Have you ever had a serious accident involving head injuries?	☐	☐
4.	Have you had any adverse response to any drugs including penicillin?	☐	☐
5.	Has a physician ever informed you that you had: A Heart Ailment?	☐	☐
6.	High blood pressure?	☐	☐
7.	Respiratory disease?	☐	☐
8.	Diabetes?	☐	☐
9.	Rheumatic fever?	☐	☐
10.	Rheumatism or arthritis?	☐	☐
11.	Tumors or growths?	☐	☐
12.	Any blood disease?	☐	☐
13.	Any liver disease?	☐	☐
14.	Any kidney disease?	☐	☐
15.	Any stomach or intestinal disease?	☐	☐
16.	Any venereal disease?	☐	☐
17.	Yellow jaundice or hepatitis?	☐	☐
18.	Do you have night sweats accompanied by weight loss or cough?	☐	☐
19.	Are you on a diet at this time?	☐	☐
20.	Are you now taking drugs or medications?	☐	☐
21.	Are you allergic to any known materials resulting—in hives, asthma, eczema, etc.?	☐	☐
22.	Are you in general good health at this time?	☐	☐
23.	Have any wounds healed slowly or presented other complications?	☐	☐
24.	Are you pregnant?	☐	☐
25.	Do you have a history of fainting?	☐	☐
26.	Have you ever had any X-RAY TREATMENTS (other than diagnostic)?	☐	☐

PATIENT DENTAL HISTORY

		Yes	No
27.	Do you have pain in or near your ears?	☐	☐
28.	Do you have any unhealed injuries or inflamed areas in or around your mouth?	☐	☐
29.	Have you experienced any growth or sore spots in your mouth?	☐	☐
30.	Does any part of your mouth hurt when clenched?	☐	☐
31.	Have you ever had Novocaine anesthetic?	☐	☐
32.	Any reactions or allergic symptoms to novocaine?	☐	☐
33.	Any difficult extractions in the past?	☐	☐
34.	Prolonged bleeding following extractions in the past?	☐	☐
35.	Trench Mouth?	☐	☐
36.	Do your gums bleed?	☐	☐
37.	Have you ever had instruction on the correct method of brushing your teeth?	☐	☐
38.	Have you ever had instructions on the care of your gums?	☐	☐
39.	Do you chew on only one side of your mouth? If so why?	☐	☐
40.	Do you at the present time have any dental complaints?	☐	☐
41.	Do you habitually clench your teeth during the night or day?	☐	☐
42.	When was your last full mouth X-RAY taken? _____ Where? _____		
43.	Any part of your mouth sore to pressures or irritants (cold, sweets, etc.)	☐	☐
	If so locate _____		

Signature _____

FORM 9879 COLWELL CO., CHAMPAIGN, ILL.

Fig. 9-7 A comprehensive medical-dental history form.

71

MEDICAL HISTORY

1. Are you in good health?_____
2. Are you under a physician's care now?_____If so, please give reason for treatment.
   _____
3. Are you taking any kind of medication at this time?_____
4. Please circle any illnesses you have ever had:

allergies	tuberculosis	anemia	kidney or liver
rheumatic fever	diabetes	heart trouble	asthma
infectious hepatitis	epilepsy	glaucoma	other

5. Have you ever had trouble with prolonged bleeding after surgery?_____
6. Have you ever had any unusual reaction to an anesthetic or drug (like penicillin)?
   _____
7. Is there any other information that should be known
   about your health?_____
   about previous dental visits?_____

   _____
   Signature

Fig. 9-8 Example of a simplified medical history form.

is confidential. Space is usually available on the medical history for the patient to circle or check any diagnosed illnesses. High blood pressure, heart ailment, respiratory disease, and allergies are probably the four medical conditions which most influence the dentist in giving dental treatment. For example, if a local anesthetic is to be given to the patient, the dentist must be aware of any of these problems as giving a particular preparation of anesthetic solution could endanger the patient's health and, sometimes, his life. Emphasize the importance of checking these questions correctly.

Questions concerning anesthetics seem to be confusing to the patient. The medical-dental history should have clearly stated questions concerning anesthetics. The question should never be, "Have you ever had an anesthetic?" It would be much clearer to ask, "Have you ever had a general anesthetic?" and "Have you ever had a local dental anesthetic?" Then, questions about any complications the patient may have had with either anesthetic should be asked.

It is very important that drug allergies be listed. *Allergies to antibiotics or pain-killing drugs can be very dangerous to the patient.* Emphasize to the patient the importance of

recording any type of allergies. Some patients are concerned about exposure to dental radiation; question him to determine when the patient has any X rays. Both medical and dental X rays should be recorded. There may be a need to give an explanation to the overly concerned patient. He may be told that X rays are safe when taken properly. Tell the patient that, because they do have a cumulative effect on the body, the office prefers not to take a full series if one has been taken elsewhere within the last few weeks. Printed pamphlets explaining dental radiation should be available to give to the patient. The American Dental Association has a variety of patient-education materials that may be helpful in explaining the various procedures to the patient. A list of these materials may be obtained by writing to the American Dental Association, 211 East Chicago Avenue, Chicago, Illinois 60611.

After the patient completes the registration form and the medical-dental history, the secretarial dental assistant should review the information carefully. Any unusual condition or known allergy should be circled in red so that the dentist may see it immediately. The secretarial dental assistant should write information such as ALLERGIC TO PENICILLIN! or ALLERGIC TO CODEINE! in red ink at the top of the patient's record. Another caution to be recorded is HEART PATIENT! Specially printed red stickers naming common allergies, such as penicillin, may be obtained from medical or dental supply companies. The method used is incidental; the important thing is that the dentist must readily see the caution and know that the problem exists.

SUMMARY

All new patients should complete two essential record forms: a registration form and a medical-dental history. The registration form is needed to make up the patient's dental record. For the safety and protection of the patient it is essential for the dental team to be aware of the general medical and dental history of the patient. Patients may need explanations of the importance of both forms. The secretarial dental assistant must be able to supply explanations and provide assistance in completing both the registration and the medical-dental history forms.

SUGGESTED ACTIVITIES

- With another classmate, role play a secretarial dental assistant helping a new patient complete registration and medical-dental history forms.
- With prior approval from the instructor, invite a dentist to talk to the group on the importance of accurate medical-dental history records.
- Write to the American Dental Association for a list of patient-education brochures available. Upon receipt, write a letter requesting two publications for use in teaching patients.

REVIEW

A. Complete the registration form as if you were a new patient in a dental office.

REGISTRATION		
Mr. Mrs. Miss	S M W D	DATE
HOME ADDRESS	HOME TEL.	
DATE OF BIRTH	SOC. SEC. NO.	
EMPLOYER	ADDRESS	
OCCUPATION	BUS. TEL.	
PREVIOUS ADDRESS	CITY	STATE
PERSON RESPONSIBLE FOR ACCOUNT		
ADDRESS		
REFERRED BY	PHYSICIAN	
DENTAL INSURANCE PROGRAM	LOCAL NO.	
PURPOSE OF CALL		
PREFERRED DAY FOR APPTS.	TIME	AM PM
REMARKS		

Form 1063 Colwell Co., Champaign, Illinois

B. Complete the comprehensive medical-dental history using personal information to answer the questions.

PATIENT MEDICAL-DENTAL HISTORY

Date _____

Name _____   Residence _____
　　Last　　　　First　　　　M. In.   Date of Birth _____

PATIENT MEDICAL HISTORY

Physician _____ Office Phone _____ Home Phone _____

Approximate date of last physical examination _____

	Yes	No
1. Are you under any medical treatment now?	☐	☐
2. Have you had any major operations? If so what?	☐	☐
3. Have you ever had a serious accident involving head injuries?	☐	☐
4. Have you had any adverse response to any drugs including penicillin?	☐	☐
5. Has a physician ever informed you that you had: A Heart Ailment?	☐	☐
6. High blood pressure?	☐	☐
7. Respiratory disease?	☐	☐
8. Diabetes?	☐	☐
9. Rheumatic fever?	☐	☐
10. Rheumatism or arthritis?	☐	☐
11. Tumors or growths?	☐	☐
12. Any blood disease?	☐	☐
13. Any liver disease?	☐	☐
14. Any kidney disease?	☐	☐
15. Any stomach or intestinal disease?	☐	☐
16. Any venereal disease?	☐	☐
17. Yellow jaundice or hepatitis?	☐	☐
18. Do you have night sweats accompanied by weight loss or cough?	☐	☐
19. Are you on a diet at this time?	☐	☐
20. Are you now taking drugs or medications?	☐	☐
21. Are you allergic to any known materials resulting—in hives, asthma, eczema, etc.?	☐	☐
22. Are you in general good health at this time?	☐	☐
23. Have any wounds healed slowly or presented other complications?	☐	☐
24. Are you pregnant?	☐	☐
25. Do you have a history of fainting?	☐	☐
26. Have you ever had any X-RAY TREATMENTS (other than diagnostic)?	☐	☐

PATIENT DENTAL HISTORY

	Yes	No
27. Do you have pain in or near your ears?	☐	☐
28. Do you have any unhealed injuries or inflamed areas in or around your mouth?	☐	☐
29. Have you experienced any growth or sore spots in your mouth?	☐	☐
30. Does any part of your mouth hurt when clenched?	☐	☐
31. Have you ever had Novocaine anesthetic?	☐	☐
32. Any reactions or allergic symptoms to novocaine?	☐	☐
33. Any difficult extractions in the past?	☐	☐
34. Prolonged bleeding following extractions in the past?	☐	☐
35. Trench Mouth?	☐	☐
36. Do your gums bleed?	☐	☐
37. Have you ever had instruction on the correct method of brushing your teeth?	☐	☐
38. Have you ever had instructions on the care of your gums?	☐	☐
39. Do you chew on only one side of your mouth? If so why?	☐	☐
40. Do you at the present time have any dental complaints?	☐	☐
41. Do you habitually clench your teeth during the night or day?	☐	☐
42. When was your last full mouth X-RAY taken? Where?		
43. Any part of your mouth sore to pressures or irritants (cold, sweets, etc.)?	☐	☐
If so locate _____		

Signature _____

FORM 9879 COLWELL CO., CHAMPAIGN, ILL.

C. State the purpose of (1) the registration card and (2) the medical-dental history.

D. Select the best answer.

1. The patient who is reluctant to complete a medical-dental history may be put at ease

   a. if he is given ample time to complete the record.

   b. if the secretarial dental assistant will watch him complete the record.

   c. if he is told that all records in the office are confidential.

   d. if the dentist sees him prior to the completion of the record.

2. The initials SMWD refer to

   a. the days of the week.

   b. the marital status of adult patients.

   c. the credit status of working patients.

   d. the general size of children's teeth.

3. The social security number of patients may be used

   a. as the patient's number in his dental records.

   b. to locate patients with overdue accounts.

   c. when referring a patient to another dentist.

   d. to send out itemized statements at the end of the month.

4. It is suggested that patients record the name of the person who referred them to the office. This source of referral may also be helpful

   a. when trying to locate new employees for the office.

   b. when trying to locate patients who have left the practice with an overdue account.

   c. in seeking new patients during "slow" months of the practice.

   d. when trying to locate patients who did not return for their routine recall visit.

5. Select the four medical conditions most likely to influence the dentist's decision about dental care for his patient.

   a. heart condition.

   b. renal problems.

   c. hormone imbalance.

   d. high blood pressure.

   e. respiratory problems.

   f. brain damage.

   g. any known allergy.

   h. blood type.

6. The dentist should be aware of any previous X-ray exposure a patient has had because

   a. the patient may be able to obtain a diagnosis from another dentist.

   b. the dentist may want to postpone the treatment.

   c. X rays have a cumulative effect.

   d. he may be able to guess correctly without exposing the patient.

7. A serious medical condition or known allergy should be

   a. circled in red for immediate attention by the dentist.

   b. written in the back of the daily log.

   c. recorded on a list and given to the dentist at the end of the day.

   d. ignored since dentistry, not medicine, is being practiced.

E. Complete the short medical history form, using personal information to answer the questions.

MEDICAL HISTORY

1. Are you in good health? _____

2. Are you under a physician's care now? _____ If so, please give reason for treatment.

   _____

3. Are you taking any kind of medication at this time? _____

4. Please circle any illnesses you have ever had:

allergies	tuberculosis	anemia	kidney or liver
rheumatic fever	diabetes	heart trouble	asthma
infectious hepatitis	epilepsy	glaucoma	other

5. Have you ever had trouble with prolonged lbeeding after surgery? _____

6. Have you ever had any unusual reaction to an anesthetic or drug (like penicillin)?

   _____

7. Is there any other information that should be known
   about your health? _____
   about previous dental visits? _____

   _____

Signature

Unit 10 Treatment Charts

OBJECTIVES

After studying this unit, the student should be able to

- List the items included on a patient's dental chart.
- Identify surfaces and teeth on the dental treatment chart.
- Write the suggested symbols used in dental charting.
- Demonstrate accurate charting of specific dental conditions and dental treatment.

There are numerous styles of dental treatment charts that may be purchased from dental supply companies. Different grades of paper are available in the selection of dental charts. Determination of the size of the chart will depend largely on the type of filing system used; they come in many sizes and types.

CHART INFORMATION

Regardless of the type of chart selected, space should be provided for:

- Full name of the patient
- Home and business address.
- Home and business telephone number.
- Brief history.
- Diagram of the deciduous (Primary) teeth.
- Diagram of the permanent (Secondary) teeth showing all surfaces.
- Treatment record.
- Financial record.

Optional features include:

- A complete history.
- Test reports such as vitality tests.
- Diet analysis.
- Recall record.

Certain charts may include three diagrams of the teeth. The first diagram is to be used to chart the existing conditions (restorations, crowns, bridges, etc.). These conditions are those observed during the first examination of the patient. The second diagram is used to chart the treatment that needs to be done. The third diagram is provided to chart the treatment completed in the dental office. The patient chart which includes three diagrams provides the most comprehensive charting of the patient.

CHARTING DENTAL CARE

Dentists use different methods of charting but regardless of the type of chart selected the charting should be uniform. The charting explained in this unit is the method most commonly used. Since dental offices differ in some routines, the secretarial dental assistant must adapt to the particular system used in the office where she works.

Charting is usually completed by the chairside assistant; however, the secretarial dental assistant should be able to read the charts. The remainder of this unit will deal with charting procedures.

The Adult Patient

The universal numbering system is usually taught in all dental-related schools. The teeth

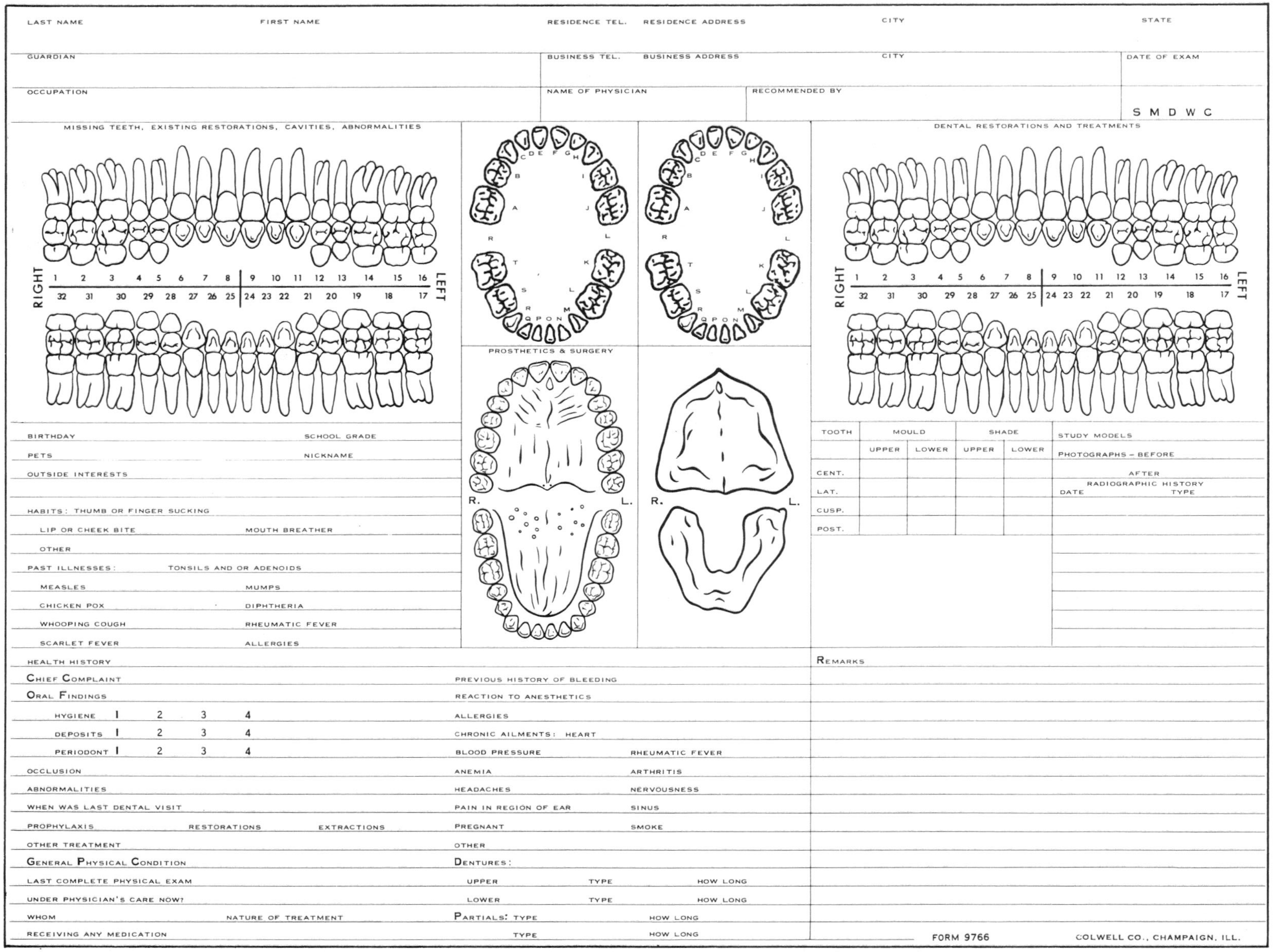

Fig. 10-1 A comprehensive dental chart.

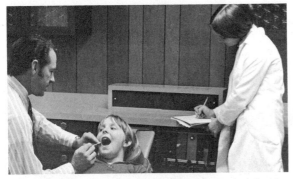

Fig. 10-2 Charting dental conditions as the dentist dictates.

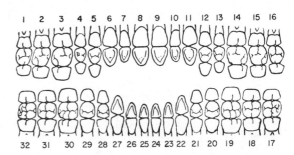

Fig. 10-3 A simplified adult dental treatment chart.

are numbered from 1-32 beginning with the third molar on the upper right, figure 10-3. The upper teeth are the maxillary teeth; the lower teeth are the mandibular teeth. The secretarial dental assistant should know all the names of the teeth and where they are located.

Number of the Teeth	Name of the tooth
1	Maxillary right third molar
2	Maxillary right second molar
3	Maxillary right first molar
4	Maxillary right second bicuspid
5	Maxillary right first bicuspid
6	Maxillary right cuspid
7	Maxillary right lateral incisor
8	Maxillary right central incisor
9	Maxillary left central incisor
10	Maxillary left lateral incisor
11	Maxillary left cuspid
12	Maxillary left first bicuspid
13	Maxillary left second bicuspid
14	Maxillary left first molar
15	Maxillary left second molar
16	Maxillary left third molar
17	Mandibular left third molar
18	Mandibular left second molar
19	Mandibular left first molar
20	Mandibular left second bicuspid
21	Mandibular left first bicuspid
22	Mandibular left cuspid
23	Mandibular left lateral incisor
24	Mandibular left central incisor
25	Mandibular right central incisor
26	Mandibular right lateral incisor
27	Mandibular right cuspid
28	Mandibular right first bicuspid
29	Mandibular right second bicuspid
30	Mandibular right first molar
31	Mandibular right second molar
32	Mandibular right third molar

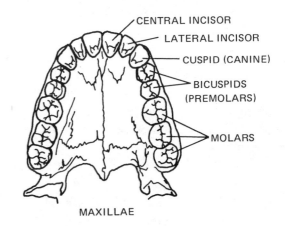

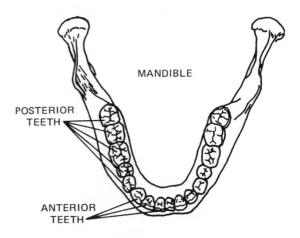

Fig. 10-4 Position of teeth in arch.

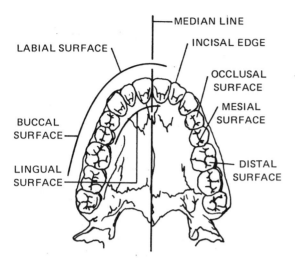

Fig. 10-5 Median line and surfaces of teeth.

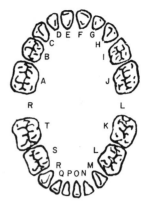

Fig. 10-6 A deciduous dental treatment chart.

The anterior teeth consist of the incisors and cuspids. The posterior teeth consist of the bicuspids and molars, figure 10-4.

Surfaces are described below and may be identified in figure 10-5.

Mesial (M) – The surface nearest to the midline. The midline is an imaginary line drawn between the maxillary centrals and the mandibular centrals.

Distal (D) – The surface furthest away from the midline.

Buccal (B) – The surface on the posterior teeth nearest to the cheek.

Labial (La) – The surface on the anterior teeth nearest to the lip.

Lingual (Li) – The surface on all teeth nearest to the tongue.

Incisal (I) – The biting edge of the anterior teeth.

Occlusal (o) – The biting surface of the posterior teeth.

The Child Patient

The primary or *deciduous* teeth number 20. The surface names of the primary teeth will be the same as for the adult teeth. However, many primary charts show only the occlusal and lingual surfaces of the primary teeth. Selection of the type of deciduous

(primary) chart may depend upon the number of child patients in the dental practice. If there are many children in the dental practice, the charting will be more comprehensive; also, the primary teeth are lettered rather than numbered to avoid confusion with the adult numbering system, figure 10-6. The lettering begins on the maxillary right.

Letter of the Tooth	Name of the tooth
A	Maxillary right primary second molar
B	Maxillary right primary first molar
C	Maxillary right primary cuspid
D	Maxillary right primary lateral incisor
E	Maxillary right primary central incisor
F.	Maxillary left primary central incisor
G	Maxillary left primary lateral incisor
H	Maxillary left primary cuspid
I	Maxillary left primary first molar
J	Maxillary left primary second molar
K	Mandibular left primary second molar
L	Mandibular left primary first molar
M	Mandibular left primary cuspid
N	Mandibular left primary lateral incisor
O	Mandibular left primary central incisor
P	Mandibular right primary central incisor
Q	Mandibular right primary lateral incisor
R	Mandibular right primary cuspid
S	Mandibular right primary first molar
T	Mandibular right primary second molar

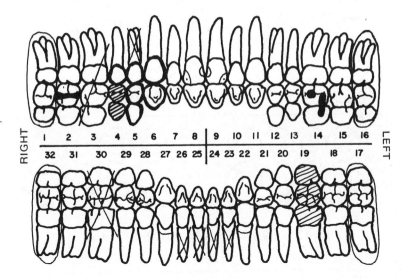

Fig. 10-7 An adult chart showing symbols that may be used in charting dental conditions.

SYMBOLS OF CHARTING

Various symbols may be used to chart dental conditions or treatments needed on either the adult or the primary chart. Keep in mind that individual dentists may have a charting method adapted to their own practice. The charting symbols illustrated in this unit are suggested symbols that may be used. These symbols are designed for use with a pencil, pen, or a colored pencil. If colored pencils are used, red should be used for carious lesions or other conditions that are in need of treatment; blue should be used for treatment procedures that have been completed in the office. For example, a carious lesion would be outlined in red. If an amalgam restoration was placed, the area may then be colored in blue, figure 10-7. Following is a list of suggested symbols:

/	Needs to be extracted
//	Tooth has been extracted
X	Tooth is missing
ⓦ	(encircle tooth) Tooth is not in evidence (Impacted)
O	Carious lesion
●	Amalgam restoration

⊙	Esthetic Restoration (acrylic, composite, etc.)
⊙	Silicate Restoration
Z	Fracture of tooth or restoration
▨	Cast gold (Inlay or crown)
▦	Chrome or stainless steel
M	Mobility exists
?	Tooth or area is questionable
$7\frac{5}{4}6$	Numbers indicate pocket depth
⌣ or ⌢	Gingival recession is present
-----	Eruption process
⌷	Indicates an esthetic facing on a bridge
———	(A line drawn above or below the lingual surface indicates a removal appliance is present.)

An alternate diagram which may be used is shown in figure 10-8, page 82.

TREATMENT RECORD

In addition to the dental chart, the treatment record is an important part of the patient's file, figure 10-9. The treatment record provides space for the date, service rendered,

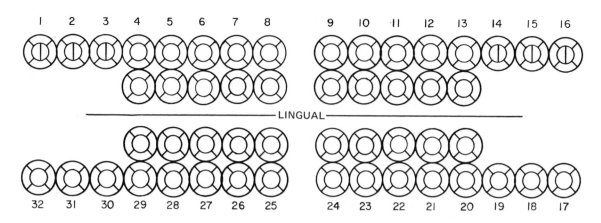

Fig. 10-8 An alternate (uncharted) dental diagram

NAME	Doe, (Miss) Mary Jane	DATE 1-4-74	AGE 33

ADDRESS 300 Nowhere St. TELEPHONE 982-8017

BUSINESS ADDRESS 189 Medical Dr. TELEPHONE 366-1405

CHARGE TO self ADDRESS 300 Nowhere St.

ESTIMATE REFERRED BY Dr. Jones

REMARKS

NAME			ADDRESS			
DATE	TOOTH	SERVICE RENDERED		CHARGE	PAID	BALANCE
1-4 74		Pro, BWxR	cash	15 00	15 00	—
2-8 74	2	#2 OL Amal.		12 00		12 00
3-1 74		RoA	ck.		12 00	—
5-6 74		#8 Imp for Cr.		NC —		
5-16 74		Seat Cr. #8	ck.	100 00	50 00	50 00
6-2 74		#12 Do Amal, #13 Mo Amal ck.		25 00	75 00	—
7-3 74		Pro.		10 00		10 00
7-16 74		#9 Cl. IV DI Adp.	ck	15 00	25 00	—
1-5 75		Pro, BWxR		15 00		15 00
1-20 75		#19 MoD Amal.		18 00		33 00

Fig. 10-9 A complete adult dental chart showing symbols charted, treatment written, and financial records recorded.

	SUGGESTED ABBREVIATIONS		
Cl. exam	Clinical examination	MO	Mesial-Occlusal Restoration or lesion.
Ext.	Extraction		
Amal. or A.	Amalgam restoration	DI	Distal-Incisal Restoration or lesion.
Cr.	Crown		
Imp.	Impression	Pro.	Prophylaxis (Cleaning)
Dent. Adj.	Denture adjustment	FMXR	Full series of radiographs
DO	Distal-Occlusal Restoration or carious lesion.	BWXR	Interproximal radiographs (Bite-wings)
MOD	Mesial-Occlusal-Distal Restoration or lesion.	R.C.	Root canal
		Apico.	Apicoectomy

and the financial record. The financial record is further broken down into a charge, paid, and balance column.

The Date column requires that the date of treatment be written to the extreme left on the treatment chart. A column may be provided to record the number of the treated tooth. However, many times the treatment involves more than one tooth. It is permissible to leave the Tooth column blank and write in the tooth number or numbers under the Services Rendered column.

Abbreviations may need to be used in recording the services rendered. The surface abbreviations are shown earlier in the unit. They may be used to denote the specific surface. The number or letter of the tooth may be used to signify the location.

The above box gives a few of the most common abbreviations used in the dental office. The dentist may list these and other abbreviations in the office manual for easy reference.

A sample treatment record is shown in figure 10-9. The Charge column is provided to write the fee for the service rendered. The Paid column denotes the amount of the fee paid on the specific date. The Balance column shows the amount the patient owes the dental office. Financial recording will be further explained in Section 5.

SUMMARY

There are many styles of dental treatment records and many methods of charting dental records. Whatever method is used, it should be uniform within the dental office. The chairside dental assistant usually is responsible for charting at the dental chair. The secretarial dental assistant should be able to read the charts; she should also be able to record on the charts from the charge slips. All dental auxiliaries should understand what is written in the patients' records.

SUGGESTED ACTIVITIES

- Role play with another student the method of charting explained in this unit. One student may act as the dentist and dictate comments about the dental examination. The second student may act as the assistant who is charting the dentist's dictation.

- Interview a chairside dental assistant. Ask her to explain the charting method used in her office.

REVIEW

A.   Answer the following questions.

1.   If the patient's dental record includes three diagrams of the teeth, how could you use each diagram effectively?

2.   The financial section of the chart-treatment form provides three columns for recording. Indicate what is included in the Charge, Paid, and Balance columns.

B.   Select the best answer.

1.   The person usually responsible for charting is the

a. secretarial dental assistant.

b. dentist.

c. chairside dental assistant.

d. registered dental hygienist.

2.   The most frequently used adult numbering system is to

a. number the teeth from 1-32 beginning with the maxillary right third molar.

b. number the teeth in each quadrant from 1-8 beginning with the third molars.

c. number the teeth in each quadrant from 1-8 beginning with the central incisors.

d. letter the teeth beginning with the maxillary right third molar.

3.   When colors are used to chart dental treatment, red is suggested for

a. dental treatment that is completed in the dental office.

b. teeth that are not in evidence.

c. conditions that need to be treated such as carious lesions.

d. a fracture of a tooth or a restoration.

4.   Using the color blue on a dental chart denotes

a. carious lesions.

b. teeth that are missing.

c. the eruption process of teeth.

d. treatment procedures that are completed in the office.

C.   Match Column I with Column II.

Column I	Column II
1. /	____ a. Esthetic restoration
2. //	____ b. Amalgam restoration
3. X	____ c. Mobility exists
4. ⊙	____ d. Needs to be extracted
5. ○	____ e. Stainless steel
6. ●	____ f. Area or tooth is questionable
7. ⊛	____ g. Tooth is missing
8. ⬭	____ h. Cast gold
9. ⬬	____ i. Carious lesion
10. ?	____ j. Tooth has been extracted
11. ⌣ or ⌢	____ k. Eruption process
12. M	____ l. Silicate restoration
13. – – – —	____ m. Gingival recession

D.   Label the following, selecting the correct word from the list given.

Mandible
Molars
Lateral Incisor
Maxillae
Anterior Teeth
Central Incisor
Bicuspids
Posterior Teeth
Cuspids (Canine)

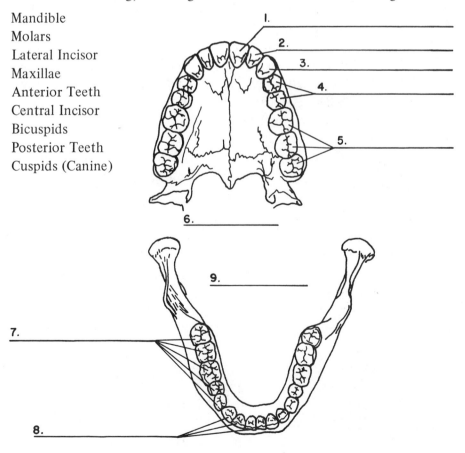

E.   Label the diagram below.   Select the appropriate word from the list.

Mesial Surface
Median Line
Lingual Surface
Occlusal Surface
Labial Surface
Incisal Edge
Distal Surface
Buccal Surface

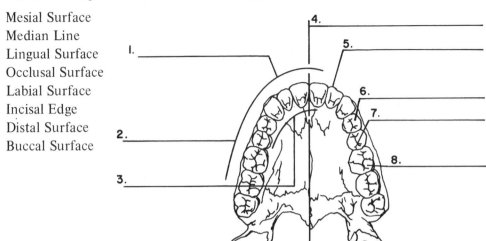

F.   Chart the following on the adult treatment chart provided below.

1.   Maxillary right second molar has a MOD amalgam restoration.
2.   Maxillary right first molar has occlusal carious lesion.
3.   Maxillary right cuspid is questionable.
4.   Maxillary right central incisor has a Distal silicate restoration.
5.   Maxillary left central incisor has a DI carious lesion.
6.   Maxillary left cuspid has gingival recession.
7.   Maxillary left second bicuspid has a DO amalgam restoration.
8.   Maxillary left first molar has been extracted.
9.   Mandibular left third molar is not in evidence.
10. Mandibular left first molar is missing.
11. Mandibular left first bicuspid has an occlusal amalgam restoration.
12. Mandibular left lateral incisor has a Mesial esthetic restoration.
13. Mandibular right cuspid has a DI carious lesion.
14. Mandibular right first molar needs to be extracted.

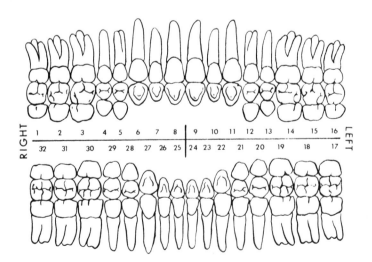

G. Chart the following conditions and treatment needed on the deciduous chart provided.

1. Maxillary right deciduous first molar has occlusal decay.
2. Maxillary right cuspid has a stainless steel crown.
3. Maxillary right central is missing.
4. Maxillary left cuspid has a stainless steel crown.
5. Maxillary left first molar has a DO amalgam restoration.
6. Maxillary left second molar has a MO amalgam restoration.
7. Mandibular left second molar is not in evidence.
8. Mandibular left first molar has a stainless steel crown.
9. Mandibular left central incisor is missing.
10. Mandibular right first molar has MOD carious lesion.

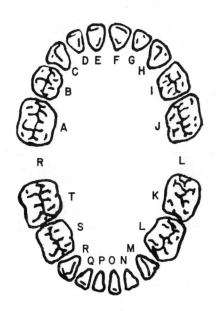

Unit 11 Radiographic and Study Model Records

OBJECTIVES

After studying this unit, the student should be able to

- Define and identify the six types of dental radiographs.
- Demonstrate the proper method of storing radiographic records.
- State methods of storing study model records.

Patient's radiographic and study model records are as important as the patient's treatment and financial records. Radiographic records include periapical, bite-wing, full mouth series, occlusal, panoramic, and cephalometric radiographs. *Periapical radiographs* are single films showing the entire tooth and bone structure of individual teeth, figure 11-1. *Bite-wing*

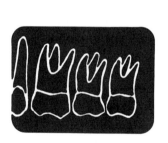

A. Periapical upper molar film

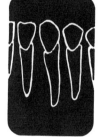

B. Periapical lower cuspid film

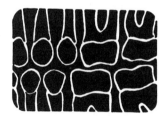

C. A bicuspid cavity-detecting film

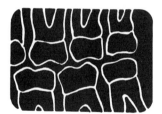

D. A molar cavity-detecting film

Fig. 11-1 Periapical and bite-wing films.

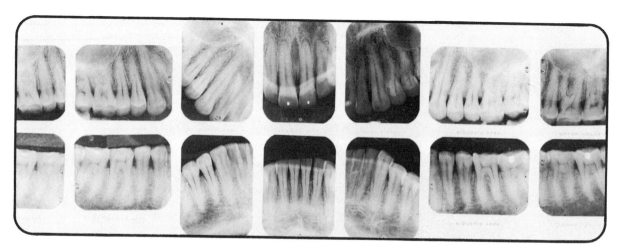

Fig. 11-2 A full series of mounted radiographs.

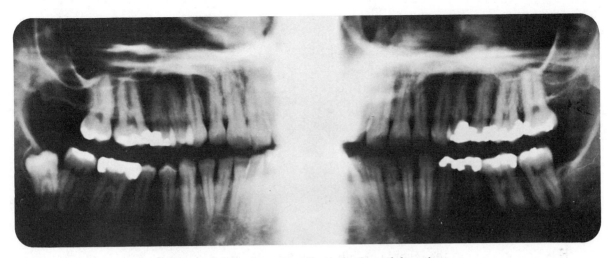

Fig. 11-3 A panoramic radiograph of an adult patient.

radiographs (sometimes called cavity-detecting radiographs) are designed to show the inter-proximal (in-between) areas of both anterior and posterior teeth. These films vary in number from two to four depending on the dental needs of the patient. A *full mouth series or survey* is a series of at least 14 films which includes periapicals of all areas of the mouth, figure 11-2. An *occlusal radiograph* is designed to show a broader view of an entire arch. This type is used for detecting conditions such as bone fractures, cysts, and salivary stones. A *panoramic survey* is an extra-oral exposure showing the maxillary and man-dibular areas in one 5 x 12 inch film, figure 11-3. A *cephalometric film* shows the bones and teeth of the head and profile. This type of film is usually used in an orthodontist's office. An *orthodontist* is a dentist with special training in preventing and correcting irregularities of the teeth and arches.

Study model records are reproductions of the maxillary and mandibular arches of a patient. Study models are obtained by taking an impression of the patient's mouth. Plaster or stone is then poured into the impression. The plaster or stone hardens after a short period of time. The model may then be separ-

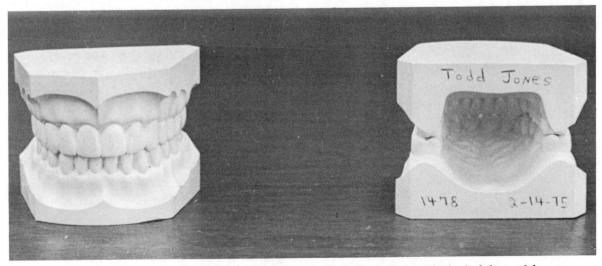

Fig. 11-4 A set of study models. Notice the information recorded on the heel of the model.

ated and trimmed. The patient's name, address, date, and model number may be written on the back (heel) of the two parts of the model, figure 11-4, page 89. Since the study model consists of both a maxillary and mandibular reproduction, they may be held together by a rubber band. The rubber band makes the models easier to handle. The dentist may study the arches and determine a treatment plan for the patient after the patient is dismissed from the dental chair. When the dentist has finished studying the models, they should be stored for future reference.

This unit deals with the records of radiographs and the study models. The secretarial dental assistant is often given the responsibility of maintaining these records; it is necessary that she understand the importance of accurate record maintanence.

RADIOGRAPHIC RECORDS

Radiographic records must be protected from excessive handling. Fingerprints should not appear on any of the radiographs used in the dental office. Radiographic mounts are available for both the bite-wing (cavity detecting) and full series films, figure 11-5. Abbreviations such as *BWXR* for bite-wing films and *FMXR* for full series films may be used. When speaking with the patient, the films should be referred to as cavity detecting and full survey radiographs; the abbreviations mean nothing to the patient. Manila envelopes are available for the panoramic and cephalometric films. Coin-sized envelopes are suggested for the single periapical films.

It is possible to attach the coin-sized envelope and the cavity detecting mounts to the treatment card for filing. However, after a period of time, the files may become very bulky. Also, the treatment cards become rather worn from the staples or paper clips. A separate radiographic filing system is suggested for the radiographic records. No mat-

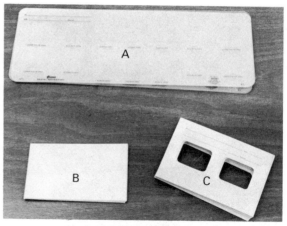

Fig. 11-5 Mounting supplies. A. A full mouth mount. B. Coin envelopes for periapical radiographs, and C. Cavity detecting mounts.

ter what method is used in the office, proper identification of the radiographs must be made. The name and date the films were *exposed* must be written on the mount or envelope. The name and date must be correct. It is possible that the wrong tooth could be extracted because the secretarial dental assistant was negligent. The date the films were developed or mounted is not important. Only the date the films were exposed should appear on the mount or envelope. Accuracy can not be overemphasized.

As suggested in Unit 9, the patient's dental record may be given a number. The patient's social security number may be used for this purpose. This number should also be written on each radiograph. The number system will simplify the filing procedures and may aid in maintaining a double check for accuracy.

Metal files of various sizes may be obtained for storing radiographic records, figure 11-6. It is suggested that the filing cabinet be of a size capable of storing all the radiographic records used in the dental office. Large 8 x 10 manila envelopes can be used to file the periapicals, cavity detecting, full surveys, panoramic and cephalometric radiographs together for each patient. The radiographs should

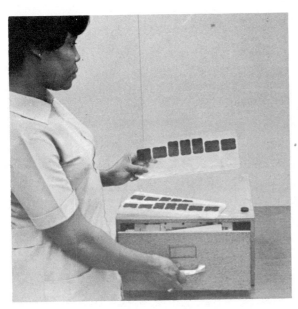

Fig. 11-6 A small stackable filing cabinet suitable for storing radiographs.

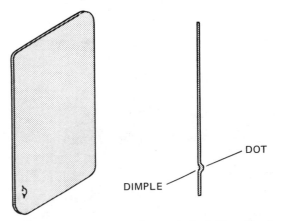

Fig. 11-7 A side view of a periapical film showing the dimple and dot of the film.

be placed systematically inside the envelope. The radiographs which were taken last should be placed near the front of the envelope as the most recent radiographs are the ones most likely to be needed from the file.

The patient's radiographic records should be filed alphabetically. The filing system should be conveniently located in order for the secretarial dental assistant to obtain the records for the dentist. Each radiograph should be kept in the office for at least five years. It may be necessary for the secretarial dental assistant to go through the files periodically and discard those films five years old or older. The *dentist should be consulted before doing this* as he may want to keep certain radiographs for a longer period.

Radiographic mounts are rather expensive; it is suggested that cavity detecting and full survey mounts be used more than once. This is possible if the secretarial dental assistant will write legibly and clearly on the mounts with pencil. After five years, the radiographs may be discarded, the information erased, and the mounts reused.

MOUNTING

Mounting radiographs may be the responsibility of the secretarial dental assistant, the chairside assistant, or the registered dental hygienist. Many times, the secretarial dental assistant may have more time for this task than others on the dental team.

The use of a rubber finger cot on the index finger is advised for ease in mounting. White cotton gloves for both hands may also be used for protection of the radiographs. In either case, the films should always be held between the edges of the fingers to avoid finger marks.

The periapical and cavity-detecting radiographs will have a dot or dimple in one corner of the film, figure 11-7. The dimple is the depressed area; the dot is the bulging area. The dots or dimples must always be turned the same way. Check with the dentist or instructor to determine which way the dots should be turned. This will vary from office to office.

To mount the films to coincide with the teeth as you look at the patient's teeth, place the dot toward you. To mount the film so that the teeth may be viewed from the lingual (tongue) side of the teeth, place the dimple toward you. The middle of the mouth corresponds with the midline of the patient's arch. Special help may be obtained from other members of the dental team for aid in determining anatomical landmarks; these landmarks will be helpful in determining the maxillary and mandibular periapicals.

STUDY MODEL RECORDS

Study model records are more difficult to store as they are very bulky and break easily. Extra care must be shown in handling study model records. Many dental offices have space problems. Not enough space is available for storage of models on very many patients. In this situation, the dentist may decide to give the patient the models to keep for future reference. Most patients like to keep their own models. Usually child patients are delighted with a reproduction of their mouths.

In an orthodontic practice, it is essential that the models be kept. When a patient is being treated for orthodontic purposes, periodic models are taken. These models are maintained for indefinite periods. During the treatment phase, the models may be compared for treatment evaluation.

The orthodontist usually has at least one person in charge of models. Most often this person is a dental laboratory technician. If a technician is not available, the dentist may train a dental assistant to perform this task. The dental laboratory is the area of the dental office most suited for storing study model records. After the impressions are poured and the models are separated and trimmed, the name and address of the patient, the date, and the model number are recorded on the heel of the model. The model number should be the same as the number used on the patient's dental record and radiographs. Having the same patient number on all the patient's records will simplify all recording procedures. The information recorded on the heel of the models should also be recorded in a filing system. Ideally, this system should be maintained in the dental laboratory. A rotary index is

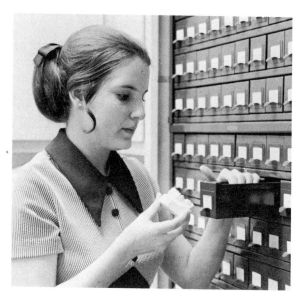

Fig. 11-8 A study model storage cabinet. If space permits in an office, this is an excellent method for storing study models.

suggested for maintaining the study model record numbers. The models are then stored in model storage cabinets, figure 11-8. If space is limited, the models may be carefully packed in boxes. The number of the models contained in the box should be recorded on the outside of the box. The numbers may be typed on 5 x 8 index cards for easy viewing. The card may then be taped to the box. Office policy will dictate the number of years to keep the study model records.

Other dental health team members are usually involved with both the radiographic and study model records. The secretarial dental assistant should be able to obtain either of the two types of records within a matter of seconds. Also, the secretarial dental assistant may be assigned the task of filing these records. Knowledge of this unit is necessary for adequate maintenance of radiographic and study model records.

SUMMARY

Radiographic and study model records are equally as important as the patient's treatment and financial records. Dental radiographs include periapical, cavity detecting, full mouth series, occlusal, panoramic, and cephalometric films. Special care should be taken in handling and filing all radiographic records. Accuracy is a must in recording the correct name and date of exposure.

Study model records are reproductions of a patient's maxillary and mandibular arches.

Information such as the patient's name, address, date, and model number should be recorded on the heel of the model. The models should be stored in specially constructed study model cabinets. Both the radiographic and study model records should be maintained efficiently. The secretarial dental assistant should be able to obtain either record within a few seconds.

SUGGESTED ACTIVITIES

- Request that a registered dental hygienist visit the class and demonstrate how to mount bite-wing and full mouth radiographs.

- Visit a local dental supply company. Note the different radiographic mounts and storage equipment available. Observe equipment used for storage of both radiographic and study model records.

- Contact a dental laboratory technician who is employed by an orthodontist and discuss what method is used to maintain study model records. Report your findings to the class.

REVIEW

A. List and define the six types of dental radiographs explained in this unit.

B. Select the best answer.

1. An orthodontist is a dentist with special postgraduate education in

   a. preventing and correcting irregularities of the teeth and arches.

   b. performing dentistry for young children.

   c. the treatment of broken bones of the entire body.

   d. constructing prosthetic appliances for the mouth.

2. Study models are helpful to a dentist because

   a. he may use the models as a gift to the adult patient in order to establish good rapport.

   b. he may study the patient's dental condition and determine a treatment plan after the patient is dismissed.

   c. charts are not as necessary if adequate study models are maintained on each patient.

   d. he does not need to have radiographs taken of the patient's mouth.

3. A separate filing cabinet is suggested for maintaining radiographic records because

   a. it is less expensive to maintain these records separately.

   b. federal law requires a separate filing of all radiographs.

   c. it is easier for the dentist to locate the radiographs after hours when the staff is away.

   d. radiographs may become worn by excessive handling especially if stapled or clipped to the treatment card.

4. The suggested way to file radiographs is to

   a. place the most recent ones last in the file.

   b. place the most recent ones first in the file.

   c. clip the radiographs directly to the treatment charts.

   d. request that the patient keep his own radiographs.

5. Fingerprints should never appear on dental radiographs. This may be avoided by

   a. using rubber finger cots or white cotton gloves.

   b. installing automatic film processing equipment.

   c. using glove powder before handling the radiographs.

   d. applying a medicated lotion to the hands prior to developing the films.

6. To properly mount the films to coincide with the teeth, as you look at the patient

   a. mount the films with the dimple toward you.

   b. mount the films with the dot toward you.

   c. turn the films either way.

   d. mount the films according to the numbers appearing in the lower left-hand corner of the film.

C.   After reading through the following statements relative to study models, place them in the proper sequence by renumbering them.

    1. Record name, address, date and model number on the heel of the model.

    2. Separate the parts of the study model.

    3. Store the study models in the storage cabinet.

    4. Pour the impressions.

    5. Trim the separated models.

    6. Record name, address, date, model number on a rotary index file.

Unit 12 Insurance and Military Records

OBJECTIVES

After studying this unit, the student should be able to

- Demonstrate how to complete the Attending Dentist Statement – Insurance Claim.

- State the difference between medicare and medicaid.

- List guidelines to follow in completing any insurance form.

- Explain the purpose of the Veterans Administration Form number 10-2570d.

During the 1930's health insurance became popular with many people. However, most of the coverage was limited to in-patient hospital visits. Since that time, medical insurance programs have become widespread but dental insurance coverage is still rather limited. Dental insurance is steadily growing in popularity and more insurance companies are including coverage for certain types of dental treatment.

Insurance records may present problems to the dental office if the secretarial dental assistant is not familiar with the various insurance forms. Completing insurance forms is not difficult if proper instructions are given with the forms. There are many different insurance companies, each with their own particular form. It is impossible in this unit to explain all the many different forms. If the secretarial dental assistant knows how to correctly complete one insurance form, she can usually figure out how to complete the others. The form explained in this unit, the Attending Dentist's Statement – Insurance Claim, is the most commonly used in dental offices. Medicaid forms and military procedures will also be mentioned.

ATTENDING DENTIST'S STATEMENT – (INSURANCE CLAIM)

Since there are so many insurance forms, an effort has been made to develop one form that could be used for many dental programs. The American Dental Association's Council on Dental Care Programs and the Health Insurance Council approved a uniform claim form in 1971, the Attending Dentist's Statement. This basic form has also been approved by the Board of Directors of the National Association of Dental Service Plans. It may be used for all types of dental insurance claims and pretreatment estimates of services to be performed.

If the insurance carrier furnishes the dental office with the form, the carrier's name and address or the policyholder's name may be printed at the top of the page. This form may also be purchased from several dental supply companies and will appear as shown in figure 12-1. The secretarial dental assistant would then indicate by checking the appropriate block if the form is being used for a pretreatment estimate or a statement of actual services.

The numbers in the following explanation correspond with the numbers on the Attending Dentist's Statement – Insurance Claim.

ATTENTING DENTIST'S STATEMENT

ATTENDING DENTIST'S STATEMENT   ADS (71)

CHECK ONE: ☐ DENTIST'S PRE-TREATMENT ESTIMATE
            ☐ DENTIST'S STATEMENT OF ACTUAL SERVICES
                    Spaced for Typewriter - Marks for Tabulator Appear on this Line

1. EMPLOYEE NAME	2. SOCIAL SECURITY NUMBER

3. ADDRESS	CITY	STATE OR PROVINCE	ZIP

4. PATIENT NAME (IF A DEPENDENT)	5. RELATIONSHIP TO EMPLOYEE	6. BIRTH DATE MO. DA. YR.	7. DATE FIRST VISIT (CURRENT SERIES)

8. EMPLOYER NAME	9. DOES PATIENT HAVE OTHER HEALTH COVERAGE? YES ☐ NO ☐ IF "YES" PLEASE IDENTIFY.

10. GROUP DENTAL PLAN NAME	11. POLICY NUMBER	12. UNION LOCAL NO.

13. DENTIST'S NAME (PRINT)	14. LICENSE NO.	15. INDIVIDUAL PRACTITIONERS - SS# ALL OTHERS - EMPLOYER I.D.#

16. ADDRESS CITY STATE OR PROVINCE ZIP	MUST BE FURNISHED UNDER AUTHORITY OF LAW

17. IS ANY OF THE TREATMENT FOR: (B) ACCIDENTAL INJURY?   (C) OCCUPATIONAL INJURY?

(A) ORTHODONTIC PURPOSES? YES ☐ NO ☐   YES ☐ NO ☐   YES ☐ NO ☐

18. IF PROSTHESIS, IS THIS INITIAL PLACEMENT? YES ☐ NO ☐   19. DATE OF PRIOR PLACEMENT?   20. ARE X-RAYS ENCLOSED?
    IF NO, REASON FOR REPLACEMENT: YES ☐ NO ☐
                                                              MO. DA. YR.   IF YES, HOW MANY?

EXAMINATION AND TREATMENT RECORD - USE CHARTING SYSTEM SHOWN

TOOTH # OR LETTER	SURFACES	DESCRIPTION OF SERVICE (INCLUDING X-RAYS, PROPHYLAXIS MATERIALS USED, ETC.)	DATE SERVICE PERFORMED MO. DA. YR.	ADA PROCEDURE NUMBER	FEE	FOR CARRIER USE ONLY

LABIAL

UPPER RIGHT PRIMARY LEFT PERMANENT LOWER

LINGUAL

INDICATE MISSING TEETH WITH AN "X"

REMARKS FOR UNUSUAL SERVICES

ORTHODONTICS: *(give diagnosis, class of malocclusion and describe appliance(s) in above treatment section)*

DATE FIRST APPLIANCE INSERTED _____

DATE LAST APPLIANCE REMOVED _____

TREATMENT PERIOD (NUMBER MONTHS) _____

TOTAL FEE $ _____

TOTAL FEE ACTUALLY CHARGED	
PATIENT PAYS	
BALANCE	
CARRIER %	
CARRIER PAYS	

I HAVE REVIEWED THE FOREGOING TREATMENT PLAN. I AUTHORIZE RELEASE OF ANY INFORMATION RELATING TO THIS CLAIM.

_____   DATE _____
SIGNED (PATIENT, OR PARENT IF MINOR)

I HEREBY CERTIFY THAT THE SERVICES LISTED ABOVE   WILL BE ☐   HAVE BEEN ☐ PERFORMED

_____   DATE _____
SIGNED (DENTIST)

I HEREBY AUTHORIZE PAYMENT DIRECTLY TO THE ABOVE-NAMED DENTIST OF THE GROUP INSURANCE BENEFITS OTHERWISE PAYABLE TO ME, BUT NOT TO EXCEED THE CHARGES SHOWN. I UNDERSTAND THAT I AM FINANCIALLY RESPONSIBLE FOR ANY CHARGES NOT COVERED BY THIS AUTHORIZATION.

_____   DATE _____
SIGNED (INSURED PERSON)

SEE INSTRUCTIONS ON REVERSE SIDE   *Form Approved by the Council on Dental Care Programs of the A.D.A. 1971*

Fig. 12-1 Attending Dentist's Statement.

1. The employee's name is printed or typed. This is the name of the person for whom the insurance policy is written. This is usually the head of the family.

2. The social security number of the employee is written. This is the social security number of the person whose name appears on line 1.

3. The address, city, state, and zip code of the employee is recorded.

4. The patient's name is recorded. The patient may be the employee or the wife, husband, or child of the employee. The full name should appear.

5. If the patient is not the same as the employee, the relationship to the employee is to be recorded.

6. The birth date of the patient is recorded.

7. The date of the first visit related to the claim is recorded.

8. The employer's name is the name of the person or company where the employee is employed.

9. If the patient has other health coverage, the "yes" block is to be checked and the name of the company providing the other coverage is written. If no other coverage is available, the "no" block is to be checked.

10. The name of the group dental plan is written.

11. The policy number is recorded. It is very important that this number be written exactly as it appears on the policy.

12. If the employee is insured through a union local, the number of the local is recorded.

13. The dentist's full name should be printed.

14. The dentist's license number is recorded. This is the number that appears on his state license.

15. The dentist's social security number is recorded on the top line. If this is a clinic or corporation situation, the identification number is recorded. This information must be recorded.

16. The complete address of the dentist or clinic is written.

17. If the treatment is for orthodontic purposes, the "yes" box must be checked. (B) and (C) parts are to be checked if the claim is due to an accidental or occupational injury.

18. Prosthesis is defined as an artificial substitute for a missing part such as a bridge, crown, or denture. If a prosthesis is being reconstructed, the "no" block should be checked. The reason for the replacement is to be stated.

19. If the "no" block was checked in no. eighteen, the date of the prior placement should be recorded.

20. Check if radiographs are enclosed with the claim. Write the number of radiographs enclosed.

The examination and treatment record is to be filled out using the charting system explained in unit 10. The information requested in the examination and treatment record is self-explanatory. The American Dental Association Procedure Number and a listing of all dental procedures may be obtained from the American Dental Association. (The Code on Dental Procedures and Nomenclature is included in the Instructor's Guide to this text.)

When the form is completed it is signed and dated by the patient, by the dentist, and by the insured person whose name appears on line 1. The patient signature is the same name as recorded on line 4. The dentist's name appears on line 13. If a question appears on a form that does not apply, write NA for nonapplicable or draw a short straight line. This tells the person reviewing the claim that the question was not ignored. No insurance form should be completed rapidly. Accuracy is a must. The form should be double checked by the secretarial dental assistant before mailing the claim. Preferably, the forms should be typed. If a typewriter is not available the names and addresses should be printed.

MISCELLANEOUS INSURANCE FORMS

There are many other insurance forms that the secretarial dental assistant may need to complete. It is suggested that a file be set up to include a sample of all insurance forms used in the dental office. If a question arises about certain forms, check in the yellow pages for a number to call for information. In most cities, there is usually a representative of major insurance companies. These company offices may have a special dental representative available to come to the dental office and explain their particular forms.

A 5 x 8 index card can be made explaining each form. The card can be attached to a sample form for easy reference. This will simplify matters when there is a change in personnel in the dental office.

FEDERALLY FUNDED PROGRAMS

Medicaid is a federally funded program that includes dental care as well as medical care. Medicaid is not to be confused with medicare. *Medicaid* is a federal and state program providing medical assistance to needy persons. A state that participates in medicaid must provide assistance in meeting certain health care costs for needy persons. *Medicare* is a federal program that helps provide medical care for people over 65 years of age. Medicare does not cover dental work.

Medicaid is formally known as Title XIX of the Social Security Act. Each state is responsible for administering its own medicaid program. In some states, the legislature has

established medicaid commisions to administer the program. In other states, the state board of health administers the program. A person is eligible for medicaid only *if* he is receiving a public assistance grant (cash assistance).

In most states, there are four programs which include specific groups of people that are eligible for public assistance grants.

- Old age assistance.
- Aid to the permanently and totally disabled.
- Aid to the blind.
- Aid to dependent children.

Most of the fifty states provide for certain dental care in their medicaid program. This care is primarily for emergency dental care in order to relieve pain and/or infection. Some states have dental programs which provide for a certain amount of restorative dental work.

Since all of the fifty states have different programs, it is impossible to explain all the various forms. A sample form from one state is shown in figure 12-2, page 100. Most of the forms are self-explanatory. The treatment and charting records will be similar in most states. If additional help is desired, consult the yellow pages of the local telephone directory for the number of the state's medicaid commission or agency. If no number is listed, contact the state board of health for information.

MILITARY FORMS

Many times the dental office may need to complete military forms. In areas where Veterans Administration Hospitals and Dental Clinics are not available, veterans may be treated by a participating dentist. A *participating dentist* is one who helps to provide dental care and treatment for veterans in conjunction with the Veterans Administration. Veterans with service-connected dental problems are eligible for this service. There are other classifications of veterans who may also be

T-12

STATE OF MISSISSIPPI MEDICAID COMMISSION

MEDICAID–TITLE XIX

DENTAL SERVICES

REGULAR

MAIL TO:
MEDICAID CLAIMS DEPARTMENT
BLUE CROSS AND BLUE SHIELD
OF MISSISSIPPI, INC.
P. O. BOX 3545
JACKSON, MS 39207

1. Patient's Name Last: First:

Patient's Address

2. Medicaid I. D. Number

_ _ _ - _ _ - _ _ _ _

3. Age or Date of Birth

4. County of patient's Welfare Record

5. Provider Name

Provider Address

6. Provider Number

7a. Any other ins? No ☐ Yes ☐ If yes give insurance and policy no.

7b. Covered by Workmans Compensation? Yes ☐ No ☐

8. Complete as required

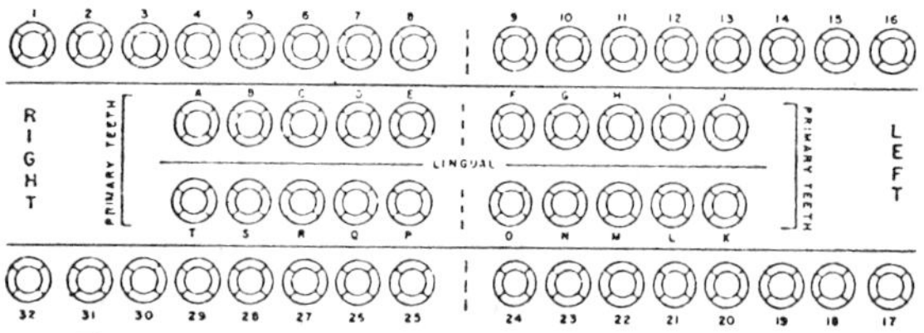

Indicates extraction on this claim

9. Patients Certification, Authorization to Release Information, and Assignment of Payment. I certify that the information given by me in applying for payment under Title XIX of the Social Security Act is correct. I authorize any holder of medical or other information about me to release to the State of Mississippi or its Fiscal Agents any information needed for this or a related Medicaid claim. I request that payment of authorized benefits be made on my behalf.

Signature ***(Patient or authorized representative)*** **Date**

10. Name of referring physician if claim is for consultation services.

11. Diagnosis

LEAVE BLANK

12. DENTAL SERVICES — **USE ONLY ONE DATE & ONE PROCEDURE PER LINE**

DATE OF SERVICE	PROCEDURE CODE	AND	DESCRIPTION OF SERVICE AND IDENTIFICATION OF TEETH	✱ PLACE OF SERVICE CODE	CHARGES

13. I certify that the foregoing information is true, accurate, and complete and that payment of eligible Title XIX benefits will be accepted as full coverage for covered services, and that notice will be given the Fiscal Agent of future receipts. I understand that payment and satisfaction of this claim will be from Federal and State funds, and that any false claims, statements, or documents, or concealment of a material fact, may be prosecuted under applicable Federal or State Laws. All services for which payment is being requested on this claim were rendered by me or under my personal direction. I am duly licensed to practice medicine or dentistry by the state in which the services were performed.

PROVIDER'S SIGNATURE:

✱ PLACE OF SERVICE: 1. Hospital In-Pat. 2. Hospital Out-Pat. 3. Nursing Home 4. Home 5. Office 6. Other

BILLING DATE ________

XIX-16 (6-73) Rev. No. 1

FISCAL AGENT COPY

Fig. 12-2 A medicaid form for dental services that is used in the state of Mississippi. Similar forms are used in other states.

NOTE – ALL ENTRIES SHOULD BE TYPEWRITTEN. IF BALLPOINT PEN MUST BE USED, APPLY HEAVY PRESSURE.

1. ISSUING OFFICE: Veterans Administration

| MEDICAL ADJUNCT CERTIFICATION | 2. DENTAL TREATMENT IS ☐ IS NOT ☐ NECESSARY AS ADJUNCT TO MEDICAL DISABILITY OF: | 3. SIGNATURE AND DATE |

4. FOR VA FISCAL USE ONLY			5. FISCAL SYMBOL 36___0160.001	6. OB. NO. AND D.S.	9. EXAMINATION AUTHORIZATION *(Authorizing Signature and Date – for services and fees listed in Items 17 and 22)*
APPROVED	VOUCHER AUDIT	DATE			
$			7. VA REGULATION	8. AUTH. EXP. DATE	

FEE DENTIST

EXAMINATION AUTHORIZATION does NOT allow for proceeding with definitive dental care. Complete all applicable Items 10 thru 21 and return (with X-rays) for TREATMENT AUTHORIZATION. After all treatment is completed return remaining packet as invoice for payment.

10. NAME AND ADDRESS OF FEE DENTIST	11 SOC. SEC. OR GROUP IRS NO.	12. LICENSE NO.
	13. SIGNATURE OF FEE DENTIST	
ZIP TELEPHONE NO.		

14. "X" OUT MISSING TEETH

ENTER ONLY ONE TOOTH NO., ONE PROCEDURE, ONE DATE OF SERVICE AND ONE FEE PER LINE.

15. TOOTH #	16. SUR-FACES (MO, DO, MOD, etc.)	17. DESCRIPTION OF SERVICE *(List treatment recommendations)*	18. DATE SERVICES PERFORMED			19. CODE NO.	20. FEE	22. FOR VA USE ONLY
			MO.	DAY	YR.			
		X-RAYS *(Type and No.)*						
		EXAMINATION *(Indicate date)* ⟶						
							23. TOTAL	

21. REMARKS *(Include significant periodontal disease, soft tissue lesions, presence and serviceability of existing prostheses, pathogenicity of impacted teeth and statement concerning teeth extracted while in service. (Attach additional sheet if necessary.)*

| 24. SERVICES NOT LINED OUT IN ITEM 17 ARE APPROVED *(Signature of Chief, Dental Service or Designee and Date)* | 25. FISCAL SYMBOL 36___0160.001 | 26. OB. NO. AND D.S. | 29. TREATMENT AUTHORIZATION *(Authorizing Signature and Date)* |
| | 27. VA REGULATION | 28. AUTH. EXP. DATE | |

| 30. PRINT BENEFICIARY'S NAME, IDENTIFICATION NO., CURRENT ADDRESS, ZIP CODE, AND TELEPHONE NO. | 31. THE SERVICES AND FEES LISTED ARE APPROVED EXCEPT – |
| | 32. SIGNATURE OF APPROVING OFFICIAL AND DATE |

VA FORM MAR 1973 **10-2570d**   DENTAL RECORD, AUTHORIZATION AND INVOICE FOR OUTPATIENT SERVICES – COPY 1

Fig. 12-3 Veterans Administration Form No. 10-2570d.

eligible. The office of the state in which the dental office is located should be consulted if the need arises.

A written authorization for an examination must be received from the Veterans Administration before any dental work is rendered by a participating dentist. The authorization is usually good for only thirty days unless an extension is requested by the dentist. A dental treatment plan is then submitted by the dentist to the Veterans Administration. If the treatment plan is approved, the dentist will receive authorization to proceed with the dental work. Treatment may then begin. VA Form Number 10-2570d is the form used for this purpose, figure 12-3, page 101.

Regardless of the type of insurance or military form used, these guidelines should be followed:

- Double check the form to make sure the information was recorded on the correct form.

- Answer all the questions. Put NA for nonapplicable or a short straight line for questions that do not apply.

- Be sure the right persons have signed the form.

- Make a copy for the office file.

- Double check all the information recorded, especially contract number, fee, amounts, and names.

- Check ahead to make sure the office has a good supply of needed forms on hand.

A good suggestion to follow is to set aside a certain time each day for completing forms. If only a limited number of claims are processed weekly, set aside a definite time each week to complete the forms. There are time limits for filing all claims. Check with the proper person to insure that the office is filing the claims on time.

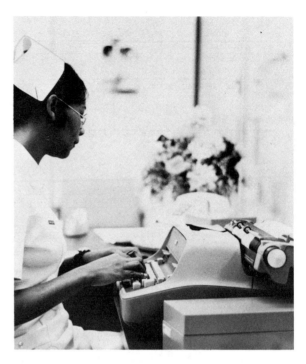

Fig. 12-4 A secretarial dental assistant typing insurance forms.

SUMMARY

In the last few years, dental insurance coverage has grown in popularity. The secretarial dental assistant is usually delegated the task of filing the insurance claims. There were so many different forms that an effort was made to construct a uniform claim for use by dentists. The Attending Dentist's Statement — Insurance Claim was approved in 1971 by the American Dental Association's Council on Dental Care Programs. The Health Insurance Council also approved the form.

Regardless of the type of insurance form used, accuracy is necessary in recording the necessary information. The forms should be typed when at all possible. A specific time should be set aside, either daily or weekly, to complete the various claim forms. All information should be double checked to insure accuracy.

SUGGESTED ACTIVITIES

- Check the yellow pages of the local telephone directory for the number of the local medicaid agency. Make arrangements for a dental representative to speak to the class concerning medicaid procedures in your state and how they apply to dental treatment.

- Collect three different insurance forms. On 5 x 8 index cards list information which will help in completing each form.

- Using a manila folder, prepare an insurance file for a dental office. Place insurance brochures and sample forms in the file.

- With another student as a medicaid patient, role play completing a medicaid insurance form. (The medicaid patient has had a severe toothache. The mandibular left first molar is to be extracted by the dentist.)

REVIEW

A. Answer the following questions.

1. Name four programs which affect specific groups that are eligible for public assistance grants in most states.

2. List six helpful guidelines to follow in completing any dental insurance or military form.

3. State the difference between medicare and medicaid.

4. State the purpose of the VA Form No. 10-2570d.

B. Select the best answer.

1. The ADA's Council on Dental Care Programs and the Health Insurance Council approved a uniform claim form in 1971. This was an effort to

    a. cut down on federal spending in insurance.

    b. provide more public assistance to needy persons.

    c. develop one form that could be used for various dental claims.

    d. place dental insurance in every home in America.

2. When a question that does not apply appears on a form, writing NA or drawing a short straight line

    a. tells the reviewer of the claim that the question was not ignored.

    b. is a signal to the dentist that other insurance forms are held by the patient.

    c. refers the reviewer to the previous line.

    d. is a method of double checking the information on the claim.

3. Medicare is a federal program that provides

    a. dental care to people over 65 years of age.

    b. public assistance grants to all needy persons.

    c. aid to the blind and disabled.

    d. medical care for people over 65 years of age.

4. Medicaid is usually administered in states by

    a. the governor's special health committee.

    b. the county or parish health department.

    c. a legislature established medicaid commission or the state board of health.

    d. a non-profit community agency.

5. Medicaid dental care is primarily approved to

    a. construct new prosthetic appliances for needy persons.

    b. provide orthodontic treatment for needy children.

    c. prevent the occurrence of dental decay by providing extensive educational programs.

    d. relieve dental pain and/or infection.

6. A Vietnam veteran is unable to travel to a Veterans Administration Center for dental work. He may be referred to

    a. a local screening agency for dental help.

    b. the state board of health in his resident state.

    c. a participating dentist who will complete a VA form for authorization to perform necessary dental treatment.

    d. The American Dental Association's Council on Dental Care Programs.

C. Complete the Attending Dentist's Statement — Insurance Claim. The patient is John Doe, who lost a maxillary central incisor as a result of an occupational injury. He has an insurance policy with Superior Insurance Company. Policy No. is 35-741321-69. His social security number is 400-00-0000. A prosthetic bridge is necessary. One dental radiograph is to be enclosed with the claim. (Any information not given may be assumed and supplied by the student.)

ATTENDING DENTIST'S STATEMENT   ADS (71)

CHECK ONE:
☐ DENTIST'S PRE-TREATMENT ESTIMATE
☐ DENTIST'S STATEMENT OF ACTUAL SERVICES

Spaced for Typewriter - Marks for Tabulator Appear on this Line

1. EMPLOYEE NAME   2. SOCIAL SECURITY NUMBER

3. ADDRESS   CITY   STATE OR PROVINCE   ZIP

4. PATIENT NAME (IF A DEPENDENT) | 5. RELATIONSHIP TO EMPLOYEE | 6. BIRTH DATE MO. DA. YR. | 7. DATE FIRST VISIT (CURRENT SERIES)

8. EMPLOYER NAME | 9. DOES PATIENT HAVE OTHER HEALTH COVERAGE? YES ☐ NO ☐ IF "YES" PLEASE IDENTIFY.

10. GROUP DENTAL PLAN NAME | 11. POLICY NUMBER | 12. UNION LOCAL NO.

13. DENTIST'S NAME (PRINT) | 14. LICENSE NO. | 15. INDIVIDUAL PRACTITIONERS - SS# | ALL OTHERS - EMPLOYER I.D.#

16. ADDRESS   CITY   STATE OR PROVINCE   ZIP
MUST BE FURNISHED UNDER AUTHORITY OF LAW

17. IS ANY OF THE TREATMENT FOR:
(A) ORTHODONTIC PURPOSES? YES ☐ NO ☐ (B) ACCIDENTAL INJURY? YES ☐ NO ☐ (C) OCCUPATIONAL INJURY? YES ☐ NO ☐

18. IF PROSTHESIS, IS THIS INITIAL PLACEMENT? YES ☐ NO ☐
IF NO, REASON FOR REPLACEMENT:
19. DATE OF PRIOR PLACEMENT? MO. DA. YR.
20. ARE X-RAYS ENCLOSED? YES ☐ NO ☐ IF YES, HOW MANY?

EXAMINATION AND TREATMENT RECORD - USE CHARTING SYSTEM SHOWN

TOOTH # OR LETTER	SURFACES	DESCRIPTION OF SERVICE (INCLUDING X-RAYS, PROPHYLAXIS MATERIALS USED, ETC.)	DATE SERVICE PERFORMED MO. DA. YR.	ADA PROCEDURE NUMBER	FEE	FOR CARRIER USE ONLY

LABIAL

UPPER RIGHT / PERMANENT / PRIMARY LEFT

LOWER

LABIAL

INDICATE MISSING TEETH WITH AN "X"

REMARKS FOR UNUSUAL SERVICES

ORTHODONTICS: *(give diagnosis, class of malocclusion and describe appliance(s) in above treatment section)*
DATE FIRST APPLIANCE INSERTED _____
DATE LAST APPLIANCE REMOVED _____
TREATMENT PERIOD (NUMBER MONTHS) _____
TOTAL FEE $ _____

TOTAL FEE ACTUALLY CHARGED
PATIENT PAYS
BALANCE
CARRIER %
CARRIER PAYS

I HAVE REVIEWED THE FOREGOING TREATMENT PLAN. I AUTHORIZE RELEASE OF ANY INFORMATION RELATING TO THIS CLAIM.

_____ SIGNED (PATIENT, OR PARENT IF MINOR)   DATE _____

I HEREBY CERTIFY THAT THE SERVICES LISTED ABOVE   WILL BE ☐   HAVE BEEN ☐ PERFORMED

_____ SIGNED (DENTIST)   DATE _____

I HEREBY AUTHORIZE PAYMENT DIRECTLY TO THE ABOVE-NAMED DENTIST OF THE GROUP INSURANCE BENEFITS OTHERWISE PAYABLE TO ME, BUT NOT TO EXCEED THE CHARGES SHOWN. I UNDERSTAND THAT I AM FINANCIALLY RESPONSIBLE FOR ANY CHARGES NOT COVERED BY THIS AUTHORIZATION.

_____ SIGNED (INSURED PERSON)   DATE _____

SEE INSTRUCTIONS ON REVERSE SIDE   *Form Approved by the Council on Dental Care Programs of the A.D.A. 1971*

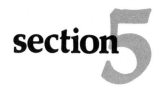

section 5

Bookkeeping Records

Unit 13 The Daily Log

OBJECTIVES

After studying this unit; the student should be able to

- State the purpose of the daily log.

- Demonstrate how to record on the daily page.

- Demonstrate recording monthly records on the Summary and Expense sheets.

- Explain how a pegboard system may be utilized in a dental office.

The daily log is a special ledger designed to reflect the business transactions in a dental practice. The financial records of patients are kept in the daily log. This includes charges made and money received on account from the patient. A sheet, called the daily page, is provided for each day of the year. At the end of each month, a monthly summary page provides space for computing the monthly totals. A yearly summary of charges and collections is included at the end of the year.

In addition to the patient's financial record, space is provided in the daily log for the following:

- Recording the expenses of the office for each month.

- Compiling a yearly summary of expenses.

- Recording employee payroll records for each quarter.

- Maintaining the doctor's personal account.

- Recording names and addresses of accounts overdue.

- Writing memos.

- Maintaining a list of checks written.

- Recording recall information on patients.

Optional features include pages for recording inoculations, surgical records, narcotics prescribed, and comparative income schedules.

The daily log is usually purchased several months prior to the first of each year. Most companies that sell daily logs supply them in attractive covers with optional looseleaf binders. This enables the dentist to select only the sheets that are necessary to maintain the records for his practice. A reorder form and a listing of all supplemental sheets available is located in the back of the daily log.

Maintaining the daily log is usually the responsibility of the secretarial dental assistant. Accuracy in recording cannot be overemphasized. Each secretarial dental assistant should develop her own system of double checking each entry. Recording the incorrect amount of a patient's fee or collection made may result in very unhappy patients. The dentist may be penalized if incorrect recording is made of records that will be used for tax purposes.

Friday   November 5

HOUR	NAME OF PATIENT	SERVICE RENDERED	CHARGE		CASH		REC'D ON ACCOUNT		√
8:00	1								
	2								
	3								
	4								
9:00	5 Mr. John Moore	#3 MOD Amalgam	18	00					✓
	6								
	7								
	8								
10:00	9 Miss Patty Sim	Seat gold Cr. ck.	75	00	25	00			✓
	10								
10:30	11 Mrs. James Douglas	Cl. exam ck.	25	00	10	00	40	00	✓
	12	FMXR, Study Models							
11:00	13								
	14								
	15								
	16								
12:00	17 Mr. C. W. Walker	ROA - cash					75	00	✓
	18								
	19								
	20								
1:00	21 Miss Marilyn Cocroft	#5 MO Amalgam ck.			30	00			✓
	22	#4 DO Amalgam							
	23								
	24								
2:00	25 Mrs. J. M. Bryan	Bridge Prep. #6-11	nc				200	00	✓
	26								
	27								
	28								
3:00	29 Mrs. David Simmons	Cr. Prep. #30	nc				100	00	✓
	30								
	31								
	32								
4:00	33 Mr. John Baxter	Prophy, Study Models ck.			35	00			✓
	34	FMXR							
	35								
	36								
5:00	37								
	38 Miss Sandra Biggs	ROA - check					10	00	✓
	39 Mr. David Callahan	ROA - money order					300	00	✓
	40 Miss Delores French	ROA - cash					100	00	✓
CARRY TOTALS FORWARD TO BUSINESS SUMMARY TOTALS			$118	00	$100	00	$825	00	✓

COLWELL CO. CHAMPAIGN. ILL.

FORM 4201

Fig. 13-1 A completed daily page from a daily log.

DAILY PAGE

The daily page provides space to record the name of the patient, the service rendered, and the amounts that are charged or paid, figure 13-1. A small check mark column is provided for a double check system. A small check mark may be placed in this column to indicate that charges and/or payments have been recorded from the daily sheet to the patient's financial record. This will eliminate many errors. Some daily pages provide space to record the hour of the patient's appointment or the number of the treatment room. The name of the patient should be recorded exactly as it is written on the appointment book. This may avoid confusion if an error is made. The services rendered should appear exactly as it is recorded on the patient's treatment card. Since the daily page is lined off in 15 minute intervals, ample space is usually available for complete recording of the service rendered. This is true because most patients have longer appointments than 15 minutes. Reference may be made to unit 10 for assistance in recording services rendered.

The charge column should show all *charges* made for the patient. This means the amount of the fee not paid for during the visit. The cash column should show all *cash* received for the services rendered on the particular day of the daily page. The cash may be in the form of currency, coins, checks, or money orders. In any form, it is monies received for the services rendered that day. The received on account column should show all monies received for services rendered prior to the day of the daily page. The services may have been performed the day before or weeks before.

Examples:

(a) Mr. John Moore's appointment was at 9:00 a.m. His Services Rendered column shows #3 MOD Amalgam. The charge was $18.00. (All charges shown in this unit do not reflect charges used in any particular office. Neither are they suggested charges. Figures are selected only to illustrate the examples.) Mr. Moore requested that he be billed for the entire amount. The $18.00 will appear in the charge column only.

(b) Miss Patty Sim's appointment was at 10:00. Her treatment was to seat a gold crown. The charge was $100.00. She was only able to pay $25.00 by check. The $25.00 should appear in the cash column. The remaining balance of $75.00 should appear in the charge column. A notation should be made that the money received was by check.

(c) Mrs. James Douglas was in the office at 10:30. Services rendered included a clinical examination, full series of radiographs, and a set of study models. The charge was $35.00. Mrs. Douglas had a previous balance of $40.00 for services performed last month. She wrote a check for $50.00. $40.00 was recorded in the received on account column, $10.00 in the cash column, and $25.00 in the charge column.

(d) Mr. C.W. Walker stopped by the office during the noon hour to pay on his account. Mr. Walker paid $75.00 in cash. His name was recorded at 12:00 noon and $75.00 was listed in the received on account column. In the services rendered column, the secretarial dental assistant should write received by cash. It may be abbreviated ROA — Cash.

(e) Miss Sandra Biggs sent a check by mail for $10.00. Her balance was $15.00 after subtracting the payment of $10.00. Her name was recorded at the bottom of the page. ROA by check was recorded in the services rendered column. $10.00 was recorded in the received on account column. Her balance of $15.00 does not appear on the daily page. It does appear on her treatment and financial record, figure 13-1, page 107.

At the bottom of the page, the secretarial dental assistant may total vertically all columns. The charge column and the cash col-

Business Summary   October

DAY OF MONTH	CHARGE BUSINESS		CASH BUSINESS		RECEIVED ON ACCOUNTS		TOTAL BUSINESS		TOTAL CASH RECEIVED	
1	320	00	200	00	1050	00	520	00	1250	00
2	175	00	400	00	3450	00	575	00	3850	00
3										
4	400	00	289	00	5360	00	689	00	5649	00
5	305	00	506	00	985	00	811	00	1491	00
6										
7										
8	425	50	300	50	675	00	726	00	975	50
9	260	00	75	00	600	00	335	00	675	00
10										
11	102	00	350	00	50	00	452	00	502	00
12	50	00	200	00	960	00	250	00	1210	00
13										
14										
15										
16										
17										
18										
19										
20										
21										
22										
23										
24										
25										
26										
27										
28										
29										
30										
31										
TOTAL FOR THE MONTH										
BROUGHT FORWARD										
GRAND TOTAL										

FORM 4202A COLWELL CO., CHAMPAIGN, ILL.

OCT

CARRY ALL **GRAND TOTALS** FORWARD TO **BUSINESS SUMMARY** OF FOLLOWING MONTH

Fig. 13-2 A business summary page.

umn added together will show the total business for the day. The cash column and the received on account column will show the total cash (money) received for the day. These totals are transferred to the monthly summary sheet.

BUSINESS SUMMARY
(MONTHLY SUMMARY)

The business or monthly summary is a summary of the total business and total cash received during the month. The daily totals should be transferred daily to this sheet. The monthly totals cannot be computed until after the last day of the month. Transfer all totals correctly! Inaccurate recording, such as transferring a wrong digit, causes many problems.

The business summary page is arranged in five columns, figure 13-2. Column I is the Charge Business column. Totals from the Charge column of the daily page are recorded here. Column II is the Cash Business column. Totals from the Cash column of the daily page are recorded here. Column III is the Received on Accounts column. Totals from the Received on Accounts column of the daily page are recorded here. Column IV is the sum of Columns I and II. Column V is the sum of Columns II and III. Each column should be added vertically. (It is suggested that each column be added twice even if using an adding machine.) These totals are recorded in the Total for the Month column. To make a quick check, see if the totals of Column I and II equal Column IV, and Column II and III equal Column V.

Totals for the previous month, if after January, should be brought forward and recorded. A running grand total for the year may then be computed by adding the Total for the Month column and the Brought Forward column. The yearly total will be the total that appears in the Grand Total column on the December business summary sheet. Accuracy is very important as the totals will be used for tax purposes.

EXPENSE SHEETS

Expense sheets are provided to record all expenses incurred by the office during any particular month, figures 13-3 and 13-4. Following is a list of expense categories for most dental offices:

- Drugs and Supplies
- Automobile Upkeep
- Salaries
- Office Rent, Upkeep
- Laundry Service
- Electricity, Gas, Water
- Telephones, Tolls
- Dues, Professional Meetings
- Office Supplies, Stamps, etc.
- Professional Insurance
- Business Taxes
- Interest Paid
- Entertainment
- Miscellaneous

All expendable dental supplies (supplies that will need to be reordered regularly such as, disposable needles, plaster, or restorative supplies) are listed under Drugs and Supplies. Dental instruments not classified as equipment may also be listed as dental supplies as they need to be replaced after a period of time.

Automobile Upkeep expenses apply only to automobiles used for professional purposes. If the automobile is also used as a family car, only the expenses relating to the professional use of the car can be listed in the expense summary. Salaries include wages paid to anyone who works in the dental office.

Dues and professional meetings are listed if they are necessary to the maintenance or success of the dental practice. Receipts of hotel bills or plane tickets should be filed separately for verification.

Office Supplies include most of the materials used by the secretarial dental assistant. Items such as treatment cards, stamps, paper, staples, and pencils are listed in this section.

June   Expense Sheet One

DRUGS AND SUPPLIES				SALARIES				DUES, MEETINGS		
DAY	ITEM	AMOUNT		DAY	ITEM	AMOUNT		DAY	ITEM	AMOUNT
3	Great Drug Co.	56	00	1	Jane Doe	325	00			
3	East Dental Co.	375	87	15	Jane Doe	325	00			
									TOTAL	
								OFFICE SUPPLIES, STAMPS ETC.		
								10	Postmaster	30	00
					TOTAL					
				OFFICE RENT, UPKEEP						
				3	ABC Realty Co.	600	00			
	TOTAL									
AUTOMOBILE UPKEEP					TOTAL					
				LAUNDRY SERVICE						
				5	Clean Laundry	56	00			
									TOTAL	
								PROFESSIONAL INSURANCE		
					TOTAL				TOTAL	
				ELECTRICITY, GAS, WATER				BUSINESS TAXES		
				3	Power Company	85	00	DO NOT INCLUDE WITHHOLDING TAX. INCLUDE ONLY ½ SOCIAL SECURITY TAX		
					TOTAL					
				TELEPHONES, TOLLS					TOTAL	
				3	A.T. & T.	45	86	INTEREST PAID		
	TOTAL				TOTAL				TOTAL	

FORM 4202B COLWELL CO., CHAMPAIGN, ILL.

Fig. 13-3 Expense Sheet One.

Expense Sheet Two   July

ENTERTAINMENT						MISCELLANEOUS		
DAY	ITEM	AMOUNT	DAY	ITEM	AMOUNT	DAY	ITEM	AMOUNT
						18	Charity Ball	100 00
	TOTAL			TOTAL				
	TOTAL			TOTAL			TOTAL	

CARRY TOTALS FORWARD TO **SUMMARY** OF **EXPENSE**

SUMMARY OF EXPENSE	AMOUNT
DRUGS AND SUPPLIES	331 87
AUTOMOBILE UPKEEP	
SALARIES	650 00
OFFICE RENT UPKEEP	600 00
LAUNDRY SERVICE	56 00
ELECTRICITY, GAS, WATER	85 00
TELEPHONES TOLLS	45 86
DUES MEETINGS	
OFFICE SUPPLIES, STAMPS, ETC.	30 00
PROFESSIONAL INSURANCE	
BUSINESS TAXES	
INTEREST PAID	
ENTERTAINMENT	
MISCELLANEOUS	100 00
TOTAL FOR PRESENT MONTH	1898 73
FORWARDED FROM PREVIOUS MONTH	10,890 00
GRAND TOTAL	12,788 73

MONTHLY BALANCES

FOR THE PRESENT MONTH

TOTAL CASH RECEIVED	
TOTAL EXPENSE	
NET EARNINGS	

FOR THE YEAR TO DATE

GRAND TOTAL CASH	
GRAND TOTAL EXPENSE	
NET EARNINGS	

EQUIPMENT (NONDEDUCTIBLE)

DAY	ITEM	AMOUNT
	* TOTAL	

* ENTER THIS TOTAL DIRECT IN **ANNUAL SUMMARY**

FORM 4203A COLWELL CO., CHAMPAIGN, ILL.

J U L Y

Fig. 13-4 Expense Sheet Two.

Magazines or materials used in the reception area may also be included.

Business Taxes are only those taxes relating to the profession. This would include the employer's share of the social security tax that is listed on the employee's earning record. This amount will be one-half of the amount of the social security tax. Money withheld from the employee's (gross) salary may not be listed as business taxes.

Interest Paid applies only to loans or installment purchases of equipment used in the dental practice. Personal interest must be listed on the personal expense sheet.

The Internal Revenue Service (IRS) may need to be contacted for an explanation of entertainment costs, figure 13-4. Entertainment costs may be listed if it is necessary for the maintenance of the practice.

Charitable donations are usually recorded in the Miscellaneous column. The remaining expense summary categories should be self-explanatory.

All of the expense categories are office-related only. The dentist's personal household expenses must never appear on this page. For record purposes, most offices pay all bills by check. The expense sheets should show the date of the check, name of person or company to whom the check is payable, and the amount.

If the expenses for March are being totaled only checks with a March date would be recorded. Even though a check written April 30 might be a March payment, the expense would be recorded in April. All of the categories are then totaled for a monthly summary. The monthly totals are carried forward to complete a year-to-date summary of expenses.

Space is also provided for recording expenses for Nondeductible Equipment. The total for this equipment should be entered directly on the Annual Summary. An additional form is provided for the Annual Summary.

EMPLOYEE'S PAYROLL RECORDS

A form is provided each month for recording payroll records. Each sheet provides space for four employees. If more than four people are employed, it will be necessary to order and use additional sheets. The payroll forms provide space for recording all information needed for tax purposes on each employee. Completion of the payroll records will be discussed in unit 15.

PERSONAL ACCOUNT

The dentist's personal account may or may not be maintained by the secretarial dental assistant. In many instances the dentist prefers to maintain these records completely separate from the office records. However, forms may be purchased for the daily log to maintain personal account records at the office, figure 13-5, page 114. Since this varies with each individual dentist, no further explanation will be given for these forms.

OTHER SUPPLEMENTAL SHEETS

The following supplemental sheets are self-explanatory according to the name of the supplement. The Accounts Due supplement provides space to list all accounts that are due. Memo sheets are printed by month and are used to record monthly reminders for the dentist or office staff. The secretarial dental assistant may use the monthly memo sheets to write reminders when local, state, or federal reports are due. For example, quarterly reports are due 30 days following the end of the last quarter.

When a dentist prefers a columnar distribution of checks written, a supplement sheet may be ordered for this purpose. The Recall Sheet provides space to maintain recall records. Other optional sheets may be purchased for recording surgical or narcotic records. Ideally, narcotic records should be

June   Personal Account

	RECEIPTS (NON-PROFESSIONAL)				DISBURSEMENTS (NON-PROFESSIONAL)				
DAY	SOURCE	AMOUNT		DAY	ITEM	WITH-DRAWALS		INVEST-MENTS	
1	Salary	2000	00	5	House Payment	215	00		
				5	Car Payment	200	00		
	TOTAL FOR PRESENT MONTH				TOTAL FOR PRESENT MONTH				
	FORWARDED (FROM PREVIOUS MONTH)				FORWARDED				
	GRAND TOTAL				GRAND TOTAL				

WITHDRAWALS AND DEPOSITS

BEGINNING CASH IN BANK . . . . $

PLUS ALL DEPOSITS THIS MONTH. . . . . . .

TOTAL TO BE ACCOUNTED FOR . . . .

LESS - OFFICE EXPENSES . . . $

NON-DEDUCT. EQUIPMENT. . .

PERSONAL WITHDRAWALS. . .

END CASH IN BANK . . . .

ACCOUNTS RECEIVABLE

BEGINNING BALANCES, OPEN ACCOUNTS . . . . $

PLUS CHARGES TO PATIENTS FOR MONTH . .

LESS RECEIPTS ON ACCOUNT . . $

DISCOUNTS AND AMOUNTS JUDGED UNCOLLECTABLE.

END BALANCES, OPEN ACCOUNTS . . . . $

FORM 4203B COLWELL CO., CHAMPAIGN, ILL.

Fig. 13-5 A Personal Account Sheet.

maintained in the daily log. Federal law requires that narcotics prescribed or used in the dental office be recorded.

PEGBOARD ACCOUNTING SYSTEMS

A new concept in dental bookkeeping is the pegboard system. This system was designed especially for professional offices. It minimizes the time that is needed for bookkeeping duties by allowing the secretarial dental assistant to write accounting records only one time. The daily log page, a charge slip, receipt slip, patient's ledger card, and a statement may be written at one time. The pegboard system cuts down on costly mistakes that are commonly made when transferring figures from one form to another. The system also gives the dentist a constant up-to-date account of cash on hand, deposits and accounts receivable. The modern pegboard system is recommended for offices where the patient load is extremely heavy. A one-girl office could certainly benefit from this system because of the time saved in recording records. At the end of the year, tax reporting is easier due to the orderly daily collection of financial information.

A lightweight aluminum pegboard may be purchased when using the pegboard system. A heavy duty binder may be purchased yearly for storing all completed pegboard forms. Forms may be ordered in the quantity the dentist desires. The following forms are available:

- punched journal daily pages sized to fit the pegboard.

- Patient ledger cards

- Punched receipt and charge slips

- Carbon paper

- Statement forms in several styles.

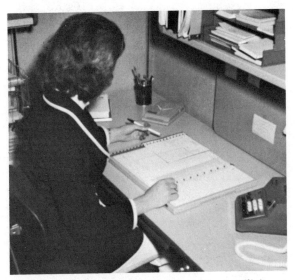

Fig. 13-6 A secretarial dental assistant utilizing a modern pegboard system.

How to Use the Pegboard System

At the beginning of each day, a daily log page is placed on the pegboard. Carbon paper is placed over the left side of the daily log page. Several receipt charge slips are then placed over the carbon. From the arriving patient's treatment card, record the patient's name, current balance, and receipt number on the charge slip. Remove the charge slip at the perforation; clip it to the patient's treatment card. The card and attached charge slip is placed conveniently for the chairside assistant to obtain when seating the patient. After dental treatment is completed, the dentist completes the charge slip which is returned to the secretarial dental assistant.

Before dismissing the patient, the account (ledger card) record is placed in alignment *under* the prenumbered receipt slip. It is even possible to place a statement form under the receipt slip. Record the date, service rendered, charge, payment (if one was made) and new balance. The daily log page, the patient's receipt, the patient's ledger card, and possibly, the statement form have all been recorded at one time. The receipt slip is given to the patient. The ledger card and statement form (if one was used) are filed. Bookkeeping is complete for the patient.

SUMMARY

The daily log is a special ledger designed to maintain most of the business records of a dental office. Financial records of patients are kept in the daily log. A sheet, called the daily page, is provided for recording daily treatments and financial records of the day. The daily log provides space to record the office expenses incurred each month. Summary sheets for the month and year provide space to record information necessary for tax records. Many supplemental sheets are available for the daily log.

A new concept in dental bookkeeping is the pegboard system. This is a new system designed to minimize the time needed for bookkeeping duties. The daily log page, a charge slip, receipt slip, patient's ledger card, and a statement may be written at one time using this system. Bookkeeping is made very simple using the pegboard method.

SUGGESTED ACTIVITIES

- Write to a dental printing company for a sample kit of dental office supplies.

- Select one aspect of the daily log and prepare a short table clinic (demonstration) on how to correctly use the area selected. Present this demonstration to the class.

- Prepare a short report on the advantages of using a pegboard bookkeeping system in the dental office.

REVIEW

A.   1.   Complete the daily page using the following information

Time	Name	Treatment	Financial Information
8:30	James King	#3 MOD Amalgam	charged $18.00
9:00	Bill Jones	Pro., BWXR	paid $14.00 by check
9:30	Mrs. Jerry Guy	#1 Ext.	charged $15.00, paid $25.00 on acct.
10:00	Mrs. C.W. Davis	Cr. Prep #7 & 8	no charge made
11:00	Micky Krellin	#8 DI Adaptic #9 M Adaptic	Total charge $24.00, paid $10.00
11:30	Rhonda Douglas	#B Pulpotomy	charged $25.00
1:15	Dudley Jacobs	Rem. Sut.	no charge
1:30	Daniel Lake	Pro. FMXR	$30.00 paid in cash
2:00	Patsy Brewer	#23 R.C. (2nd visit)	charged $10.00
2:30	Todd Dixon	#2 DO Amalgam #3 MOD Amalgam	charged $30.00 paid $15.00
3:00	Mrs. Ben Smith	Cl. Exam. #5 PA X ray	$10.00 paid by check
3:30	Mr. Tom Acey	Pro. BWXR	charged $14.00, paid $53.00 on account
4:00	Cindy Beck	#5 Ext.	charged $10.00

The following persons paid on account.

C.M. Crook	paid $78.00 on account by check
Samuel Miller	paid $50.00 on his wife, Linda's account in cash
T.M. Gilmore	paid $25.00 on account by money order
David Monk	paid $100.00 by check to apply to his son, John's account
Lester Prestwood	paid $25.00 on account by cash
Lamar Smith	paid $93.50 on account by check

Friday   July 9

HOUR	NAME OF PATIENT	SERVICE RENDERED	CHARGE	CASH	REC'D ON ACCOUNT	√
1						
2						
3						
4						
5						
6						
7						
8						
9						
10						
11						
12						
13						
14						
15						
16						
17						
18						
19						
20						
21						
22						
23						
24						
25						
26						
27						
28						
29						
30						
31						
32						
33						
34						
35						
36						
37						
38						
39						
40						
CARRY TOTALS FORWARD TO **BUSINESS SUMMARY** TOTALS						

COLWELL CO. CHAMPAIGN, ILL.

FORM 4201

2. Complete the Expense Sheets from the list of checks on pages 118 and 119.

Check Number	Date	Paid to	Amount
#1468	Jan. 3	Acme Dental Supply	$39.56
#1469	Jan. 3	Rx Drug Co.	29.60
#1470	Jan. 3	Superior Dental Supply	103.46
#1471	Jan. 3	A.T. & T.	64.50
#1472	Jan. 3	Clean Laundry Co.	32.75
#1473	Jan. 3	State Power and Light Co.	63.90
#1474	Jan. 3	State Gas Co.	19.60
#1475	Jan. 3	City Water Works	8.73
#1476	Jan. 3	Medical Arts – rent	250.00

January   Expense Sheet One

JAN

DRUGS AND SUPPLIES			SALARIES			DUES, MEETINGS		
DAY	ITEM	AMOUNT	DAY	ITEM	AMOUNT	DAY	ITEM	AMOUNT
							TOTAL	
							OFFICE SUPPLIES, STAMPS ETC.	
				TOTAL				
				OFFICE RENT, UPKEEP				
	TOTAL							
	AUTOMOBILE UPKEEP							
				TOTAL				
				LAUNDRY SERVICE				
							TOTAL	
							PROFESSIONAL INSURANCE	
				TOTAL			TOTAL	
				ELECTRICITY, GAS, WATER			BUSINESS TAXES	
							DO NOT INCLUDE WITHHOLDING TAX, INCLUDE ONLY ½ SOCIAL SECURITY TAX	
				TOTAL				
				TELEPHONES, TOLLS			TOTAL	
							INTEREST PAID	
	TOTAL			TOTAL			TOTAL	

FORM 42028 COLWELL CO., CHAMPAIGN, ILL.

#	Date	Payee	Amount
#1477	Jan. 3	Mary Jones, R.D.H.	883.00
#1478	Jan. 3	Linda Barret, C.D.A.	692.78
#1479	Jan. 3	Clare Rayfield, C.D.A.	692.78
#1480	Jan. 3	Marvin Gray, C.D.T.	710.78
#1481	Jan. 10	ADA Relief Fund	100.00
#1482	Jan. 15	Postmaster — stamps	16.00
#1483	Jan. 15	Central District — Dental Seminar	50.00
#1484	Jan. 15	Great Dental Laboratory	569.10
#1485	Jan. 16	Better Homes and Garden (subscription)	8.10
#1486	Jan. 30	Internal Revenue Service	478.32

Expense Sheet Two   January

JAN

ENTERTAINMENT						MISCELLANEOUS		
DAY	ITEM	AMOUNT	DAY	ITEM	AMOUNT	DAY	ITEM	AMOUNT
	TOTAL			TOTAL				
	TOTAL			TOTAL			TOTAL	

CARRY TOTALS FORWARD TO **SUMMARY** OF **EXPENSE**

SUMMARY OF EXPENSE			MONTHLY BALANCES		
	AMOUNT				
DRUGS AND SUPPLIES			FOR THE PRESENT MONTH		
AUTOMOBILE UPKEEP					
SALARIES			TOTAL CASH RECEIVED		
OFFICE RENT UPKEEP			TOTAL EXPENSE		
LAUNDRY SERVICE			NET EARNINGS		
ELECTRICITY, GAS, WATER			FOR THE YEAR TO DATE		
TELEPHONES TOLLS					
DUES MEETINGS			GRAND TOTAL CASH		
OFFICE SUPPLIES, STAMPS, ETC.			GRAND TOTAL EXPENSE		
PROFESSIONAL INSURANCE			NET EARNINGS		
BUSINESS TAXES			EQUIPMENT (NONDEDUCTIBLE)		
INTEREST PAID					
ENTERTAINMENT			DAY	ITEM	AMOUNT
MISCELLANEOUS					
TOTAL FOR PRESENT MONTH					
FORWARDED FROM PREVIOUS MONTH			*TOTAL		
GRAND TOTAL			* ENTER THIS TOTAL DIRECT IN **ANNUAL SUMMARY**		

FORM 4203A COLWELL CO., CHAMPAIGN, ILL.

3. Complete the Business Summary page shown.

Business Summary   May

DAY OF MONTH	CHARGE BUSINESS		CASH BUSINESS		RECEIVED ON ACCOUNTS		TOTAL BUSINESS		TOTAL CASH RECEIVED	
1	203	50	135	00	1, 347	50				
2	106	00	50	00	984	00				
3	679	50	268	50	1, 072	00				
4	345	70	35	00	865	00				
5	308	50	450	00	650	00				
6	Saturday									
7	Sunday									
8	145	00	800	00	875	00				
9	297	50	25	00	543	00				
10	346	00	75	00	645	00				
11	178	00	650	00	135	00				
12	267	25	250	00	78	00				
13	Saturday									
14	Sunday									
15	378	00	35	00	1, 357	50				
16	206	35	86	50	975	25				
17	175	00	750	50	753	00				
18	700	00	20	00	389	00				
19	137	00	350	00	10	00				
20	Saturday									
21	Sunday									
22	168	50	250	00	25	00				
23	467	00	5	00	76	00				
24	146	75	350	00	35	50				
25	654	00	65	00	10	00				
26	207	00	205	00	–					
27	Saturday									
28	Sunday									
29	135	50	785	75	25	00				
30	359	00	5	00	50	00				
31										
TOTAL FOR THE MONTH										
BROUGHT FORWARD										
GRAND TOTAL										

CARRY ALL **GRAND TOTALS** FORWARD TO **BUSINESS SUMMARY** OF FOLLOWING MONTH

FORM 4202A COLWELL CO. CHAMPAIGN, ILL.

MAY

B.   State the function of the following items:

1.   Daily Log.

2.   Employee's Earning Record.

3.   Pegboard System.

C.   Select the best answers.

1.   The items recorded on the daily page are

a. the service rendered.
b. the name of the patient.
c. the number of injections given.
d. the study model record numbers.
e. the number of radiographs recommended by the dentist.
f. the amounts that are charged or paid.

2.   The monthly summary sheet is used to show the total of

a. the business and cash received in a month.
b. the number of patients seen in a month's time.
c. the number of employees that received wages during the month.
d. all expenses for the office.

3.   Expense sheets are provided to record

a. the patients that owe money to the office.
b. the amount of money owed to the office by patients.
c. all expenses incurred by the office during the month.
d. the dental supplies purchased for the month.

4.   Select the items that are expendable supplies.

a. plaster
b. cement
c. dental chair
d. model trimmer
e. restorative supplies
f. air compressor
g. disposable needles

5.   A pegboard accounting system is practical because

a. it is the most inexpensive of all dental accounting systems.
b. the dentist may do all the accounting by himself.
c. it automatically records the bookkeeping records.
d. it minimizes time as all of the accounting records can be written at one time.

Unit 14 Banking Records

OBJECTIVES

After studying this unit, the student should be able to

- Correctly write a check.
- Properly complete a check stub.
- Make out a bank deposit slip.
- Demonstrate reconciling a bank statement.
- List items to check when a mistake occurs in reconciling a bank statement.
- Define petty cash.

In many dental offices, the secretarial dental assistant is delegated the task of keeping bank records. These records include writing checks, making deposits, and reconciling bank statements. Because banking records involve all the money taken in and issued out of the

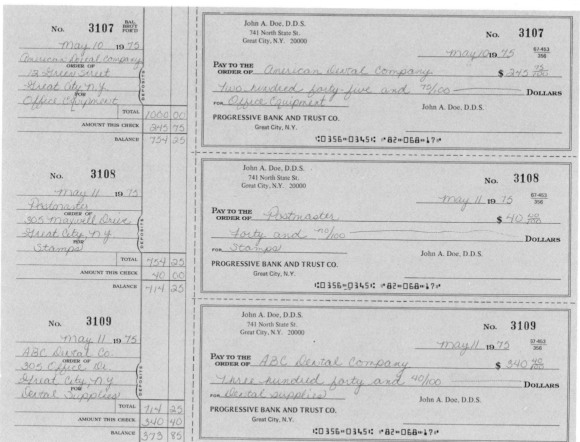

Fig. 14-1 Properly written check and stub on a page of a business, multiple-checkbook.

office, the secretarial dental assistant must be proficient in maintaining these records. Bank records are used in compiling monthly, quarterly, and yearly income tax reports. They must be accurate. Mistakes made by the secretarial dental assistant may be very embarrassing to the office and, also, may require valuable time in making corrections. Transferring figures from one bank record to another must always be done carefully and accurately.

WRITING CHECKS

Checks must be written properly to insure the correct payment to the proper party. Checks not written properly may result in serious problems for the office. Printed checks for the office should include the name and address of the dentist or dental clinic in the upper left-hand corner as shown in figure 14-1. They should be reordered in ample time to allow for printing before the supply is depleted. It is suggested that printed checks be ordered at least one month in advance of the supply depletion.

Always write checks using an ink pen or ballpoint pen. Never should a check be written in pencil! Pencil written checks can easily be altered by an unscrupulous person. *Write legibly!*

Check stubs should always be completed at the time the check is written. Postponing this task may result in forgetting the name and the amount of the check. Get in the habit of completing the check stub before writing the check. Never remove a check from a checkbook without completing the stub.

The amount of the check, the date, and the name of the person to whom the check is payable is written on the stub. Directly under the name line on the stub is a line for recording the purpose of the check. The balance brought forward from the last check written is recorded in the figures column. Any money deposited since the last check was written should be recorded and added to the balance brought forward. Next, write the amount of the check. Subtract this amount from the total of the balance brought forward and the deposit. The new balance should be carried to the balance brought forward of the next check.

The check is now ready to be written. Write the name of the payee (the person to whom the check is written) at the extreme left of the line which reads "Pay to the order of." Do not allow room for anyone to write or change the name. The figure amount is written to the right of the payee's name. Again, write the figure as close as possible to the dollar sign. Do not allow room where a digit may be added. It takes very little space for someone to add a single digit, thus changing the amount of the check. The amount, $100.00 could easily be changed to read $1000.00. Be very careful in the placement of the decimal point. The amount of cents may be written as a fraction such as 75/100. This eliminates the need for a decimal point.

The second line of the check is used to write out the amount of the check. Again, start writing at the extreme left of the line. The cents amount should be written as a fraction of 100. If it is an even dollar amount, write the word "no" where the cents amount is normally written. Draw a solid straight line from the last letter or figure to the word "Dollars." The check is now ready for the dentist's signature, figure 14-1.

Unless the dentist has authorized the bank to accept the secretarial dental assistant's signature on his checks, the dentist is the only person allowed to sign office checks. Usually the dentist prefers to sign his own checks. Time can be saved if the secretarial dental assistant has properly made the check out in advance. A rubber stamp of the dentist's signature *must not* be used for signing checks.

It is advisable for the dental office to purchase a check-writing machine. This can elim-

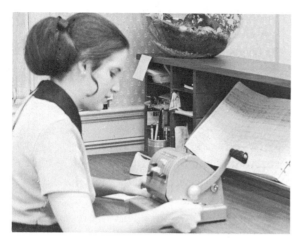

Fig. 14-2 Using a check writer.

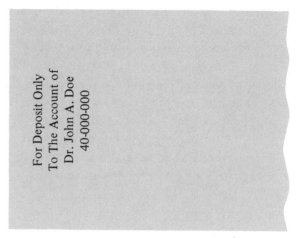

Fig. 14-3 A properly endorsed check.

inate costly mistakes. The amount of the check is selected in buttons on the check-writing machine. The blank check is inserted and a lever pulled to inscribe the correct amount on the checks. A check-writing machine ensures that the amount of the check will not be changed. If a large number of checks are written in the office, a check-writing machine is recommended.

MAKING DEPOSITS

Money that is received in the dental office from patients should be deposited in the bank as soon as practical. It is suggested that a deposit be made daily. With this method, the daily bank deposit should agree with the total cash received for the day. Most banks provide services for deposits to be made after hours. It is not advisable to leave money or checks in the office after closing hours. If they must be left, they should be locked in a safe place.

Before a deposit can be made, two procedures must take place: (1) the checks must be properly endorsed, (2) a deposit slip must be completed. (Don't forget to credit the patient's account with the proper amount.) There are several ways that a check may be endorsed. Turning the check over, the dentist may sign his name along the left end of the

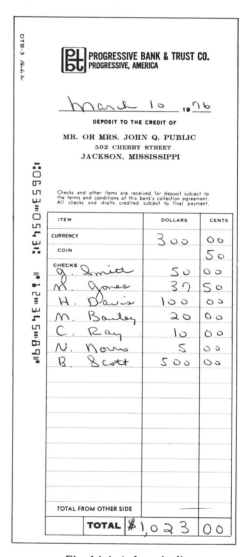

Fig. 14-4 A deposit slip.

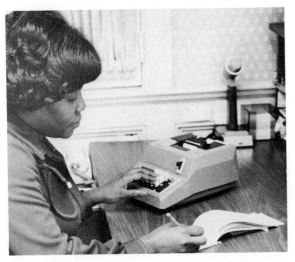

Fig. 14-5 The secretarial dental assistant has bookkeeping and banking duties.

back of the check. If he endorses the check in this manner, anyone may cash it. The dentist may endorse the check by indicating the party to whom he is transferring the right to cash the check. For example: "Pay to the order of The City Bank, or John Doe, D.D.S." Although this method is safe, it is rather time-consuming for the dentist with a large practice. The safest and most practical method is to endorse the checks with a restriction by writing the words, "For Deposit Only." A rubber stamp may be purchased which reads: "For Deposit Only, To the Account of John Doe, D.D.S., Account No. 40-400-00," figure 14-3. This endorsement restriction indicates the check must be deposited to the dentist's account. With this method, the secretarial dental assistant may stamp any check and proceed with the deposit slip without bothering the dentist.

The deposit slip is merely a matter of listing coins, currency, and checks. Most banks require the use of preprinted computerized deposit slips. The name of the dentist or office and the account number is printed on the deposit slip. After the date is recorded, list any coins or currency. Currency refers to cash bills. Next, list each check separately by

writing the name of the person who signed the check, figure 14-4. It is usually permissible to write just the last name. List the names alphabetically as this becomes especially helpful when a need arises to determine whether a check was deposited, or a patient wishes to know about an amount he thought had been paid. The deposit slip will verify the financial record of the patient's treatment card.

Total the figures column. Double check to make sure the amounts were transferred correctly. Check to make sure all the checks were endorsed. The deposit is now ready for the bank. The deposit total should be recorded immediately in the checkbook.

RECONCILING THE BANK STATEMENT

One way to maintain cancelled checks (checks that have cleared the bank) is to tape them back to the check stubs. Since the used up checkbook is maintained for at least three to five years, the checks may be filed in the checkbook. This method simplifies filing and saves space; there is no bulky bank statement envelope to file in the filing cabinet. The statement sheet from the bank may be filed in a manila folder or it may be taped to the back of the last three checks for the particular month. This may even make reconciling the bank statement easier.

Once a month the bank sends the dental office a bank statement, figure 14-6, page 126. The bank statement shows all checks that have cleared the bank since the last statement. All deposits made since the previous statement are also shown. Service charges, if any, are denoted with the initials "S.C." written by the amount of the service charge. (The amount of the service charge *must* be subtracted from the checkbook balance.) The dates the checks or deposits were recorded at the bank appears in the left-hand column. The bank statement should be reconciled as soon as practical after it arrives in the dental office.

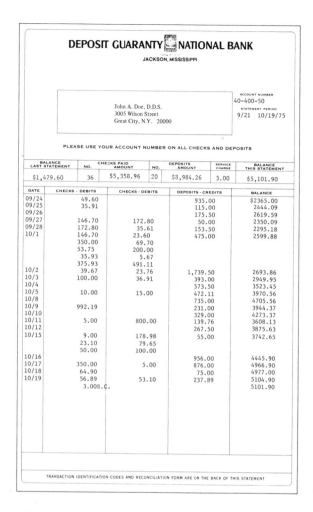

Fig. 14-6 A typical bank statement from a dental office.

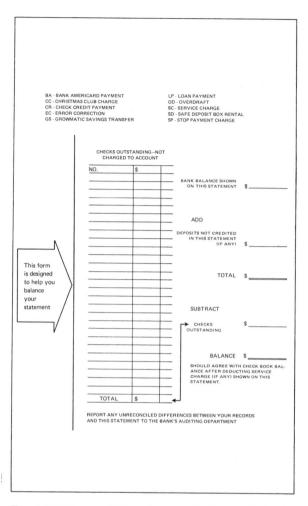

Fig. 14-7 Reconciliation form on the back of a bank statement.

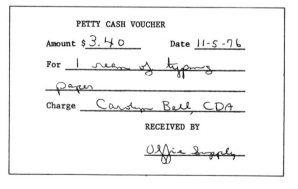

Fig. 14-8 A completed petty cash voucher.

Most banks supply a reconciliation form on the back of the bank statement, figure 14-7. This is very convenient for the secretarial dental assistant. Following the suggested form may increase the speed of reconciling the statement. The first procedure is to check the cancelled checks against the written check stubs in the checkbook. A small check mark may be placed in the upper left-hand corner of each check stub. Any written check that has not cleared the bank is called an *outstanding check*. The outstanding checks should be listed in a column on the back of the statement. The check number and the amount should be recorded. All of the outstanding checks should be added together to obtain a total. This total is the outstanding check total.

Next, check to see if all the deposits have been listed on the statement; there may be deposits in transit which did not reach the bank before the statement was prepared. Starting with the balance figure listed on the statement, add any deposits not listed. From this total subtract the total of outstanding checks. The balance arrived at should agree with the checkbook balance after deducting from the checkbook any service charges shown on the statement. If the balance agrees, the statement has been reconciled. The balance in the checkbook that agrees with the reconciled bank balance should be marked with an asterisk. The next month's reconciliation will begin from this asterisk.

A common mistake made by the secretarial dental assistant is to forget to enter and deduct service charges from the checkbook. This will result in a problem the next month when attempts are made to reconcile the bank statement.

If the figures from the bank statement and the checkbook do not agree, start checking for errors. It may be wise to first check with the dentist to make sure he did not write a check that was not recorded. Make sure the addition and subtraction used in the reconciliation is correct. Check to see if any of the patient's checks were returned to the office because of nonsufficient funds. The nonsufficient fund checks are returned to the payee and the amount deducted from the payee's deposit slip. Check to see if the number of deposits and the deposit figures shown on the bank statement agree with the checkbook. Next, check to make sure the figures on the stub and the corresponding checks agree. If the mistake has still not been discovered, check the addition and subtraction on the check stubs. It is possible that an error was made when transferring the balance from one check stub to another.

If further checking is needed, check the figures on the checks against the figures on the statement. Double check to make sure that the service charges were subtracted from the

checkbook last month. Hopefully, the mistake may be found after rechecking all these items. If there is still a problem, put all the bank records away. After a brief rest, start checking again. If all else fails, consult the bank. Most banks list a special number in the telephone directory for customer service. The bank will have trained persons to help you find the error.

PETTY CASH

Although not a banking record, petty cash does involve money transactions and, therefore, records. *Petty cash* is a small amount of cash kept in the office to purchase inexpensive, miscellaneous supplies for the office. The amount will be determined by the dentist or the office needs. The secretarial dental assistant is usually responsible for maintaining this small fund. Items such as coffee, pencils, and erasers may be purchased from this fund. Many items purchased from the petty cash fund will be under one dollar in price.

An accurate record should be kept of all money used from petty cash. Special petty cash vouchers may be secured for maintaining petty cash records, figure 14-8. An alternate method is to purchase a small ring binder notebook to use for keeping the records. The date, name of the purchase, and the amount of the purchase should be listed in the record book. Sales slips of purchases should be kept near the record book. It is suggested that a small lockable cash box be purchased. The cash, record book, and sales slips may be kept safely in the cash box. The box should be kept in an inconspicuous place in the office.

SUMMARY

Dental banking records include writing checks, making deposits, and reconciling bank statements. All the money taken in and issued out of the dental office is channeled through the banking records. They are also used in compiling tax reports for the dental office. The secretarial dental assistant must be proficient in handling banking records.

Checks should be written carefully to ensure that the figures cannot be changed by a dishonest person. Check to make sure all balances are transferred correctly. Double check the addition or subtraction on check stubs, deposit slips, and when reconciling bank statement. Mistakes made with banking records may be very embarrassing to the dental office. The secretarial dental assistant must be very careful in working with all banking figures.

SUGGESTED ACTIVITIES

- Request that the class secretary write to a company that sells check writers and request brochures for the class stating the advantages of a check writer.

- Invite a bank representative from a local bank to speak to the class on "Efficient Banking Procedures."

- Set up a petty cash container and record file. Any file or small container is permissible.

REVIEW

A. Complete a deposit slip from the following list of financial deposits.

Checks from:	Amount
David Jones	$ 25.00
Bill Buckley	5.00
Nancy Seago	55.00
Mrs. Jerry Dill	10.00
Mr. J. C. Vest	53.00
Mr. E. C. Daigle	22.50
Mrs. Mary Hand	25.00
Safe Insurance Co.	600.00
Currency	350.00

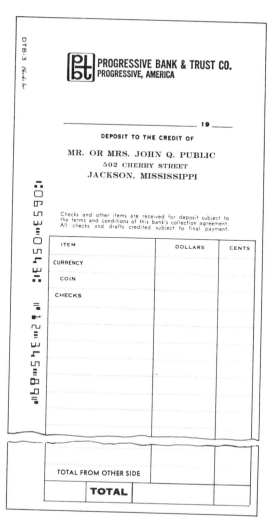

B. Write the following checks and check stubs.

Date	Payee	Amount	Purpose
June 1, 1975	Best Dental Supplies	$146.70	Supplies
June 1, 1975	Dental-Medical Bldg.	472.80	Rent
June 1, 1975	Superior Drug Co.	23.60	Drugs

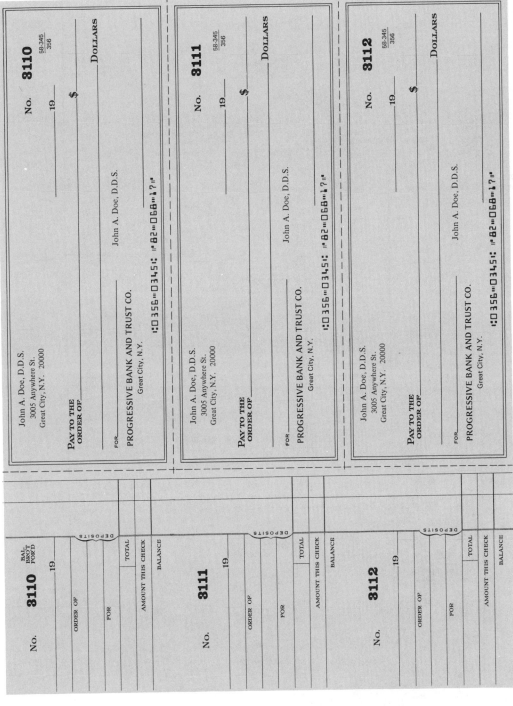

C. Reconcile a bank statement using the following information. Dr. John Doe's bank statement is shown in figure 14-6. The bank balance that appears in the checkbook is $4,831.90. The outstanding checks total $573.00. The amount of $300.00 was deposited after the bank statement was prepared at the bank. A service charge of $3.00 is shown on the bank statement. Proceed with the reconciliation.

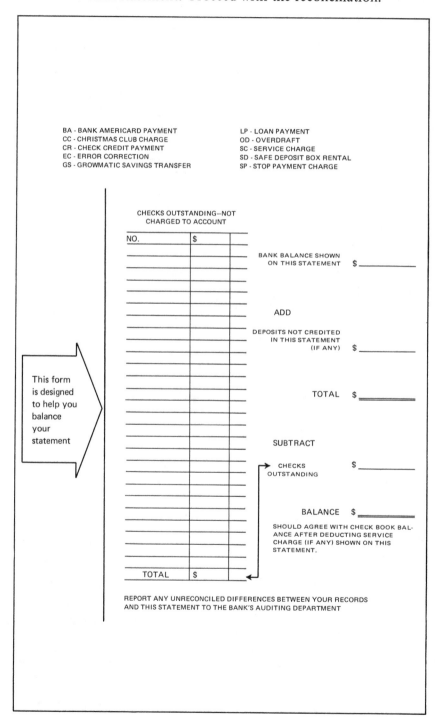

D. Select the best answer.

1. Check stubs should be completed

    a. after making the bank deposit.
    b. after removing the check from the checkbook.
    c. as soon as practical.
    d. prior to writing the check.

2. Checks should never be written in pencil because

    a. pencil writing is hard for the bank computer to pick up.
    b. a pencil check may be changed by a dishonest person.
    c. the dentist always prefers an ink pen.
    d. the professional image of the dental office is important.

3. The amount of the check is written out on the second line of the check. This writing should start

    a. at the extreme left of the line.
    b. at the extreme right of the line.
    c. directly under the payee's name.
    d. as close as possible to the dollar sign.

4. A rubber stamp with the dentist's signature

    a. may be used to sign the office checks.
    b. must never be used to sign the office checks.
    c. may be used only in extreme emergencies.
    d. may be used only when the dentist is out of town.

5. The most practical method for check endorsement is

    a. for the dentist to endorse each check.
    b. for the dentist to indicate who he is transferring the right to cash the check.
    c. for the secretarial dental assistant to stamp, "For Deposit Only, To the Account of . . . "
    d. for the secretarial dental assistant to endorse the check by signing the dentist's name by her name.

6. An outstanding check is

    a. a check written for an outstanding amount.
    b. a check returned to the office due to nonsufficient funds.
    c. a written check that has not cleared the bank.
    d. a check written for expensive equipment to be used in the dental treatment area.

7. Petty cash is

    a. a substantial amount of money used to purchase dental supplies.
    b. a small amount of cash used to purchase inexpensive, miscellaneous supplies for the dental office.
    c. the amount of cash recorded in the daily log for a particular day.
    d. the amount of cash listed on the daily bank deposit slip.

Unit 15 Payroll Forms and Employee Records

OBJECTIVES

After studying this unit, the student should be able to

- Demonstrate how to complete an Employee's Withholding Allowance Certificate.
- Compute a payroll using both the FICA and withholding tax tables.
- Explain the difference between FICA and withholding taxes.
- Complete an employee's earning record.

There are many rewarding compensations received when working in a dental office as a member of the dental health team. One such compensation is monetary payment, commonly referred to as a paycheck. Paychecks are given to employees in a dental office at regular periods of time, which have been decided upon by the dentist. Some paychecks may be written once a week; others may be written once every two weeks, or once a month. The dentist may wish to write these checks personally. However, he may delegate this task to the secretarial dental assistant. If the secretarial dental assistant does write the payroll checks. she must do so in the strictest of confidence. She must not discuss salaries with other members of the dental team. The secretarial dental assistant does not decide what the office salaries will be. She receives instructions from the dentist concerning the amount of the salaries.

There is no set salary for any person in the dental office. Salaries are decided by the dentist and discussed with the employee prior to employment. There may or may not be a definite salary schedule in the dental office. Again, the dentist will make this decision. If raises are given in the dental office on a regular basis, the dentist will instruct the secretarial dental assistant how this is to be carried out.

Salaries may be computed on an hourly, daily, weekly, or monthly basis. If computed on an hourly basis, the secretarial dental assistant may keep a time record on each employee. Otherwise, paychecks will be computed daily, weekly, or monthly. Whatever the method, the secretarial dental assistant must maintain a record of the salaries paid to each employee in the dental office. A special form for keeping records can be found in the daily log. (The form, Employee's Earning Record, figure 15-5, will be discussed later in this unit.)

An employee in a dental office must have a social security number. If for some reason, a new employee does not have a social security number, it must be applied for immediately. The local social security office should be contacted for the proper form. It is rare for an applicant to apply for a position and not have a social security number; however, an applicant from another country may not have a number. NOTE: The payroll forms and records explained in this unit as well as the examples given in the remainder of the section show wages, taxes and withholding amounts *which may vary through the years.* The student must not consider the figures or even the format of the forms as standard items. The student must focus learning on *how* and *what* to do, using the tables as guides.

Form W–4 (Revised April 1975)
Employee's Withholding Allowance Certificate
(Use for wages paid after April 30, 1975 and before January 1, 1976)

The explanatory material below will help you determine your correct number of withholding allowances, and will assist you in completing the Form W–4 at the bottom of this page.

Avoid Overwithholding or Underwithholding

By claiming the proper number of withholding allowances you are entitled to, you can fit the amount of tax withheld from your wages to your tax liability. In addition to the allowances for personal exemptions to be claimed in items (a) through (g) below, be sure you claim any additional allowances you are entitled to in item (h) "Special withholding allowance," and item (i) "Allowance(s) for itemized deductions." While these allowances may be claimed on Form W–4 for withholding purposes, they are not to be claimed under "Exemptions" on your tax return Form 1040 or Form 1040A.

You may claim the special withholding allowance if you are single with only one employer, or married with only one employer and your spouse is not employed. If you have unusually large itemized deductions, you may claim the allowance(s) for itemized deductions to avoid having too much income tax withheld from your wages. On the other hand, if you and your spouse are both employed or you have more than one employer, you should take steps to assure that enough has been withheld. If you find that you need more withholding, claim fewer exemptions or ask for additional withholding. If you are currently claiming additional withholding allowances based on itemized deductions, check the table on the back to see that you are claiming the proper number of allowances.

How Many Withholding Allowances May You Claim?

Please use the schedule below to determine the number of allowances you may claim for tax withholding purposes. In determining the number, keep in mind these points: If you are single and hold more than one job, you may not claim the same allowances with more than one employer at the same time; or if you are married and both you and your spouse are employed, you may not claim the same allowances with your employers at the same time. A nonresident alien, other than a resident of Canada, Mexico, or Puerto Rico, may claim only one personal allowance.

Figure Your Total Withholding Allowances Below

(a) Allowance for yourself—enter 1 . . . . _____

(b) Allowance for your spouse—enter 1 . . . . _____

(c) Allowance for your age—if 65 or over—enter 1 . . . . _____

(d) Allowance for your spouse's age—if 65 or over—enter 1 . . . . _____

(e) Allowance for blindness (yourself)—enter 1 . . . . _____

(f) Allowance for blindness (spouse's)—enter 1 . . . . _____

(g) Allowance(s) for dependent(s)—you are entitled to claim an allowance for each dependent you will be able to claim on your Federal income tax return. Do not include yourself or your spouse * _____

(h) Special withholding allowance—if you are single with only one employer, or married with only one employer and your spouse is not employed—enter 1** . . . . _____

(i) Allowance(s) for itemized deductions—if you do plan to itemize deductions on your income tax return, enter the number from the table on back** . . . . _____

(j) Total—add lines (a) through (i) above. Enter here and on line 1, Form W–4 below . . . . _____

* If you are in doubt as to whom you may claim as a dependent, see the instructions which came with your last Federal income tax return or call your local Internal Revenue Service office.

** This allowance is used solely for purposes of figuring your withholding tax, and cannot be claimed when you file your tax return.

See Table on Back if You Plan to Itemize Your Deductions

Completing Form W–4.—If you find that you are entitled to one or more allowances in addition to those which you are now claiming, increase your number of allowances by completing the form below and filing it with your employer. If the number of allowances you previously claimed decreases, you must file a new Form W–4 within 10 days. (Should you expect to owe more tax than will be withheld, you may use the same form to increase your withholding by claiming fewer or "0" allowances on line 1, or by asking for additional withholding on line 2, or both.)

▼ Give the bottom part of this form to your employer; keep the upper part for your records and information ▼

.... Cut along this line ....

Form **W-4**
(Rev. April 1975)
Department of the Treasury
Internal Revenue Service

Employee's Withholding Allowance Certificate
(This certificate is for income tax withholding purposes only; it will remain in effect until you change it.)

Type or print your full name | Your social security number

Home address (Number and street or rural route)

Marital status
☐ Single   ☐ Married
(If married but legally separated, or spouse is a nonresident alien, check the single block.)

City or town, State and ZIP code

1 Total number of allowances you are claiming . . . . _____

2 Additional amount, if any, you want deducted from each pay (if your employer agrees) . . . . $ _____

I certify that to the best of my knowledge and belief, the number of withholding allowances claimed on this certificate does not exceed the number to which I am entitled.

Signature ▶ .... Date ▶ ...., 19 ....

Fig. 15-1 Employee's Withholding Allowance Certificate, Form W-4.

On the first day of employment, the new employee completes an *Employee's Withholding Allowance Certificate,* figure 15-1 (often referred to as form W-4), from the Department of Treasury – Internal Revenue Service. The name, address, and social security number are filled out by the new employee; the marital status should be checked on the form. If legally separated, divorced, widowed, or if the spouse is a nonresident alien, the *single* status should be checked. If single and not responsible for anyone else, only one exemp-

tion may be claimed. If an employee is married and the mother of children, the husband and wife must decide how they will claim the exemptions. Both may not claim each other and the children. If a person expects to owe more tax than the amount to be withheld, it is permissible to claim fewer exemptions. After determining the number of exemptions, the date and signature are written on the form. The W-4 form should be filed for future use.

In brief, the W-4 form authorizes the employer to deduct the tax from the em-

SINGLE Persons — SEMIMONTHLY Payroll Period

And the wages are—		And the number of withholding allowances claimed is—										
At least	But less than	0	1	2	3	4	5	6	7	8	9	10 or more
		The amount of income tax to be withheld shall be—										
$260	$270	$39.00	$32.30	$26.00	$19.80	$13.70	$8.70	$3.70	$0	$0	$0	$0
270	280	41.30	34.30	28.00	21.80	15.50	10.30	5.30	.30	0	0	0
280	290	43.60	36.40	30.00	23.80	17.50	11.90	6.90	1.90	0	0	0
290	300	45.90	38.70	32.00	25.80	19.50	13.50	8.50	3.50	0	0	0
300	320	49.30	42.10	35.00	28.80	22.50	16.30	10.90	5.90	.90	0	0
320	340	53.90	46.70	39.50	32.80	26.50	20.30	14.10	9.10	4.10	0	0
340	360	58.50	51.30	44.10	36.90	30.50	24.30	18.00	12.30	7.30	2.30	0
360	380	63.10	55.90	48.70	41.50	34.50	28.30	22.00	15.80	10.50	5.50	.50
380	400	67.70	60.50	53.30	46.10	39.00	32.30	26.00	19.80	13.70	8.70	3.70
400	420	72.00	65.10	57.90	50.70	43.60	36.40	30.00	23.80	17.50	11.90	6.90
420	440	76.20	69.70	62.50	55.30	48.20	41.00	34.00	27.80	21.50	15.30	10.10
440	460	80.40	73.90	67.10	59.90	52.80	45.60	38.40	31.80	25.50	19.30	13.30
460	480	84.60	78.10	71.50	64.50	57.40	50.20	43.00	35.80	29.50	23.30	17.00
480	500	88.80	82.30	75.70	69.10	62.00	54.80	47.60	40.40	33.50	27.30	21.00
500	520	93.00	86.50	79.90	73.30	66.60	59.40	52.20	45.00	37.80	31.30	25.00
520	540	97.70	90.70	84.10	77.50	71.00	64.00	56.80	49.60	42.40	35.30	29.00
540	560	102.90	94.90	88.30	81.70	75.20	68.60	61.40	54.20	47.00	39.80	33.00
560	580	108.10	100.00	92.50	85.90	79.40	72.80	66.00	58.80	51.60	44.40	37.20
580	600	113.30	105.20	97.00	90.10	83.60	77.00	70.40	63.40	56.20	49.00	41.80
600	620	118.70	110.40	102.20	94.30	87.80	81.20	74.60	68.00	60.80	53.60	46.40
620	640	124.70	115.60	107.40	99.30	92.00	85.40	78.80	72.30	65.40	58.20	51.00
640	660	130.70	121.30	112.60	104.50	96.40	89.60	83.00	76.50	69.90	62.80	55.60
660	680	136.70	127.30	118.00	109.70	101.60	93.80	87.20	80.70	74.10	67.40	60.20
680	700	142.70	133.30	124.00	114.90	106.80	98.70	91.40	84.90	78.30	71.80	64.80
700	720	148.70	139.30	130.00	120.60	112.00	103.90	95.70	89.10	82.50	76.00	69.40
720	740	154.70	145.30	136.00	126.60	117.20	109.10	100.90	93.30	86.70	80.20	73.60
740	760	160.70	151.30	142.00	132.60	123.20	114.30	106.10	98.00	90.90	84.40	77.80
760	780	167.90	157.30	148.00	138.60	129.20	119.80	111.30	103.20	95.10	88.60	82.00
780	800	175.10	163.90	154.00	144.60	135.20	125.80	116.50	108.40	100.30	92.80	86.20
800	820	182.30	171.10	160.00	150.60	141.20	131.80	122.50	113.60	105.50	97.40	90.40
820	840	189.50	178.30	167.00	156.60	147.20	137.80	128.50	119.10	110.70	102.60	94.60
840	860	196.70	185.50	174.20	163.00	153.20	143.80	134.50	125.10	115.90	107.80	99.60
860	880	203.90	192.70	181.40	170.20	159.20	149.80	140.50	131.10	121.70	113.00	104.80
880	900	211.10	199.90	188.60	177.40	166.10	155.80	146.50	137.10	127.70	118.30	110.00
900	920	218.30	207.10	195.80	184.60	173.30	162.10	152.50	143.10	133.70	124.30	115.20
920	940	225.50	214.30	203.00	191.80	180.50	169.30	158.50	149.10	139.70	130.30	121.00
940	960	232.70	221.50	210.20	199.00	187.70	176.50	165.20	155.10	145.70	136.30	127.00
960	980	239.90	228.70	217.40	206.20	194.90	183.70	172.40	161.20	151.70	142.30	133.00
980	1,000	247.10	235.90	224.60	213.40	202.10	190.90	179.60	168.40	157.70	148.30	139.00
1,000	1,020	254.30	243.10	231.80	220.60	209.30	198.10	186.80	175.60	164.30	154.30	145.00
1,020	1,040	261.50	250.30	239.00	227.80	216.50	205.30	194.00	182.80	171.50	160.30	151.00
1,040	1,060	268.70	257.50	246.20	235.00	223.70	212.50	201.20	190.00	178.70	167.50	157.00
1,060	1,080	275.90	264.70	253.40	242.20	230.90	219.70	208.40	197.20	185.90	174.70	163.40
1,080	1,100	283.10	271.90	260.60	249.40	238.10	226.90	215.60	204.40	193.10	181.90	170.60
1,100	1,120	290.30	279.10	267.80	256.60	245.30	234.10	222.80	211.60	200.30	189.10	177.80
1,120	1,140	297.50	286.30	275.00	263.80	252.50	241.30	230.00	218.80	207.50	196.30	185.00
1,140	1,160	304.70	293.50	282.20	271.00	259.70	248.50	237.20	226.00	214.70	203.50	192.20
1,160	1,180	311.90	300.70	289.40	278.20	266.90	255.70	244.40	233.20	221.90	210.70	199.40
1,180	1,200	319.10	307.90	296.60	285.40	274.10	262.90	251.60	240.40	229.10	217.90	206.60
1,200	1,220	326.30	315.10	303.80	292.60	281.30	270.10	258.80	247.60	236.30	225.10	213.80
1,220	1,240	333.50	322.30	311.00	299.80	288.50	277.30	266.00	254.80	243.50	232.30	221.00
1,240	1,260	340.70	329.50	318.20	307.00	295.70	284.50	273.20	262.00	250.70	239.50	228.20
1,260	1,280	347.90	336.70	325.40	314.20	302.90	291.70	280.40	269.20	257.90	246.70	235.40
1,280	1,300	355.10	343.90	332.60	321.40	310.10	298.90	287.60	276.40	265.10	253.90	242.60
1,300	1,320	362.30	351.10	339.80	328.60	317.30	306.10	294.80	283.60	272.30	261.10	249.80
$1,320 and over		36 percent of the excess over $1,320 plus—										
$1,320 and over		365.90	354.70	343.40	332.20	320.90	309.70	298.40	287.20	275.90	264.70	253.40

Fig. 15-2 Single Persons — Semimonthly Withholding Tax Table.

ployee's salary. It also informs the office of the number of exemptions claimed by the employee.

The federal government requires that all employers deduct certain items from an employee's pay. Federal law requires that Income Tax (Withholding) and Social Security Tax (FICA) be withheld from each employee. The initials, FICA, indicate *Federal Insurance Contribution Act.* Many states require a certain amount of state tax to be withheld also. This amount or rate will vary from state to state.

Other deductions may include group insurance policy premiums. Occasionally, the dentist will offer the employee a retirement plan and a certain amount may be withheld for this. It is possible for there to be other deductions; however, dental offices usually do not deduct anything other than those amounts required by federal and state laws.

WITHHOLDING TAX

All employees in the dental office must file a personal income tax report by April 15

MARRIED Persons—MONTHLY Payroll Period

And the wages are—		And the number of withholding allowances claimed is—										
At least	But less than	0	1	2	3	4	5	6	7	8	9	10 or more
		The amount of income tax to be withheld shall be—										
$420	$440	$59.00	$49.00	$39.00	$29.00	$19.00	$10.00	$1.30	$0	$0	$0	$0
440	460	62.20	52.20	42.20	32.20	22.20	12.80	4.10	0	0	0	0
460	480	65.40	55.40	45.40	35.40	25.40	15.60	6.90	0	0	0	0
480	500	68.60	58.60	48.60	38.60	28.60	18.60	9.70	.90	0	0	0
500	520	71.80	61.80	51.80	41.80	31.80	21.80	12.50	3.70	0	0	0
520	540	75.00	65.00	55.00	45.00	35.00	25.00	15.30	6.50	0	0	0
540	560	78.20	68.20	58.20	48.20	38.20	28.20	18.20	9.30	.60	0	0
560	580	81.40	71.40	61.40	51.40	41.40	31.40	21.40	12.10	3.40	0	0
580	600	84.60	74.60	64.60	54.60	44.60	34.60	24.60	14.90	6.20	0	0
600	640	89.40	79.40	69.40	59.40	49.40	39.40	29.40	19.40	10.40	1.60	0
640	680	95.80	85.80	75.80	65.80	55.80	45.80	35.80	25.80	16.00	7.20	0
680	720	102.20	92.20	82.20	72.20	62.20	52.20	42.20	32.20	22.20	12.80	4.10
720	760	109.20	98.60	88.60	78.60	68.60	58.60	48.60	38.60	28.60	18.60	9.70
760	800	117.20	105.00	95.00	85.00	75.00	65.00	55.00	45.00	35.00	25.00	15.30
800	840	125.20	112.70	101.40	91.40	81.40	71.40	61.40	51.40	41.40	31.40	21.40
840	880	133.20	120.70	108.20	97.80	87.80	77.80	67.80	57.80	47.80	37.80	27.80
880	920	141.30	128.70	116.20	104.20	94.20	84.20	74.20	64.20	54.20	44.20	34.20
920	960	150.90	136.70	124.20	111.70	100.60	90.60	80.60	70.60	60.60	50.60	40.60
960	1,000	160.50	145.50	132.20	119.70	107.20	97.00	87.00	77.00	67.00	57.00	47.00
1,000	1,040	170.10	155.10	140.20	127.70	115.20	103.40	93.40	83.40	73.40	63.40	53.40
1,040	1,080	179.70	164.70	149.70	135.70	123.20	110.70	99.80	89.80	79.80	69.80	59.80
1,080	1,120	189.30	174.30	159.30	144.30	131.20	118.70	106.20	96.20	86.20	76.20	66.20
1,120	1,160	198.90	183.90	168.90	153.90	139.20	126.70	114.20	102.60	92.60	82.60	72.60
1,160	1,200	208.50	193.50	178.50	163.50	148.50	134.70	122.20	109.70	99.00	89.00	79.00
1,200	1,240	218.10	203.10	188.10	173.10	158.10	143.10	130.20	117.70	105.40	95.40	85.40
1,240	1,280	227.70	212.70	197.70	182.70	167.70	152.70	138.20	125.70	113.20	101.80	91.80
1,280	1,320	237.30	222.30	207.30	192.30	177.30	162.30	147.30	133.70	121.20	108.70	98.20
1,320	1,360	246.90	231.90	216.90	201.90	186.90	171.90	156.90	141.90	129.20	116.70	104.60
1,360	1,400	256.50	241.50	226.50	211.50	196.50	181.50	166.50	151.50	137.20	124.70	112.20
1,400	1,440	266.80	251.10	236.10	221.10	206.10	191.10	176.10	161.10	146.10	132.70	120.20
1,440	1,480	278.00	260.70	245.70	230.70	215.70	200.70	185.70	170.70	155.70	140.70	128.20
1,480	1,520	289.20	271.70	255.30	240.30	225.30	210.30	195.30	180.30	165.30	150.30	136.20
1,520	1,560	300.40	282.90	265.40	249.90	234.90	219.90	204.90	189.90	174.90	159.90	144.90
1,560	1,600	311.60	294.10	276.60	259.50	244.50	229.50	214.50	199.50	184.50	169.50	154.50
1,600	1,640	322.80	305.30	287.80	270.30	254.10	239.10	224.10	209.10	194.10	179.10	164.10
1,640	1,680	334.00	316.50	299.00	281.50	264.00	248.70	233.70	218.70	203.70	188.70	173.70
1,680	1,720	345.20	327.70	310.20	292.70	275.20	258.30	243.30	228.30	213.30	198.30	183.30
1,720	1,760	356.40	338.90	321.40	303.90	286.40	268.90	252.90	237.90	222.90	207.90	192.90
1,760	1,800	367.90	350.10	332.60	315.10	297.60	280.10	262.60	247.50	232.50	217.50	202.50
1,800	1,840	380.70	361.30	343.80	326.30	308.80	291.30	273.80	257.10	242.10	227.10	212.10
1,840	1,880	393.50	373.50	355.00	337.50	320.00	302.50	285.00	267.50	251.70	236.70	221.70
1,880	1,920	406.30	386.30	366.30	348.70	331.20	313.70	296.20	278.70	261.30	246.30	231.30
1,920	1,960	419.10	399.10	379.10	359.90	342.40	324.90	307.40	289.90	272.40	255.90	240.90
1,960	2,000	431.90	411.90	391.90	371.90	353.60	336.10	318.60	301.10	283.60	266.10	250.50
2,000	2,040	444.70	424.70	404.70	384.70	364.80	347.30	329.80	312.30	294.80	277.30	260.10
2,040	2,080	457.50	437.50	417.50	397.50	377.50	358.50	341.00	323.50	306.00	288.50	271.00
2,080	2,120	470.30	450.30	430.30	410.30	390.30	370.30	352.20	334.70	317.20	299.70	282.20
2,120	2,160	484.60	463.10	443.10	423.10	403.10	383.10	363.40	345.90	328.40	310.90	293.40
2,160	2,200	499.00	476.50	455.90	435.90	415.90	395.90	375.90	357.10	339.60	322.10	304.60
2,200	2,240	513.40	490.90	468.70	448.70	428.70	408.70	388.70	368.70	350.80	333.30	315.80
2,240	2,280	527.80	505.30	482.80	461.50	441.50	421.50	401.50	381.50	362.00	344.50	327.00
2,280	2,320	542.20	519.70	497.20	474.70	454.30	434.30	414.30	394.30	374.30	355.70	338.20
2,320	2,360	556.60	534.10	511.60	489.10	467.10	447.10	427.10	407.10	387.10	367.10	349.40
2,360	2,400	571.00	548.50	526.00	503.50	481.00	459.90	439.90	419.90	399.90	379.90	360.60
2,400	2,440	585.40	562.90	540.40	517.90	495.40	472.90	452.70	432.70	412.70	392.70	372.70
2,440	2,480	599.80	577.30	554.80	532.30	509.80	487.30	465.50	445.50	425.50	405.50	385.50
2,480	2,520	614.20	591.70	569.20	546.70	524.20	501.70	479.20	458.30	438.30	418.30	398.30
2,520	2,560	628.60	606.10	583.60	561.10	538.60	516.10	493.60	471.10	451.10	431.10	411.10
2,560	2,600	643.00	620.50	598.00	575.50	553.00	530.50	508.00	485.50	463.90	443.90	423.90
2,600	2,640	657.40	634.90	612.40	589.90	567.40	544.90	522.40	499.90	477.40	456.70	436.70
2,640	2,680	671.80	649.30	626.80	604.30	581.80	559.30	536.80	514.30	491.80	469.50	449.50
2,680	2,720	686.20	663.70	641.20	618.70	596.20	573.70	551.20	528.70	506.20	483.70	462.30
2,720	2,760	700.60	678.10	655.60	633.10	610.60	588.10	565.60	543.10	520.60	498.10	475.60
		36 percent of the excess over $2,760 plus—										
$2,760 and over		707.80	685.30	662.80	640.30	617.80	595.30	572.80	550.30	527.80	505.30	482.80

Fig. 15-3 Married Persons — Monthly Withholding Tax Table.

each year. This report covers the income received in the preceding year.

Withholding tax is deducted regularly from paychecks so that employees will not have to pay a large sum at the end of the year. The amount deducted depends on how much the employee is paid and the number of exemptions claimed by the employee. Deduction tables are available for determining the amount to be withheld. Before referring to the deduction tables, the secretarial dental assistant must check the W-4 form to obtain the marital status and the number of exemptions claimed. It is also necessary to know if the employee is being paid by the day, the week, biweekly, semimonthly or monthly in order to select the proper tax table. Two sample tables are shown in figure 15-2 and figure 15-3. The tables are found in the Circular E, Employer's Tax Guide, which is a publication of the Internal Revenue Service. Every office should have a current copy of this publication. The secretarial dental assistant will have to consult it frequently for up-to-date information about federal taxes.

Referring to figures 15-2 and 15-3, the two left-hand columns indicate *At least* and *But less than*. The amount of the gross pay (the total amount of the salary before any deductions are made) is found in these two columns. If the amount is $275.00, the line that reads, *at least $272.00 but less than $280.00,* would be the proper line. Using a soft lead pencil as a guide, trace this line over to the top column corresponding to the number of exemptions withheld. This will be the amount to deduct for withholding income tax. This amount is to be recorded on the employee's earning record (figure 15-5) under withholding tax.

FICA (SOCIAL SECURITY TAX)

FICA tax is a required amount of money to be withheld from the employee's gross pay. It is commonly referred to as *social security,* an insurance program designed to help persons over 62, families of deceased persons, and disabled persons. It also provides medical insurance in the form of Medicare to persons over 65 years of age.

The number of exemptions *are not needed* for computing FICA tax because the amount is deducted from the gross amount of the salary, regardless of the claimed exemptions. The social security tables are located in the back of the Circular E publication of the Internal Revenue Service. The amount of the gross pay is the only information needed to figure the amount of the FICA tax, figure 15-4. FICA tax deductions are always a certain percentage of the employee's income. In 1974, the percentage rate amounted to 5.85. Each year the percentage rate may be subject to change by law. There is also a maximum amount of wages subject to FICA taxes. This amount is also likely to change from year to year. The 1975 maximum amount of wages subject to FICA taxes was $14,100. The amount of FICA taxes to withhold is calcu-

lated from the FICA tax tables. The amount of tax may be double-checked by multiplying the amount of the gross pay by the annual percentage rate. Record the FICA tax amount in the proper column on the employee's earning record.

THE EMPLOYEE'S EARNING RECORD

After the withholding and FICA amount of deductions have been recorded, *the employee's earning record* may be completed. This employee's earning record may be kept in the daily log on a special form. Four employee's earning records may be recorded on one sheet if the Colwell Form no. 4233 is used, figure 15-5. The name of the employee, the social security number, and the number of exemptions are written at the top of the individual form. The date the payroll is computed is recorded in the left-hand column. Hours and rate of pay may be recorded if desired in the next two columns. The fourth column is for the gross amount of the employee's pay. Gross pay is the amount of the salary before any deductions are withheld. The withholding column is for recording the amount of income tax withheld. This is the amount computed from the tables in Circular E. The amount of the pay and the number of exemptions are needed before computing this tax. The FICA column is for recording the amount of social security taxes. This is the amount also computed from the social security (FICA) tables in Circular E. Only the amount of gross pay is needed to compute this tax. Two columns are provided for any additional deductions. State income tax, if any, is withheld and recorded in one of the blank columns. Hospitalization or retirement funds may be withheld and recorded in the second blank column. Other deductions may vary from office to office. The state income tax deductions will vary from state to state. Subtract all of the deductions from the gross pay to obtain the

Social Security Employee Tax Table—Continued

5.85 percent employee tax deductions

Wages At least	Wages But less than	Tax to be withheld	Wages At least	Wages But less than	Tax to be withheld	Wages At least	Wages But less than	Tax to be withheld	Wages At least	Wages But less than	Tax to be withheld
$266.59	$266.76	$15.60	$277.70	$277.87	$16.25	$288.81	$288.98	$16.90	$299.92	$300.09	$17.55
266.76	266.93	15.61	277.87	278.04	16.26	288.98	289.15	16.91	300.09	300.26	17.56
266.93	267.10	15.62	278.04	278.21	16.27	289.15	289.32	16.92	300.26	300.43	17.57
267.10	267.27	15.63	278.21	278.38	16.28	289.32	289.49	16.93	300.43	300.60	17.58
267.27	267.44	15.64	278.38	278.55	16.29	289.49	289.66	16.94	300.60	300.77	17.59
267.44	267.61	15.65	278.55	278.72	16.30	289.66	289.83	16.95	300.77	300.95	17.60
267.61	267.78	15.66	278.72	278.89	16.31	289.83	290.00	16.96	300.95	301.12	17.61
267.78	267.95	15.67	278.89	279.06	16.32	290.00	290.18	16.97	301.12	301.29	17.62
267.95	268.12	15.68	279.06	279.24	16.33	290.18	290.35	16.98	301.29	301.46	17.63
268.12	268.30	15.69	279.24	279.41	16.34	290.35	290.52	16.99	301.46	301.63	17.64
268.30	268.47	15.70	279.41	279.58	16.35	290.52	290.69	17.00	301.63	301.80	17.65
268.47	268.64	15.71	279.58	279.75	16.36	290.69	290.86	17.01	301.80	301.97	17.66
268.64	268.81	15.72	279.75	279.92	16.37	290.86	291.03	17.02	301.97	302.14	17.67
268.81	268.98	15.73	279.92	280.09	16.38	291.03	291.20	17.03	302.14	302.31	17.68
268.98	269.15	15.74	280.09	280.26	16.39	291.20	291.37	17.04	302.31	302.48	17.69
269.15	269.32	15.75	280.26	280.43	16.40	291.37	291.54	17.05	302.48	302.65	17.70
269.32	269.49	15.76	280.43	280.60	16.41	291.54	291.71	17.06	302.65	302.83	17.71
269.49	269.66	15.77	280.60	280.77	16.42	291.71	291.89	17.07	302.83	303.00	17.72
269.66	269.83	15.78	280.77	280.95	16.43	291.89	292.06	17.08	303.00	303.17	17.73
269.83	270.00	15.79	280.95	281.12	16.44	292.06	292.23	17.09	303.17	303.34	17.74
270.00	270.18	15.80	281.12	281.29	16.45	292.23	292.40	17.10	303.34	303.51	17.75
270.18	270.35	15.81	281.29	281.46	16.46	292.40	292.57	17.11	303.51	303.68	17.76
270.35	270.52	15.82	281.46	281.63	16.47	292.57	292.74	17.12	303.68	303.85	17.77
270.52	270.69	15.83	281.63	281.80	16.48	292.74	292.91	17.13	303.85	304.02	17.78
270.69	270.86	15.84	281.80	281.97	16.49	292.91	293.08	17.14	304.02	304.19	17.79
270.86	271.03	15.85	281.97	282.14	16.50	293.08	293.25	17.15	304.19	304.36	17.80
271.03	271.20	15.86	282.14	282.31	16.51	293.25	293.42	17.16	304.36	304.53	17.81
271.20	271.37	15.87	282.31	282.48	16.52	293.42	293.59	17.17	304.53	304.71	17.82
271.37	271.54	15.88	282.48	282.65	16.53	293.59	293.77	17.18	304.71	304.88	17.83
271.54	271.71	15.89	282.65	282.83	16.54	293.77	293.94	17.19	304.88	305.05	17.84
271.71	271.89	15.90	282.83	283.00	16.55	293.94	294.11	17.20	305.05	305.22	17.85
271.89	272.06	15.91	283.00	283.17	16.56	294.11	294.28	17.21	305.22	305.39	17.86
272.06	272.23	15.92	283.17	283.34	16.57	294.28	294.45	17.22	305.39	305.56	17.87
272.23	272.40	15.93	283.34	283.51	16.58	294.45	294.62	17.23	305.56	305.73	17.88
272.40	272.57	15.94	283.51	283.68	16.59	294.62	294.79	17.24	305.73	305.90	17.89
272.57	272.74	15.95	283.68	283.85	16.60	294.79	294.96	17.25	305.90	306.07	17.90
272.74	272.91	15.96	283.85	284.02	16.61	294.96	295.13	17.26	306.07	306.24	17.91
272.91	273.08	15.97	284.02	284.19	16.62	295.13	295.30	17.27	306.24	306.42	17.92
273.08	273.25	15.98	284.19	284.36	16.63	295.30	295.48	17.28	306.42	306.59	17.93
273.25	273.42	15.99	284.36	284.53	16.64	295.48	295.65	17.29	306.59	306.76	17.94
273.42	273.59	16.00	284.53	284.71	16.65	295.65	295.82	17.30	306.76	306.93	17.95
273.59	273.77	16.01	284.71	284.88	16.66	295.82	295.99	17.31	306.93	307.10	17.96
273.77	273.94	16.02	284.88	285.05	16.67	295.99	296.16	17.32	307.10	307.27	17.97
273.94	274.11	16.03	285.05	285.22	16.68	296.16	296.33	17.33	307.27	307.44	17.98
274.11	274.28	16.04	285.22	285.39	16.69	296.33	296.50	17.34	307.44	307.61	17.99
274.28	274.45	16.05	285.39	285.56	16.70	296.50	296.67	17.35	307.61	307.78	18.00
274.45	274.62	16.06	285.56	285.73	16.71	296.67	296.84	17.36	307.78	307.95	18.01
274.62	274.79	16.07	285.73	285.90	16.72	296.84	297.01	17.37	307.95	308.12	18.02
274.79	274.96	16.08	285.90	286.07	16.73	297.01	297.18	17.38	308.12	308.30	18.03
274.96	275.13	16.09	286.07	286.24	16.74	297.18	297.36	17.39	308.30	308.47	18.04
275.13	275.30	16.10	286.24	286.42	16.75	297.36	297.53	17.40	308.47	308.64	18.05
275.30	275.48	16.11	286.42	286.59	16.76	297.53	297.70	17.41	308.64	308.81	18.06
275.48	275.65	16.12	286.59	286.76	16.77	297.70	297.87	17.42	308.81	308.98	18.07
275.65	275.82	16.13	286.76	286.93	16.78	297.87	298.04	17.43	308.98	309.15	18.08
275.82	275.99	16.14	286.93	287.10	16.79	298.04	298.21	17.44	309.15	309.32	18.09
275.99	276.16	16.15	287.10	287.27	16.80	298.21	298.38	17.45	309.32	309.49	18.10
276.16	276.33	16.16	287.27	287.44	16.81	298.38	298.55	17.46	309.49	309.66	18.11
276.33	276.50	16.17	287.44	287.61	16.82	298.55	298.72	17.47	309.66	309.83	18.12
276.50	276.67	16.18	287.61	287.78	16.83	298.72	298.89	17.48	309.83	310.00	18.13
276.67	276.84	16.19	287.78	287.95	16.84	298.89	299.06	17.49	310.00	310.18	18.14
276.84	277.01	16.20	287.95	288.12	16.85	299.06	299.24	17.50	310.18	310.35	18.15
277.01	277.18	16.21	288.12	288.30	16.86	299.24	299.41	17.51	310.35	310.52	18.16
277.18	277.36	16.22	288.30	288.47	16.87	299.41	299.58	17.52	310.52	310.69	18.17
277.36	277.53	16.23	288.47	288.64	16.88	299.58	299.75	17.53	310.69	310.86	18.18
277.53	277.70	16.24	288.64	288.81	16.89	299.75	299.92	17.54	310.86	311.03	18.19

Fig. 15-4 Social Security Employee Tax Table. For wages not shown on this table, use 5.85% to compute the social security tax deduction. (continued on page 138)

Social Security Employee Tax Table—Continued
5.85 percent employee tax deductions

Wages At least	But less than	Tax to be withheld	Wages At least	But less than	Tax to be withheld	Wages At least	But less than	Tax to be withheld	Wages At least	But less than	Tax to be withheld
$311.03	$311.20	$18.20	$322.14	$322.31	$18.85	$333.25	$333.42	$19.50	$344.36	$344.53	$20.15
311.20	311.37	18.21	322.31	322.48	18.86	333.42	333.59	19.51	344.53	344.71	20.16
311.37	311.54	18.22	322.48	322.65	18.87	333.59	333.77	19.52	344.71	344.88	20.17
311.54	311.71	18.23	322.65	322.83	18.88	333.77	333.94	19.53	344.88	345.05	20.18
311.71	311.89	18.24	322.83	323.00	18.89	333.94	334.11	19.54	345.05	345.22	20.19
311.89	312.06	18.25	323.00	323.17	18.90	334.11	334.28	19.55	345.22	345.39	20.20
312.06	312.23	18.26	323.17	323.34	18.91	334.28	334.45	19.56	345.39	345.56	20.21
312.23	312.40	18.27	323.34	323.51	18.92	334.45	334.62	19.57	345.56	345.73	20.22
312.40	312.57	18.28	323.51	323.68	18.93	334.62	334.79	19.58	345.73	345.90	20.23
312.57	312.74	18.29	323.68	323.85	18.94	334.79	334.96	19.59	345.90	346.07	20.24
312.74	312.91	18.30	323.85	324.02	18.95	334.96	335.13	19.60	346.07	346.24	20.25
312.91	313.08	18.31	324.02	324.19	18.96	335.13	335.30	19.61	346.24	346.42	20.26
313.08	313.25	18.32	324.19	324.36	18.97	335.30	335.48	19.62	346.42	346.59	20.27
313.25	313.42	18.33	324.36	324.53	18.98	335.48	335.65	19.63	346.59	346.76	20.28
313.42	313.59	18.34	324.53	324.71	18.99	335.65	335.82	19.64	346.76	346.93	20.29
313.59	313.77	18.35	324.71	324.88	19.00	335.82	335.99	19.65	346.93	347.10	20.30
313.77	313.94	18.36	324.88	325.05	19.01	335.99	336.16	19.66	347.10	347.27	20.31
313.94	314.11	18.37	325.05	325.22	19.02	336.16	336.33	19.67	347.27	347.44	20.32
314.11	314.28	18.38	325.22	325.39	19.03	336.33	336.50	19.68	347.44	347.61	20.33
314.28	314.45	18.39	325.39	325.56	19.04	336.50	336.67	19.69	347.61	347.78	20.34
314.45	314.62	18.40	325.56	325.73	19.05	336.67	336.84	19.70	347.78	347.95	20.35
314.62	314.79	18.41	325.73	325.90	19.06	336.84	337.01	19.71	347.95	348.12	20.36
314.79	314.96	18.42	325.90	326.07	19.07	337.01	337.18	19.72	348.12	348.30	20.37
314.96	315.13	18.43	326.07	326.24	19.08	337.18	337.36	19.73	348.30	348.47	20.38
315.13	315.30	18.44	326.24	326.42	19.09	337.36	337.53	19.74	348.47	348.64	20.39
315.30	315.48	18.45	326.42	326.59	19.10	337.53	337.70	19.75	348.64	348.81	20.40
315.48	315.65	18.46	326.59	326.76	19.11	337.70	337.87	19.76	348.81	348.98	20.41
315.65	315.82	18.47	326.76	326.93	19.12	337.87	338.04	19.77	348.98	349.15	20.42
315.82	315.99	18.48	326.93	327.10	19.13	338.04	338.21	19.78	349.15	349.32	20.43
315.99	316.16	18.49	327.10	327.27	19.14	338.21	338.38	19.79	349.32	349.49	20.44
316.16	316.33	18.50	327.27	327.44	19.15	338.38	338.55	19.80	349.49	349.66	20.45
316.33	316.50	18.51	327.44	327.61	19.16	338.55	338.72	19.81	349.66	349.83	20.46
316.50	316.67	18.52	327.61	327.78	19.17	338.72	338.89	19.82	349.83	350.00	20.47
316.67	316.84	18.53	327.78	327.95	19.18	338.89	339.06	19.83	350.00	350.18	20.48
316.84	317.01	18.54	327.95	328.12	19.19	339.06	339.24	19.84	350.18	350.35	20.49
317.01	317.18	18.55	328.12	328.30	19.20	339.24	339.41	19.85	350.35	350.52	20.50
317.18	317.36	18.56	328.30	328.47	19.21	339.41	339.58	19.86	350.52	350.69	20.51
317.36	317.53	18.57	328.47	328.64	19.22	339.58	339.75	19.87	350.69	350.86	20.52
317.53	317.70	18.58	328.64	328.81	19.23	339.75	339.92	19.88	350.86	351.03	20.53
317.70	317.87	18.59	328.81	328.98	19.24	339.92	340.09	19.89	351.03	351.20	20.54
317.87	318.04	18.60	328.98	329.15	19.25	340.09	340.26	19.90	351.20	351.37	20.55
318.04	318.21	18.61	329.15	329.32	19.26	340.26	340.43	19.91	351.37	351.54	20.56
318.21	318.38	18.62	329.32	329.49	19.27	340.43	340.60	19.92	351.54	351.71	20.57
318.38	318.55	18.63	329.49	329.66	19.28	340.60	340.77	19.93	351.71	351.89	20.58
318.55	318.72	18.64	329.66	329.83	19.29	340.77	340.95	19.94	351.89	352.06	20.59
318.72	318.89	18.65	329.83	330.00	19.30	340.95	341.12	19.95	352.06	352.23	20.60
318.89	319.06	18.66	330.00	330.18	19.31	341.12	341.29	19.96	352.23	352.40	20.61
319.06	319.24	18.67	330.18	330.35	19.32	341.29	341.46	19.97	352.40	352.57	20.62
319.24	319.41	18.68	330.35	330.52	19.33	341.46	341.63	19.98	352.57	352.74	20.63
319.41	319.58	18.69	330.52	330.69	19.34	341.63	341.80	19.99	352.74	352.91	20.64
319.58	319.75	18.70	330.69	330.86	19.35	341.80	341.97	20.00	352.91	353.08	20.65
319.75	319.92	18.71	330.86	331.03	19.36	341.97	342.14	20.01	353.08	353.25	20.66
319.92	320.09	18.72	331.03	331.20	19.37	342.14	342.31	20.02	353.25	353.42	20.67
320.09	320.26	18.73	331.20	331.37	19.38	342.31	342.48	20.03	353.42	353.59	20.68
320.26	320.43	18.74	331.37	331.54	19.39	342.48	342.65	20.04	353.59	353.77	20.69
320.43	320.60	18.75	331.54	331.71	19.40	342.65	342.83	20.05	353.77	353.94	20.70
320.60	320.77	18.76	331.71	331.89	19.41	342.83	343.00	20.06	353.94	354.11	20.71
320.77	320.95	18.77	331.89	332.06	19.42	343.00	343.17	20.07	354.11	354.28	20.72
320.95	321.12	18.78	332.06	332.23	19.43	343.17	343.34	20.08	354.28	354.45	20.73
321.12	321.29	18.79	332.23	332.40	19.44	343.34	343.51	20.09	354.45	354.62	20.74
321.29	321.46	18.80	332.40	332.57	19.45	343.51	343.68	20.10	354.62	354.79	20.75
321.46	321.63	18.81	332.57	332.74	19.46	343.68	343.85	20.11	354.79	354.96	20.76
321.63	321.80	18.82	332.74	332.91	19.47	343.85	344.02	20.12	354.96	355.13	20.77
321.80	321.97	18.83	332.91	333.08	19.48	344.02	344.19	20.13	355.13	355.30	20.78
321.97	322.14	18.84	333.08	333.25	19.49	344.19	344.36	20.14	355.30	355.48	20.79

Fig. 15-4

Payroll   December

NAME: Janice E. Smith   **SOC. SEC. NO.** 427-93-6103   **NUMBER OF EXEMPTIONS** 3

DATE	HOURS	RATE	GROSS PAY	WITHHOLDING	F.I.C.A.			NET PAY
12-1		500/mo	500 00	41 80	29 25	7 08		421 87
		TOTALS	500 00	41 80	29 25	7 08		421 87
QUARTER	BROUGHT FWD.		1000 00	83 60	58 50	14 16		843 74
	TO DATE		1500 00	125 40	87 75	21 24		1265 61
YEAR	BROUGHT FWD.		4500 00	376 20	263 25	63 72		3796 83
	TO DATE		6000 00	501 60	351 00	84 96		5062 44

NAME: Mary M. Doe   **SOC. SEC. NO.** 425-79-5100   **NUMBER OF EXEMPTIONS** 1

DATE	HOURS	RATE	GROSS PAY	WITHHOLDING	F.I.C.A.			NET PAY
12-1		480/mo	480 00	61 80	28 08	15 90		374 22
		TOTALS	480 00	61 80	28 08	15 90		374 22
QUARTER	BROUGHT FWD.		960 00	123 60	56 16	31 80		748 44
	TO DATE		1440 00	185 40	84 24	47 70		1122 66
YEAR	BROUGHT FWD.		4320 00	556 20	252 72	143 10		3367 98
	TO DATE		5760 00	741 60	336 96	190 80		4490 64

NAME: Rebecca M. Dudley   **SOC. SEC. NO.** 419-77-5421   **NUMBER OF EXEMPTIONS** 1

DATE	HOURS	RATE	GROSS PAY	WITHHOLDING	F.I.C.A.			NET PAY
12-1		600/mo	600 00	79 40	35 10	22 23		463 27
		TOTALS	600 00	79 40	35 10	22 23		463 27
QUARTER	BROUGHT FWD.		1200 00	158 80	70 20	44 46		926 54
	TO DATE		1800 00	238 20	105 30	66 69		1389 81
YEAR	BROUGHT FWD.		5400 00	714 60	315 90	200 07		4169 43
	TO DATE		7200 00	952 80	421 10	266 76		5559 24

NAME: Sarah L. Doe   **SOC. SEC. NO.** 418-97-1032   **NUMBER OF EXEMPTIONS** 2

DATE	HOURS	RATE	GROSS PAY	WITHHOLDING	F.I.C.A.			NET PAY
12-1		525/mo	525 00	55 00	30 71	17 80		421 49
		TOTALS	525 00	55 00	30 71	17 80		421 49
QUARTER	BROUGHT FWD.		1050 00	110 00	61 42	35 60		842 98
	TO DATE		1575 00	165 00	92 13	53 40		1264 47
YEAR	BROUGHT FWD.		4725 00	495 00	276 39	160 20		3793 41
	TO DATE		6300 00	660 00	368 52	213 60		5057 88

FORM 4233   COLWELL CO. CHAMPAIGN, ILL.   **DEC**

Fig. 15-5 An example of an Employee's Earning Record.

net pay. The net pay is the amount frequently referred to as "take home pay." This is the amount for which the payroll check is written.

At the end of the month all of the columns should be totaled on the employee's earning record. The totals from the previous months, if after January, should be brought forward. At the end of each quarter the totals, to date, may be used in compiling the quarterly income tax report. A yearly total may also be kept at the bottom of each individual employee's form.

Remittance to the federal government of the employee's deductions will be explained in detail in units 16 through 18.

SUMMARY

The secretarial dental assistant may be given the task of compiling payroll amounts and writing payroll checks. Payroll must be figured accurately from tables supplied by the Internal Revenue Service. The secretarial dental assistant must also maintain a record of the salaries paid to the employees in the dental office.

The first day of employment, the new employee must complete an Employee's Withholding Allowance Certificate declaring the number of exemptions to be claimed. Income Tax (Withholding tax) is deducted regularly from the paycheck so that the employee will not have to pay a large sum at the end of the year. The amount deducted depends on how much the employee is paid and the number of exemptions claimed. Social Security Tax (FICA) is figured on an annual percentage rate. This amount is computed from the gross pay of the employee. The percentage rate of social security deductions is likely to change from year to year. The Employer's Tax Guide, Circular E, published yearly by the Internal Revenue Service must be consulted and used to compute all payroll records.

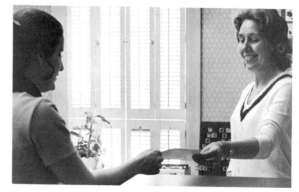

Fig. 15-6   A paycheck being received by a member of the dental office staff.

SUGGESTED ACTIVITIES

- Prepare index cards on the following subjects:

    a. How to complete a W-4 form.
    b. Withholding Tax Information
    c. FICA Tax Requirements.

- Obtain a copy of a Circular E, Employer's Tax Guide. Review the tables used in payroll computation.

REVIEW

A.   Define the following

   1. Gross Pay.

   2. Net pay.

   3. Withholding Tax.

   4. FICA Tax.

B.   Using the withholding and FICA tax tables in this unit, figure the payroll for the following:

   1. Mary Jean Bailey, is single and receives her paycheck every two weeks. Her social security number is 427-51-6857. She receives $260.00 gross pay each pay period. Her paycheck without any other deductions would be _____

   2. Bart Clark is married and receives his paycheck on a monthly basis. He claims a total of 4 exemptions including himself. His monthly salary is $650.00; social security number is 427-97-4410. His paycheck without any other deductions would be _____

3. Martha Jones is married and claims only herself. She is paid monthly at the rate of $800.00. Her social security number is 329-57-6179. Her paycheck without further deductions would be _____

4. Jennifer Callahan is divorced but is responsible for herself and her three children. She receives her paycheck semi-monthly. Her gross pay is $600.00 per month. Her social security number is 427-77-4489. Her paycheck without further deductions would be _____

C. Using the payroll information given in B, complete the Employee's Earning Record on all four employees.

Payroll August

NAME:				SOC. SEC. NO.			NUMBER OF EXEMPTIONS				
DATE	HOURS	RATE	GROSS PAY	WITHHOLDING	F.I.C.A.					NET PAY	
		TOTALS									
QUARTER	BROUGHT FWD.										
	TO DATE										
YEAR	BROUGHT FWD.										
	TO DATE										

NAME:				SOC. SEC. NO.			NUMBER OF EXEMPTIONS				
DATE	HOURS	RATE	GROSS PAY	WITHHOLDING	F.I.C.A.					NET PAY	
		TOTALS									
QUARTER	BROUGHT FWD.										
	TO DATE										
YEAR	BROUGHT FWD.										
	TO DATE										

NAME:				SOC. SEC. NO.			NUMBER OF EXEMPTIONS				
DATE	HOURS	RATE	GROSS PAY	WITHHOLDING	F.I.C.A.					NET PAY	
		TOTALS									
QUARTER	BROUGHT FWD.										
	TO DATE										
YEAR	BROUGHT FWD.										
	TO DATE										

AUG

NAME:				SOC. SEC. NO.			NUMBER OF EXEMPTIONS				
DATE	HOURS	RATE	GROSS PAY	WITHHOLDING	F.I.C.A.					NET PAY	
		TOTALS									
QUARTER	BROUGHT FWD.										
	TO DATE										
YEAR	BROUGHT FWD.										
	TO DATE										

FORM 4233   COLWELL CO., CHAMPAIGN, ILL.

D.   Complete a W-4 form as if you were the new employee.

Form W–4 (Revised April 1975)
Employee's Withholding Allowance Certificate
(Use for wages paid after April 30, 1975 and before January 1, 1976)

The explanatory material below will help you determine your correct number of withholding allowances, and will assist you in completing the Form W–4 at the bottom of this page.

Avoid Overwithholding or Underwithholding

By claiming the proper number of withholding allowances you are entitled to, you can fit the amount of tax withheld from your wages to your tax liability. In addition to the allowances for personal exemptions to be claimed in items (a) through (g) below, be sure you claim any additional allowances you are entitled to in item (h) "Special withholding allowance," and item (i) "Allowance(s) for itemized deductions." While these allowances may be claimed on Form W–4 for withholding purposes, they are not to be claimed under "Exemptions" on your tax return Form 1040 or Form 1040A.

You may claim the special withholding allowance if you are single with only one employer, or married with only one employer and your spouse is not employed. If you have unusually large itemized deductions, you may claim the allowance(s) for itemized deductions to avoid having too much income tax withheld from your wages. On the other hand, if you and your spouse are both employed or you have more than one employer, you should take steps to assure that enough has been withheld. If you find that you need more withholding, claim fewer exemptions or ask for additional withholding. If you are currently claiming additional withholding allowances based on itemized deductions, check the table on the back to see that you are claiming the proper number of allowances.

How Many Withholding Allowances May You Claim?

Please use the schedule below to determine the number of allowances you may claim for tax withholding purposes. In determining the number, keep in mind these points: If you are single and hold more than one job, you may not claim the same allowances with more than one employer at the same time; or if you are married and both you and your spouse are employed, you may not claim the same allowances with your employers at the same time. A nonresident alien, other than a resident of Canada, Mexico, or Puerto Rico, may claim only one personal allowance.

Figure Your Total Withholding Allowances Below

(a) Allowance for yourself—enter 1 . . . . _____

(b) Allowance for your spouse—enter 1 . . . . _____

(c) Allowance for your age—if 65 or over—enter 1 . . . . _____

(d) Allowance for your spouse's age—if 65 or over—enter 1 . . . . . _____

(e) Allowance for blindness (yourself)—enter 1 . . . . _____

(f) Allowance for blindness (spouse's)—enter 1 . . . . _____

(g) Allowance(s) for dependent(s)—you are entitled to claim an allowance for each dependent you will be able to claim on your Federal income tax return. Do not include yourself or your spouse * . . . . _____

(h) Special withholding allowance—if you are single with only one employer, or married with only one employer and your spouse is not employed—enter 1** . . . . _____

(i) Allowance(s) for itemized deductions—if you do plan to itemize deductions on your income tax return, enter the number from the table on back** . . . . _____

(j) Total—add lines (a) through (i) above. Enter here and on line 1, Form W–4 below . . . . _____

* If you are in doubt as to whom you may claim as a dependent, see the instructions which came with your last Federal income tax return or call your local Internal Revenue Service office.

** This allowance is used solely for purposes of figuring your withholding tax, and cannot be claimed when you file your tax return.

See Table on Back if You Plan to Itemize Your Deductions

Completing Form W–4.—If you find that you are entitled to one or more allowances in addition to those which you are now claiming, increase your number of allowances by completing the form below and filing it with your employer. If the number of allowances you previously claimed decreases, you must file a new Form W–4 within 10 days. (Should you expect to owe more tax than will be withheld, you may use the same form to increase your withholding by claiming fewer or "0" allowances on line 1, or by asking for additional withholding on line 2, or both.)

▼ **Give the bottom part of this form to your employer; keep the upper part for your records and information** ▼

-- Cut along this line --

Form **W-4** (Rev. April 1975) Department of the Treasury Internal Revenue Service	# Employee's Withholding Allowance Certificate (This certificate is for income tax withholding purposes only; it will remain in effect until you change it.)
Type or print your full name	Your social security number
Home address (Number and street or rural route)	Marital status ☐ Single ☐ Married
City or town, State and ZIP code	(If married but legally separated, or spouse is a nonresident alien, check the single block.)

1 Total number of allowances you are claiming . . . . _____

2 Additional amount, if any, you want deducted from each pay (if your employer agrees) . . . . $ _____

I certify that to the best of my knowledge and belief, the number of withholding allowances claimed on this certificate does not exceed the number to which I am entitled.

Signature ▶ .... Date ▶ .... , 19 ....

E. Select the best answer(s).

1. The form used to maintain salary records of employees is called

    a. Employee's Withholding Allowance Certificate.
    b. Employee's Earning Record.
    c. Employer's Federal Quarterly Tax Return.
    d. Employer's Tax Guide.

2. The W-4 Form, Employee's Withholding Allowance Certificate

    a. authorizes the employer to deduct tax from the employee's salary.
    b. states the amount of withholding tax to deduct from the employee's salary.
    c. requires the employer to deduct certain amounts for state income tax.
    d. informs the office of the number of exemptions claimed by the employee.

3. Withholding tax is deducted regularly from paychecks according to

    a. the amount the employee desires to have deducted.
    b. the marital status of the employee only.
    c. the number of days the employee worked during the month.
    d. the amount of the gross salary and the number of claimed exemptions.

4. The initials FICA mean

    a. Federal Income Contribution Act.
    b. Federal Insurance Contribution Act.
    c. Federal Internal Cooperation Act.
    d. Federal Insurance Cooperation Act.

5. FICA, commonly referred to as social security, is an insurance program designed to

    a. aid families of deceased persons.
    b. provide housing benefits for elderly people.
    c. aid persons over 62.
    d. aid disabled persons.
    e. provide medical care for persons on medicare.
    f. provide insurance and dental care to persons under 65.
    g. aid in providing educational opportunities for the handicapped.

6. An employee's net pay is the

    a. amount of the salary before any deductions are made.
    b. total amount of the deductions required of employees.
    c. maximum amount of wages subject to FICA taxes.
    d. amount of the paycheck after all necessary deductions are made.

Unit 16 Social Security (FICA)

OBJECTIVES

After studying this unit, the student should be able to

- State how FICA deductions are made.

- Give examples of benefits provided by Social Security.

- List kinds of proof required of applicants for social security benefits.

FICA tax (Social Security) was discussed in the preceding unit as it related to payroll deductions. However, many dental team members do not understand the importance of FICA taxes. They do not realize what social security can mean to a person or family. In a group dental practice where 17 dental assistants were employed, a survey was taken. It was found that only the two bookkeepers were knowledgeable about social security. Since others have indicated that similar situations exist, an entire unit is devoted to an explanation of these taxes for the personal benefit of the secretarial dental assistant as well as to add to her job performance.

The social security program became a law in 1935. Many amendments have been added since then. Now a wage earner (male or female) may apply for social security at age 62 and receive a reduced monthly benefit or file at age 65 for a larger amount. Both young and old people receive many benefits from the program. The percentage of social security payments have increased. Likewise, the social security benefits have increased. New types of benefits have been added. Eligibility requirements have modified so that more people are eligible.

Approximately 90% of all working people are protected under the social security law. Both employees and employers pay into the social security fund. This fund is actually a federal insurance program designed to aid aged persons, families of deceased persons, disabled persons, and to provide medical assistance to persons 65 years of age and over. Employees pay social security contributions into trust funds during all of their working years. When employees who have sufficient social security coverage are no longer working because of retirement or disability, periodic cash payments may be made to the employee. If an employee dies, cash payments are made to the surviving family members. Social security may help provide the employee with hospital and medical insurance protection. This medical help is called Medicare.

The social security protection you earn stays with you even if you change jobs. In fact, a person may move from one state to another, and the protection remains with the person. Neither does it matter how many different jobs a person may have during his working years. Most jobs are covered by social security. Earnings from a private business may also be covered.

Every employee must have a social security number. Application for the number may be made any time after a child's birth. Figure 16-1 shows the proper form to complete when applying for a social security number. A social security number will be assigned and a card issued by the local office of the Social Security Administration, a part of the

```
ID                  CN                      DO
APPLICATION FOR A SOCIAL SECURITY NUMBER                              ┌                        ┐
  See Instructions on Back.         Print in Black or Dark Blue Ink or Use Typewriter.        └─ DO NOT WRITE IN THE ABOVE SPACE ─┘
```

| 1 | Print FULL NAME YOU WILL USE IN WORK OR BUSINESS | (First Name) | (Middle Name or Initial – if none, draw line ___) | (Last Name) |

2 Print FULL NAME GIVEN YOU AT BIRTH

6 YOUR DATE OF BIRTH   (Month) (Day) (Year)

3 PLACE OF BIRTH   (City)   (County if known)   (State)

7 YOUR PRESENT AGE (Age on last birthday)

4 MOTHER'S FULL NAME AT HER BIRTH (Her maiden name)

8 YOUR SEX   MALE □   FEMALE □

5 FATHER'S FULL NAME (Regardless of whether living or dead)

9 YOUR COLOR OR RACE   WHITE □   NEGRO □   OTHER □

10 HAVE YOU EVER BEFORE APPLIED FOR OR HAD A SOCIAL SECURITY, RAILROAD, OR TAX ACCOUNT NUMBER?   NO □   DON'T KNOW □   YES □   (If "YES" Print STATE in which you applied and DATE you applied and SOCIAL SECURITY NUMBER if known)

11 YOUR MAILING ADDRESS   (Number and Street, Apt. No., P.O. Box, or Rural Route)   (City)   (State)   (Zip Code)

12 TODAY'S DATE

14 NOTICE: Whoever, with intent to falsify his or someone else's true identity, willfully furnishes or causes to be furnished false information in applying for a social security number, is subject to a fine of not more than $1,000 or imprisonment for up to 1 year, or both.

13 TELEPHONE NUMBER

Sign YOUR NAME HERE (Do Not Print)

TREASURY DEPARTMENT Internal Revenue Service   □ RESCREEN   □ ASSIGN   □ DUP ISSUED   Return completed application to nearest SOCIAL SECURITY ADMINISTRATION OFFICE
FORM SS-5 (2-73)

Fig. 16-1 An application for a Social Security Number (Form SS-5).

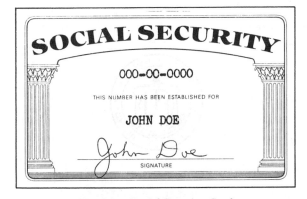

Fig. 16-2 Social Security Card.

U.S. Department of Health, Education and Welfare, figure 16-2. The secretarial dental assistant can contact the local office by checking the phone directory under United States Government when there are questions about social security benefits, including Medicare.

The social security number issued to a person is the number he keeps throughout his or her life. If the card should become lost or stolen, a duplicate one may be obtained; the originally assigned number will always remain the same. If a woman marries and changes her name, only the name will be changed on the card. The local security office would have to be contacted by the person (wage earner) who needs a duplicate card to replace a lost one or to reflect a name change.

Today, the social security number may be used for various records. Some states use the person's social security number for the driver's license number. Many colleges and universities use the social security number for the student number. This simplifies record keeping.

The social security card should be shown on the first day of employment each time a person changes jobs. The card is usually requested when the Employee's Withholding Allowance Certificate is given to the new employee. The social security number is also needed for income tax purposes. Any person or agency that pays dividends, interest, or other income reportable to the Internal Revenue Service will need the social security number for reporting purposes.

Year	For retirement, survivors, and disability insurance	For hospital insurance	Total
1974-1977	4.95%	.90%	5.85%
1978-1980	4.95	1.10	6.05
1981-1985	4.95	1.35	6.30
1986-1998	4.95	1.50	6.45
1999-2010	4.95	1.50	6.45
2011 & later	5.95	1.50	7.45

The amount of yearly earnings on which employers and employees pay social security contributions is $17,700 in 1978. This amount may be increased for the years following 1978.

Fig. 16-3 Social Security Contribution Rate schedule for employers and employees.

SOCIAL SECURITY DEDUCTIONS

Social security benefits are paid for by contributions; these are based on the employee's covered earnings. The contributions are deducted from the employee's salary each time a paycheck is written and the employer matches the amount of the deduction. *Both the employee and the employer pay equal amounts for the employee's contribution.* A self-employed person, such as a dentist, contributes about three-fourths of the combined employee-employer rate for retirement, survivors, and disability insurance. The medical insurance contribution rate is the same for employees, employers, or self-employed persons.

There is a maximum amount of yearly earnings on which employers and employees pay social security contributions. Social security tax is not paid on money earned over the maximum amount. The maximum amount for 1978 is $17,700. An employee making over that amount would not pay social security contributions on earnings over $17,700. Figure 16-3 shows a contribution rate schedule for employees or employers. Notice that the percent of covered earnings becomes higher every few years. This is necessary to provide

more social security benefits as wages go higher. The rate for 1978 is 6.05%.

SOCIAL SECURITY FORMS

At the end of each year all employers are required by law to furnish each employee with a W-2 form (Wage and Tax Statement). This form shows the amount of the employee's earnings and tax deductions for the year, including the amount of FICA taxes paid. This form may be given earlier if a person leaves a place of employment before the end of the year.

The employer's Quarterly Tax Return (941) is used to report employee earnings to the Social Security Administration. Magnetic tapes are used to maintain all the social security records; they are maintained in the Social Security Administration's central office. One single reel of tape may hold the lifetime earning records of 100,000 people. There is also a duplicate record maintained in the event the originals are destroyed.

It is possible to periodically obtain a statement of one's social security earnings. The statement will show the total amount of earnings an employee has reported beginning with 1937. It is suggested that individuals check their statement of earnings record from time to time; a postcard form may be obtained from the local social security office for this purpose. The postcard must be completed, signed and sent to the Baltimore office. The card asks for the date of birth. If an individual also wishes to know the number of credits she has already earned and the number of credits required for future benefits, the Baltimore office will supply the information; a brief request for this information must be written on the card. As social security records are confidential, no one can obtain another's record.

If the individual's statement of earnings seems to be in error, the local social security office should be contacted immediately for help in solving the differences. All errors must be reported within 3 years, 3 months, and 15 days after the period covered by the report.

SOCIAL SECURITY BENEFITS

To become eligible for social security benefits an employee must have worked under social security covered employment for a certain length of time. The credit may have been earned any time after 1936. A person with a total of 10 years of work credit is considered fully insured if social security contributions were made during that period. The *number of credits required depends on the wage earner's date of birth;* however, no one is considered to be fully insured with less than 1 1/2 years of covered employment.

Most employees get credit for one-fourth of a year of work if they have received at least $50.00 in a three month period. A self-employed person receives a full year of credit if his self-employment *net* income is at least $400.00 per year. Any one who earns the maximum wages creditable for social security in a year receives a full year's credit. This person may have worked only part of the year.

An employee is *currently insured* if he has received credit for having worked at least 1 1/2

years of work within the 3 year period *before disability began or death occurred.* Certain kinds of benefits may be payable to the wage earner and/or his dependents if he was currently insured, regardless of age at the time of disability or death. The number of credits does not determine the amount of the monthly benefits; they simply establish eligibility to receive a benefit. The amount of the monthly payment will depend on the amount of *earnings* one has received during his working years.

In short, eligibility to receive benefits depends on the credits *earned,* based on the *time* a person worked. Eligibility must be established first. Then, the earnings record is used to determine the amount to be paid.

Monthly payments may be made to an eligible person who is disabled, is 62 or over, or is a widow, widower, parent, or dependent child. A disabled person is one who cannot work because of a severe physical or mental handicap that has lasted (or is expected to last) twelve months or longer. When disability benefits are applied for, proof must be submitted to support the claim that a physical or mental handicap does exist. The final determination is made by the Social Security Administration.

A death benefit check may be issued to whoever paid the funeral expenses of a wage earner who died (if he had sufficient wage credits) regardless of his age at the time of death.

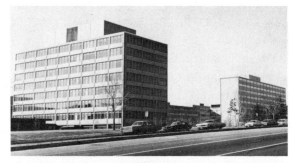

Fig. 16-4 The Social Security Administration's central office in Baltimore, Maryland.

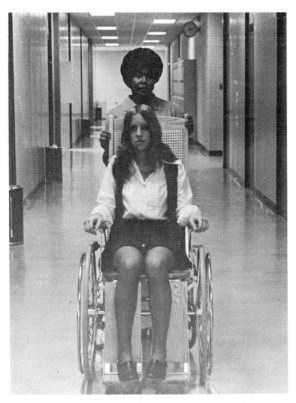

Fig. 16-5 Even a young person may qualify for benefits if she meets the requirements established by the Social Security laws.

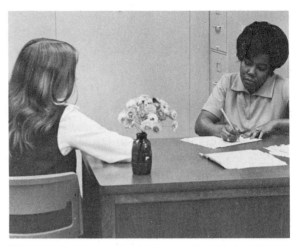

Fig. 16-6   An application must be filed with the local social security office before benefits can be received.

An application must be filed with a local social security office before benefits can be received. When applying for social security benefits proof of eligibility will be needed. The employee's social security number and proof of age are items needed by the social security office. Birth certificates will verify the ages of anyone in the family eligible to collect monthly social security benefits. Some evidence such as the W-2 form or a copy of the previous year's income tax return will provide evidence of work and earnings which may not have yet been recorded in Baltimore, and could affect the amount of benefit.

When applying for survivors benefits, a death certificate will be needed. Marriage certificates or divorce decrees may be requested for certain types of benefits.

Every employed person in the dental office should know these basic facts about social security. For questions not explained in this unit, contact the local social security office. There are more than 850 local social security offices in the United States. The trained personnel who are employed in these offices are very helpful to anyone wanting information or applying for monthly benefits.

SUMMARY

Many people in the dental field are unaware of the purpose of social security. Social security (FICA) is a federal insurance program providing monthly benefits to the aged, disabled, survivors of wage earners and medical assistance to persons age 62 and older. Sufficient credits must be earned by an employee before he or she is eligible to receive social security benefits. An employee contributes a certain percentage of his salary regularly into the social security fund; this amount is matched by the employer. Then, when employment stops due to death, retirement, or disability, monthly payments may be made to the employee or the family. Medicare, the medical insurance supplement of social security, helps to provide the employee with adequate hospital or medical protection after he reaches the age of 65.

SUGGESTED ACTIVITIES

- Visit the nearest social security office and obtain pamphlets for the class to read.
- After studying the pamphlets, make posters explaining the social security benefits available.

REVIEW

A.   Select the best answer.

1.   The social security program became a law in the year
   a. 1960.
   b. 1924.
   c. 1859.
   d. 1935.

2.   Medicare is that part of the social security program that helps provide
   a. disabled employees with medical aid.
   b. financial aid to the families of deceased persons.
   c. hospital and medical insurance to persons over 65 years of age.
   d. medical and dental care to dependent children.

3.   Social security protection remains with a person
   a. even if one changes jobs or moves to a different state.
   b. unless he moves to another state.
   c. only if the employee owns his own business.
   d. unless he changes jobs.

4.   Application for a social security number may be made
   a. after one becomes of legal age.
   b. any time after birth.
   c. at the beginning of one's first employment.
   d. after one becomes 12 years of age.

5.   Based on covered earnings, social security (FICA) contributions are made by the employee and by
   a. the employer deducting a certain amount from the net income.
   b. the employer matching the amount.
   c. the employer deducting a certain amount from the gross income.
   d. the federal government matching the amount of the employee's deduction.

6. The retirement, survivors, and disability contribution rate for self-employed persons is about

   a. one/half of the combined employee-employer rate.

   b. one/third of the combined rate.

   c. two/thirds of the combined rate.

   d. three/fourths of the combined rate.

7. The central office of the Social Security Administration is located in

   a. Baltimore, Maryland.

   b. San Francisco, California.

   c. Washington, D.C.

   d. Atlanta, Georgia.

8. A wage and tax statement known as the W-2 form is

   a. issued to the employer by the federal government to show taxes that are due and payable.

   b. given to the employee to verify the number of exemptions claimed.

   c. a form the employer prepares for the federal government for unemployment taxes.

   d. furnished to the employee to show the amount of yearly earnings and tax deductions.

9. Before monthly social security benefits may be received, it is necessary to have

   a. credit for a certain amount of covered employment.

   b. worked until retirement age.

   c. current employment.

   d. worked for someone who has paid federal unemployment tax.

B. Select the best answers. More than one reply is correct.

1. Monthly payments may be made to the following eligible persons

   a. disabled.

   b. under 62 years of age.

   c. over 65 years of age.

   d. a widow or widower.

   e. an employed person.

   f. a dental cripple.

   g. a dependent child.

2. Proof of eligibility must be made to the social security office when application is made for benefits. The applicant should be prepared to furnish his or her

a. social security number.

b. birth certificate(s) or other acceptable proof of age.

c. evidence of earnings for the preceding year.

d. death and marriage certificates, possible divorce decrees.

C. Briefly answer the following questions.

1. What should be done if a co-worker tells the secretarial dental assistant that, because of marriage, her name is different than that shown on her social security card?

2. Who pays for the employee's FICA deductions?

3. How can a person find out the amount of earnings credited to her account and how many credits of coverage she will need to qualify for benefits?

Unit 17 Monthly and Quarterly Income Tax Forms

OBJECTIVES

After studying this unit, the student should be able to

- Complete an application form for an employer identification number.
- State the four payment rules that determine if taxes are to be paid monthly or quarterly.
- Complete a Federal Tax Deposit.
- Complete a Quarterly Federal Tax Return.

There are several federal income tax forms that the dental office is required to complete, such as monthly, quarterly, or yearly tax reports. These forms must be completed accurately and mailed by certain dates. The secretarial dental assistant must be familiar with each form as failure to complete tax reports may result in serious problems for the dentist.

Every dentist or dental clinic must have an employer identification number. Every person who pays wages to one or more persons is required to have this identification number. Do not confuse this number with the social security number. The social security number is an employee number; this is an employer number. An application for an employer identification number should be filed immediately at the start of any new business. It should be filed no later than the end of the first week of business. The application form comes in two parts and is generally self-explanatory, figure 17-1. (Note question #5, "Organization, check type." Most dental offices would be checked as *individual* as the dentist is requesting the number.) When applying for an employer identification number, use the Internal Revenue Service Form SS-4. This form is correctly filled out and then mailed to the United States Internal Revenue office servicing the area; the addresses are shown on

the form. The federal tax returns for the area are filed in these centers. The IRS Circular E, which is the Employer's Tax Guide lists the addresses of the states and the area offices. The Circular E publication should be consulted frequently for answers to federal income tax questions.

After the employer's identification number has been received, preinscribed federal forms and the current Circular E will be automatically sent to the dentist's office. If additional forms are needed, the IRS area office is contacted by the secretarial dental assistant.

MONTHLY AND QUARTERLY PAYMENTS

The federal government has provided a method for employers to pay federal taxes periodically during the year. This method eliminates the need for a large lump sum to be paid by the employer at the end of the year. Federal taxes are payable either monthly or quarterly during the year. The dental office does not have a choice of whether the payments will be made monthly or quarterly. The amount of taxes that are due will determine when the payment is to be made:

- If the total amount of taxes due at the end of the quarter is less than $200, a monthly deposit of taxes is not required.

FORM SS-4 (3-69)
PART 1   U.S. TREASURY DEPARTMENT—INTERNAL REVENUE SERVICE
APPLICATION FOR EMPLOYER IDENTIFICATION NUMBER

1. NAME (*TRUE name as distinguished from TRADE name.*)

John Melvin Doe, D.D.S.

2. TRADE NAME, IF ANY (*Enter name under which business is operated, if different from item 1.*)

3. ADDRESS OF PRINCIPAL PLACE OF BUSINESS (*No. and Street, City, State, Zip Code*)

300 Dental Drive, Anywhere, USA 39000

4. COUNTY OF BUSINESS LOCATION

Smith

5. ORGANIZATION Check Type

[X] Individual   [ ] Partnership   [ ] Corporation   [ ] Other (*specify e.g. estate, trust, etc.*)
[ ] Governmental   [ ] Nonprofit Organization
   (See Instr. 5)   (See Instr. 5)

6. Ending Month of Accounting year

December

7. REASON FOR APPLYING (*If "other" specify such as "Corporate structure change," "Acquired by gift or trust," etc.*)

[X] Started new business   [ ] Purchased going business   [ ] Other

8. Date you acquired or started business (*Mo., day, year*)

January 1, 1975

9. First date you paid or will pay wages (*Mo., day, year*)

January 15

10. NATURE OF BUSINESS (*See Instructions*)

Dental Practice

11. NUMBER OF EMPLOYEES → IF "NONE" ENTER "0"

Non-agricultural	Agricultural
2	

12. If nature of business is MANUFACTURING, list in order of their importance the principal products manufactured and the estimated percentage of the total value of all products which each represents.

A _____ %

B _____ %   C _____ %

PLEASE LEAVE BLANK

R	DO	TA
FR		FRC

13. Do you operate more than one place of business?   [ ] Yes   [X] No

If "Yes," attach a list showing for each separate establishment:
a. Name and address.   b. Nature of business   c. Number of employees.

14. To whom do you sell most of your products or services?

[ ] Business establishments   [X] General public   [ ] Other (*Specify*)

PLEASE LEAVE BLANK →

Geo.	Ind.	Class	Size	Reas. for Appl.	Bus. Bir. Date

FORM SS-4 (3-69)
PART 2

DO NOT DETACH ANY PART OF THIS FORM. SEND ALL COPIES TO INTERNAL REVENUE SERVICE

PLEASE LEAVE BLANK

NAME AND COMPLETE ADDRESS

1. NAME (*TRUE name as distinguished from TRADE name.*)

John Melvin Doe, D.D.S.

2. TRADE NAME, IF ANY (*Enter name under which business is operated, if different from item 1.*)

3. ADDRESS OF PRINCIPAL PLACE OF BUSINESS (*No. and Street*)

300 Dental Drive

(*City, State, Zip Code*)

Anywhere, USA 39000

4. COUNTY OF BUSINESS LOCATION

Smith

5. ORGANIZATION Check Type

[X] Individual   [ ] Partnership   [ ] Corporation   [ ] Other (*specify e.g. estate, trust, etc.*)
[ ] Governmental   [ ] Nonprofit Organization
   (See Instr. 5)   (See Instr. 5)

6. Ending Month of Accounting year

December

7. REASON FOR APPLYING (*If "other" specify such as "Corporate structure change," "Acquired by gift or trust," etc.*)

[X] Started new business   [ ] Purchased going business   [ ] Other

8. Date you acquired or started business (*Mo., day, year*)

January 1, 1975

9. First date you paid or will pay wages (*Mo., day, year*)

January 15

10. NATURE OF BUSINESS (*See Instructions*)

Dental Practice

11. NUMBER OF EMPLOYEES → IF "NONE" ENTER "0"

Non-agricultural	Agricultural
2	

12. Have you ever applied for an identification number for this or any other business?   [X] No   [ ] Yes

If "Yes," enter name and trade name (if any). Also enter the approximate date, city, and state where you first applied and previous number if known. →

DATE _____   SIGNATURE _____   TITLE _____

Fig. 17-1 An application for employer identification number (SS-4). Note that it is a two-part form.

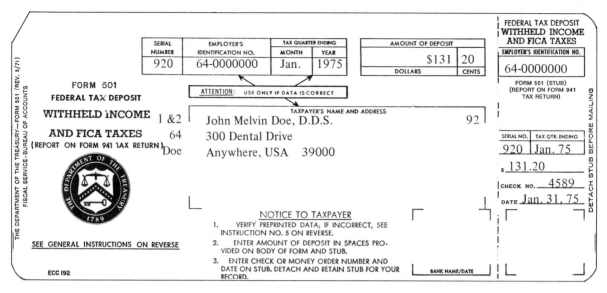

Fig. 17-2 Monthly federal tax deposit Form 501.

- If the total amount of taxes due at the end of the quarter is $200 or more, a monthly deposit must be made. This deposit must be made on or before the last day of the next month.

- If the total amount of taxes due at the end of the month is $200 or more, a monthly deposit must be made within 15 days after the end of the month.

- If the total amount of taxes due at the end of the month is more than $2,000, a deposit must be made within three days after the end of the month (sometimes referred to as quarter).

Monthly deposits are made with a Federal Reserve bank or with an authorized commercial bank. If in doubt, a telephone call is made to the bank with whom the dental office does business. The quarterly payments are made to the regional Internal Revenue Service office. The monthly form is Form 501; the quarterly form is Form 941. It is important to note that if any of the previously mentioned dates should fall on a Saturday, Sunday, or a legal holiday, the next regular workday is to be substituted. For example, if the date falls on a Saturday, the following Monday would be the deadline unless the particular Monday is a legal holiday.

If taxes are to be paid quarterly, they must be paid on or before April 30, July 31, October 31, and January 31. These dates should be circled on the calendar. A notation should be made either on the appointment book or daily log approximately 10 days before these dates as a reminder that the quarterly form should be prepared. If the taxes are to be paid monthly, the quarterly report, Form 941, must still be prepared. Making monthly deposits does not cancel the requirement for filing a quarterly report. The difference is that no money will be sent with the quarterly report. The Internal Revenue Service does not accept forgetfulness as a reasonable excuse for being late with the tax payment or report. Penalties are imposed for failure to pay taxes when due. This could be an additional charge of five percent. Criminal and civil penalties may be initiated for failure to file a report or for filing false information on the reports.

If a mistake is made in completing either the monthly or quarterly reports, space is provided on the forms for an adjustment. The next form completed must show the adjustment. If an adjustment is necessary, an attached duplicated statement must accompany the form showing the adjustment. If too few taxes are withheld from an employee's paycheck, the corrected withholdings may be deducted from later paychecks. However, the employer is responsible for any payment under the correct amount. This matter is to be settled between the employer and the employee. If too much money is withheld from an employee's paycheck, the employee should be reimbursed by the employer. A written receipt from the employee should be maintained stating the date and the amount of the repayment.

Most of the federal forms have an employer's copy, commonly labeled "your copy." These copies must be maintained in an up-to-date file. It is suggested that a file be made for each form. If the Internal Revenue Service should need to check office records, time would not be lost in searching for the individual forms. All federal tax records should be kept at least four years. After four years, the files may be discarded. However, most dental offices prefer to keep federal tax reports for a longer period of time.

FEDERAL TAX DEPOSITS (FORM 501)

Federal Tax Form 501 is provided for employers to make monthly tax deposits, figure 17-3. Since these deposit forms automatically come to the dental office preinscribed (after a deposit form has once been filed), very little writing is necessary to complete this form. The taxpayer's name and address are preprinted on the form. At the top of the form, the serial number, employer's identification number, and the date are also preprinted. The right portion of the form (stub) may be detached as a receipt for the dental office. Be sure to correctly complete the receipt before detaching it from the original form. The main portion of the form will

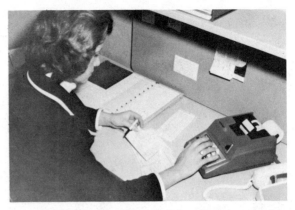

Fig. 17-3 A secretarial dental assistant preparing monthly deposit form (#501) to be deposited at a local bank.

not be returned to the dental office. The deposit stub will be the record receipt to keep in the file. The date and the number of the office check used in paying the deposit must be recorded on the stub. The amount of the deposit must also be written directly above the check number on the stub.

Figuring the amount of the deposit will be the most important part of completing the form. Turn to 'the preceding month's employee earning record located in the daily log. The withholding and FICA taxes are added together for this deposit. Reminder: Withholding taxes are only those taxes withheld from the employee. FICA (social security) taxes are those taxes withheld from the employee and matched by the employer. For each employee who has received wages during the month, write the amount of the withholding tax on a slip of paper. Multiply the FICA tax withheld from the employee by the figure 2. Add this amount to the withholding tax. This will be the amount to deposit for one employee. Figure all employee deposits in this same manner. Add all the employee deposits together to give the total amount of the deposit. Write a check for this amount, have the dentist check your records and sign the check. Finally, attach the check to Form 501 before making the bank deposit.

Form **941**
(Rev. April 1975)
Department of the Treasury
Internal Revenue Service

**Employer's Quarterly
Federal Tax Return**

Schedule A—Quarterly Report of Wages Taxable under the Federal Insurance Contributions
Act—FOR SOCIAL SECURITY

List for each nonagricultural employee the WAGES taxable under the FICA which were paid during
the quarter. If you pay an employee more than $14,100 in a calendar year report only the first $14,100
of such wages. In the case of "Tip Income" see instructions on page 4. IF WAGES WERE NOT TAX-
ABLE UNDER THE FICA MAKE NO ENTRIES IN ITEMS 1 THROUGH 9 AND 14 THROUGH 18.

SSA Use Only

F ☐ 2 ☐ U ☐ E ☐
S ☐ 1 ☐ L ☐ T ☐
X ☐ 0 ☐ V ☐ A ☐

1. Total pages of this return including this page and any pages of Form 941a ▶	2. Total number of employees listed ▶	3. (First quarter only) Number of employees (except household) employed in the pay period including March 12th ▶
1	*2*	*2*

4. EMPLOYEE'S SOCIAL SECURITY NUMBER	5. NAME OF EMPLOYEE (Please type or print)	6. TAXABLE FICA WAGES Paid to Employee in Quarter (Before deductions)	7. TAXABLE TIPS REPORTED (See page 4)
000 00 0000		Dollars · Cents	Dollars · Cents
427 71 7896	*Mary Jane Smith*	*1800 00*	
427 73 8754	*Sally Ann Jones*	*1000 00*	

If you need more space for listing employees, use Schedule A continuation sheets, Form 941a.
Totals for this page—Wage total in column 6 and tip total in column 7 ⟶ *$2800.00*

8. **TOTAL WAGES TAXABLE UNDER FICA PAID DURING QUARTER.** $ *$2800.00*   ◁
(Total of column 6 on this page and continuation sheets.) Enter here and in item 14 below.

9. **TOTAL TAXABLE TIPS REPORTED UNDER FICA DURING QUARTER.** $ *none*   ◁
(Total of column 7 on this page and continuation sheets.) Enter here and in item 15 below. (If no tips reported, write "None.")

Employer's name, address, employer identification number, and calendar quarter. (If not correct, please change)

Name (as distinguished from trade name)
John Melvin Doe, D.D.S.

Date quarter ended
March 30, 1975

Trade name, if any

Employer Identification No.
64-0000000

Address and ZIP code
300 Dental Drive, Anywhere, USA 39000

Entries must be made both above and below this line; if address different from previous return check here ☐

Name (as distinguished from trade name)

Date quarter ended

Trade name, if any

Employer Identification No.

Address and ZIP code

	T		FP
	FF		I
	FD		TOT

10. Total Wages And Tips Subject To Withholding Plus Other Compensation . . . . . ⟶	$2800	00
11. Amount Of Income Tax Withheld From Wages, Tips, Annuities, etc. (See instructions) . . .	331	80
12. Adjustment For Preceding Quarters Of Calendar Year		
13. Adjusted Total Of Income Tax Withheld . . . . ⟶	331	80
14. Taxable FICA Wages Paid (Item 8) . . $ *2800.00* multiplied by 11.7% =TAX	327	60
15. Taxable Tips Reported (Item 9) . . . $ multiplied by 5.85% =TAX	none	
16. Total FICA Taxes (Item 14 plus Item 15) . . . . ⟶	327	60
17. Adjustment (See instructions)	none	
18. Adjusted Total Of FICA Taxes . . . . ⟶	327	60
19. Total Taxes (Item 13 plus Item 18)	659	40
20. TOTAL DEPOSITS FOR QUARTER (INCLUDING FINAL DEPOSIT MADE FOR QUARTER) AND OVERPAYMENT FROM PREVIOUS QUARTER LISTED IN SCHEDULE B (See instructions on page 4)	659	40

Note: If undeposited taxes at the end of the quarter are $200 or more, the full amount must be deposited with an authorized commercial bank or a Federal Reserve bank. This deposit must be entered in Schedule B and included in item 20.

21. Undeposited Taxes Due (Item 19 Less Item 20—This Should Be Less Than $200). Pay To Internal Revenue Service And Enter Here . . . . ⟶

22. If Item 20 Is More Than Item 19, Enter Excess Here ▶ $ And Check If You Want It ☐ Applied To Next Return, Or ☐ Refunded.

23. If not liable for returns in succeeding quarters write "FINAL" here ▶   and enter date of final payment of taxable wages here ▶

Under penalties of perjury, I declare that I have examined this return, including accompanying schedules and statements, and to the best of my knowledge and belief it is true, correct and complete.

Date _____   Signature _____   Title (Owner, etc) _____

Form 941 (Rev. 4-75)

Fig. 17-4 A completed Employer's Quarterly Federal Tax Return. Form 941.

EMPLOYER'S QUARTERLY FEDERAL TAX RETURN (FORM 941)

The quarterly report must be filed by all employers whether or not monthly deposits are made, figure 17-4. If monthly deposits are not made, a check for the taxes due must be mailed with this form. **Reminder:** Form 941 is due on or before 30 days after the end of the quarter; it should be typed if possible. The deadline dates again are April 30, July 31, October 31, and January 31.

The following explanation is given for the quarterly report. The numbers used in the explanation correspond with the numbers on the form.

1. The total pages used in the completion of the form are to be listed. However, in most dental practices only one page is necessary. If a continuing page is needed, Form 941a is available from the Internal Revenue Service for this purpose.

2. The total number of employees listed in the report is recorded.

3. If the report is being prepared for the first quarter, January, February, and March of the specific year, the number of employees employed in the dental office including the March 12 pay period must be written.

4. For each employee to be listed on Item 5, the social security number of the employee is to be written. The social security number is always a 9 digit number with a hyphen after the first three digits and after the next 2 digits. It will appear as 000-00-0000.

5. The name of the employee that corresponds with the social security number in Item 4 is to be typed or printed. The name of the employee must appear exactly as it appears on their social security card.

6. The total amount of wages paid to the employee during the quarter is to be written. This is the amount before any deductions were made, usually referred to as gross pay. If an employee's salary is $600.00 per month, then the figure $1800.00 would appear on this line. Remember at all times during the completion of this report, that this is a quarterly or three-month-period report. Total the figures in the space provided.

7. This column is for reporting taxable tips. It should be blank for dental offices. Tips should not be accepted by the dental team from dental patients. Since column 7 is blank, no total will appear for column 7.

8. Simply, bring the total figures in Column 6 down to Item 8. This will be the total amount of taxable wages paid during the quarter by the dental office.

9. NONE should be written to show that no tips were reported.

The next portion of the form is usually preinscribed with the dentist's name, address, employer identification number, and the quarter date. Space is provided directly below to correct any error that might appear in the preprinted information. An address change may also be noted in this space.

10. This figure is a total of columns 6 and 7. In most dental practices this will be a total of column 6. This figure is the total amount of wages subject to federal taxes.

11. The amount of income tax withheld is recorded in this space. This will be the total amount of withholding taxes withheld from each employee. Refer to the employee's earning record in the daily log for this information. If the earning records have been completed properly, these figures will already be totaled for the quarter on each employee. Simply, add the individual employee totals together.

12. This line provides space for making an adjustment for a previous quarter.

13. The adjusted total of income tax is recorded. If no adjustment is necessary in Item 12, Item 13 will be the same as Item 11.

14. The amount of FICA (Social Security) taxes payable is to be written. This is the *total* amount withheld from the employee's paycheck and matched by the employer. Each 941 form will state the percentage that is to be withheld for the specific year. This percentage is to be multiplied by the figure that appears in Item 8.

15. Only the employee pays FICA taxes on tips. The percentage figure would be half the percentage figure in Item 14. The word, none, should again be written here to show that tips were not made to the dental employees.

16. Add Items 14 and 15 for a total amount of FICA taxes. Since 15 is normally blank, this amount will be the same as Item 14.

17. Adjustment space.

18. If no adjustment appears in Item 17, transfer the figure in Item 16 to this item.

19. The total taxes due from the dental office is to be written. This total will be Item 13 plus Item 18. Total taxes include withholding taxes and FICA taxes from both the employee and the employer.

20. This item is for reporting the amount of monthly deposits made on forms 501. The total amount deposited from the three months period should be written. If monthly deposits were not made, write the word, none. **Reminder:** taxes totaling more than $200.00 for the quarter, should be deposited monthly. Taxes totaling less than $200.00 may be paid with the 941 form.

21. The amount of undeposited taxes due is to be entered. A check for this amount must accompany this 941 report. The check should be made payable to the Internal Revenue Service.

22. If an overpayment has been made, check the proper box if the excess is to be refunded or applied as credit on the next return.

23. This item applies only to closing a dental practice. If the practice has terminated during the quarter for any reason, write the word, FINAL, and enter the date the last taxable wages were paid.

The date, signature and title of the person signing appears at the extreme bottom of the form. Double check each item for errors. Make sure the figures were added correctly from the employee's earning record. After rechecking, the form and a check, if necessary, is mailed to the area district Internal Revenue Service office.

If a question should arise about any of the forms mentioned in this unit, contact the nearest IRS service center. They have a publication, "Tax Guide for Small Businesses" (current each year) which gives a detailed explanation of how to start, operate, or dispose of a business. The publication explains how Federal income, excise, and employment taxes apply to sole proprietorships, partnerships, and corporations.

SUMMARY

Every dentist or dental office must have an employer identification number before filing federal tax returns. To obtain this number, Form SS-4 should be filed before the end of the first week of practice. Federal taxes may be paid periodically during the year. This eliminates the need for the dental office to pay a large sum at the end of the year. Federal taxes are due either monthly or quarterly, depending on the amount of taxes due. If more than $200 in taxes is due at the end of the quarter, a monthly deposit (Form 501) must be made. If less than $200 is due at the end of the quarter, the taxes may be paid with the quarterly report. Making monthly deposits does not cancel the need for the quarterly report. The quarterly report (Form 941) must be completed by all dental offices. The secretarial dental assistant must be very proficient in completing these forms. Failure to do so may result in penalties for the dental office.

SUGGESTED ACTIVITIES

- Prepare index cards stating deadlines, where to file, and how to complete the form, for all forms explained in this unit.

- Make arrangements to invite a representative from the Internal Revenue Service to speak to the class on federal forms that apply to the operation of a dental office.

REVIEW

A. Match the form with the description.

_____ 1. Form SS-4

_____ 2. Form 501

_____ 3. Form 941

_____ 4. Form W-2

    a. employer's quarterly federal tax return.

    b. is used to obtain an employer identification number.

    c. wage and tax statement.

    d. monthly tax deposit form.

B. From Column II select the form which matches the federal tax payment shown in Column I.

Column I

_____ 1. Less than $200 due at end of quarter.
_____ 2. More than $200 due at end of quarter.
_____ 3. More than $200 due at end of month.
_____ 4. More than $2000 due at end of month or quarter.

Column II

a. Form 501 within 15 days after the end of the month.

b. Form 501 within 3 days after end of the month or quarter.

c. Form 501 before the last day of the next month.

d. Form 941 due at the end of the quarter and before the last day of the next month.

C. List the four payment rules.

1.

2.

3.

4.

D. Select the best answer.

1. An application for an employer identification number, Form SS-4, should be filed before
   a. the end of the first month of practice.
   b. the end of the first week of practice.
   c. the end of the first quarter.
   d. the employer files his first federal income tax return.

2. The dental office makes either monthly or quarterly payments of taxes according to
   a. the number of employees.
   b. the salary of the owner of the office.
   c. the percentage rate of FICA taxes.
   d. the amount of taxes due from the dental office.

3. The employer's quarterly federal tax return is made
   a. only if monthly deposits are not made.
   b. only if taxes due amount to more than $200.
   c. if the employer desires not to pay a large lump sum at the end of the year.
   d. by any dental office that employs one or more persons.

4. Federal tax records must be kept for at least
   a. five years.   c. ten years.
   b. four years.   d. three years.

5. The monthly federal tax deposit (Form 501) is figured by adding the
   a. FICA taxes of the employees.
   b. withholding taxes of all employees.
   c. withholding and FICA taxes of the employees and the FICA taxes paid by the employer.
   d. withholding taxes of the employer and the employees.

6. The employer's quarterly tax return (Form 941) is due
   a. on or before 30 days after the end of the quarter.
   b. on or before 30 days after the end of the month.
   c. on or before the last working day of the month.
   d. on or before the last working day of the quarter.

7. If there is insufficient space for listing all employees on Form 941, the form which should be used is
   a. Form 940.   c. Form 941a.
   b. Form 601.   d. Form 9411.

8. The name of the employee is to be written on Form 941
   a. as it appears on the payroll check.
   b. as it appears on the employee's social security card.
   c. as it appears on the employee's birth certificate.
   d. as it may appear on the employee's marriage certificate.

9. Item 20 on the Employer's Quarterly Federal Tax Return (Form 941) is used to report

    a. any taxable tips reported by the employee.

    b. the amount of FICA taxes paid by the employee and matched by the employer.

    c. an overpayment made to the Internal Revenue Service.

    d. the amount of monthly deposits already made on Form 501.

E.   1. Complete the monthly tax deposit using the following information.

Employee	S.S. Number	Federal Wages (gross)	Withholding	FICA
Mary E. Jones	427-71-7714	$600.00	$108.30	$35.10
Dick M. Smith	427-73-8765	$700.00	$ 82.20	$40.95
Jane Williams	427-75-4567	$450.00	$ 32.20	$26.33

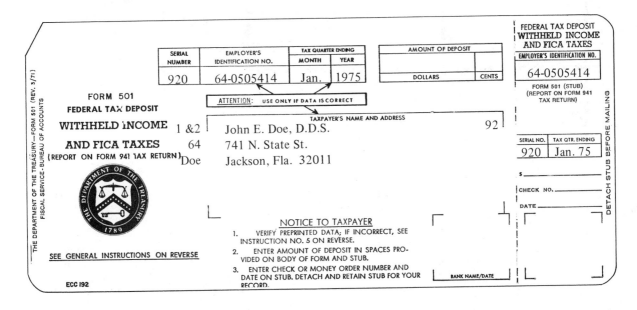

2. Complete the Employer's Quarterly Federal Tax Return (Form 941) using the information given in E-1. All three employees received the same wages for the three month period. Assume that two more monthly deposits were made.

| Form **941** (Rev. April 1975) Department of the Treasury Internal Revenue Service | **Employer's Quarterly Federal Tax Return** |

Schedule A—Quarterly Report of Wages Taxable under the Federal Insurance Contributions Act—FOR SOCIAL SECURITY

List for each nonagricultural employee the WAGES taxable under the FICA which were paid during the quarter. If you pay an employee more than $14,100 in a calendar year report only the first $14,100 of such wages. In the case of "Tip Income" see instructions on page 4. IF WAGES WERE NOT TAXABLE UNDER THE FICA MAKE NO ENTRIES IN ITEMS 1 THROUGH 9 AND 14 THROUGH 18.

SSA Use Only

F ☐ 2 ☐ U ☐ E ☐
S ☐ 1 ☐ L ☐ T ☐
X ☐ 0 ☐ V ☐ A ☐

| 1. Total pages of this return including this page and any pages of Form 941a ▶ | 2. Total number of employees listed ▶ | 3. (First quarter only) Number of employees (except household) employed in the pay period including March 12th ▶ |

4. EMPLOYEE'S SOCIAL SECURITY NUMBER	5. NAME OF EMPLOYEE (Please type or print)	6. TAXABLE FICA WAGES Paid to Employee in Quarter (Before deductions)	7. TAXABLE TIPS REPORTED (See page 4)
000 00 0000	▼	Dollars Cents	Dollars Cents

If you need more space for listing employees, use Schedule A continuation sheets, Form 941a.
Totals for this page—Wage total in column 6 and tip total in column 7 ⟶

8. TOTAL WAGES TAXABLE UNDER FICA PAID DURING QUARTER. $ ◁
(Total of column 6 on this page and continuation sheets.) Enter here and in item 14 below.

9. TOTAL TAXABLE TIPS REPORTED UNDER FICA DURING QUARTER. $ ◁
(Total of column 7 on this page and continuation sheets.) Enter here and in item 15 below. (If no tips reported, write "None.")

Employer's name, address, employer identification number, and calendar quarter. (If not correct, please change) ▶

Name (as distinguished from trade name)
Trade name, if any   **John E. Doe, D.D.S.**
Address and ZIP code   **741 N. State St.**
Jackson, Fla. 32011

Date quarter ended   **Jan. 1975**
Employer Identification No.   **64-0505414**

Entries must be made both above and below this line; if address different from previous return check here ☐

Name (as distinguished from trade name)   Date quarter ended
Trade name, if any   Employer Identification No.
Address and ZIP code

T	FP
FF	I
FD	TOT

10. Total Wages And Tips Subject To Withholding Plus Other Compensation . . . . . ⟶
11. Amount Of Income Tax Withheld From Wages, Tips, Annuities, etc. (See instructions) . . .
12. Adjustment For Preceding Quarters Of Calendar Year . . . .
13. Adjusted Total Of Income Tax Withheld . . . . ⟶
14. Taxable FICA Wages Paid (Item 8) . . $............... multiplied by 11.7%—TAX
15. Taxable Tips Reported (Item 9) . . . $............... multiplied by 5.85%—TAX
16. Total FICA Taxes (Item 14 plus Item 15) . . . . ⟶
17. Adjustment (See instructions) . . . .
18. Adjusted Total Of FICA Taxes . . . . ⟶
19. Total Taxes (Item 13 plus Item 18) . . . . ⟶
20. TOTAL DEPOSITS FOR QUARTER (INCLUDING FINAL DEPOSIT MADE FOR QUARTER) AND OVERPAYMENT FROM PREVIOUS QUARTER LISTED IN SCHEDULE B (See instructions on page 4) . . . .
Note: If undeposited taxes at the end of the quarter are $200 or more, the full amount must be deposited with an authorized commercial bank or a Federal Reserve bank. This deposit must be entered in Schedule B and included in item 20.
21. Undeposited Taxes Due (Item 19 Less Item 20—This Should Be Less Than $200). Pay To Internal Revenue Service And Enter Here . . . . ⟶
22. If Item 20 Is More Than Item 19, Enter Excess Here ▶ $ And Check If You Want It ☐ Applied To Next Return, Or ☐ Refunded.
23. If not liable for returns in succeeding quarters write "FINAL" here ▶   and enter date of final payment of taxable wages here ▶

Under penalties of perjury, I declare that I have examined this return, including accompanying schedules and statements, and to the best of my knowledge and belief it is true, correct and complete.

Date .... Signature .... Title (Owner, etc) ....

Form 941 (Rev. 4-75)

Unit 18 Annual Tax Preparation

OBJECTIVES

After studying this unit, the student should be able to

- Differentiate between Wage and Tax Statement (W-2) and Transmittal of Income and Tax Statements (W-3) forms.
- Correctly complete a W-2 and a W-3 form.
- State information relating to the Employer's Annual Federal Unemployment Tax Return.
- Explain how the secretarial dental assistant may help prepare for the state and federal income tax returns.

In January each year, there are several forms that must be submitted to the federal government for the preceding year. The secretarial dental assistant should be knowledgeable in preparing these annual forms for the dental office.

The W-2 form is a Wage and Tax Statement prepared for each employee that was on the payroll during the year. The W-3 form is a Transmittal of Income and Tax Statements. The W-2 and W-3 forms are completed on or before January 31 of each year for the pre-

ceding year. These two forms are required in all dental offices.

A third form which may be required is the Employer's Annual Federal Unemployment Tax Return (Form 940). The fourth form is the Annual Income Tax Return (Form 1040 Series) that must be filed each year on or before April 15. The dentist files a return for the dental office and a personal return.

Each state also has its own income tax requirements. The dental office must file state tax forms according to the particular

Wage and Tax Statement 1975				
64-0000000 John Melvin Doe, D.D.S. 300 Dental Drive Anywhere, USA 39000		Type or print EMPLOYER'S name, address, ZIP code and Federal identifying number.	Copy D For employer	
			Employer's State identifying number 64-0000000	
Employee's social security number 427-73-8765	1 Federal income tax withheld $832.80	2 Wages, tips, and other compensation $7200.00	3 FICA employee tax withheld $402.99	4 Total FICA wages $7200.00
Type or print Employee's name, address, and ZIP code below. Jane Ellen Doe 901 Nowhere Street Anywhere, USA 3900		5 Was employee covered by a qualified pension plan, etc.?	6	7
		8 State or local tax withheld $119.00	9 State or local wages $7200.00	10 State or locality USA
		11 State or local tax withheld	12 State or local wages	13 State or locality

Form **W-2**   Department of the Treasury—Internal Revenue Service

Fig. 18-1 Example of a Wage and Tax Statement.

state requirements. Since tax requirements of each state differs, they will not be discussed in depth in this unit. The secretarial dental assistant must contact the specific state office for further information.

WAGE AND TAX STATEMENT (FORM W-2)

The statement of wages paid and taxes withheld from the employee is often called the W-2 form. A W-2 form must be completed for each person employed for any part of the year. After the first of each year, the secretarial dental assistant may start completing W-2 forms for the employees. The W-2 statements must be completed so that the employee receives it no later than January 31. It covers the income received during the previous year. However, if an employee permanently leaves the practice before the end of the calendar year, the W-2 form should be given to him no later than 30 days after final payment. The statement may be mailed to his home address.

Form W-2 is simple to complete if adequate earning records have been kept on each employee. The W-2 form supplied by the Internal Revenue Service is a six-part form. Carbon paper may be inserted so that all six parts are completed at one time. A typewriter should be used to complete the forms so that all copies will be legible. If a typewriter is not available, print the answers and check all the copies to make sure they are legible. The first copy is Copy A which is for the Internal Revenue Service. The second copy is Copy 1 for the state tax department. Copy B is the third copy and is to be filed with the employees' federal tax return. Copy C is the fourth copy which is kept by the employee for his own records. The fifth copy is Copy 2 which is for the employee to file with the local income tax return if required. Some cities require an income tax return to be filed, in addition to the state and federal returns.

The last copy is Copy D which is for the employer to retain in his file.

The employee receives Copies B, C, 1 and 2. The employer sends Copy A to the proper federal office and Copy D is filed as a record in the dental office.

In the upper left-hand corner, the *employer's* federal identification number, name, and address is typed or printed. The employer's state identification number is placed in the block to the right of the employer's name. (This identification number remains the same).

The *employee's* social security number is recorded as well as the employee's name and address. Tax information requested is divided into federal income tax information and social security information. Referring to Form W-2 from left to right the following entries are made:

- This block asks the amount of income tax withheld from the employee for the entire year.

- The gross amount of wages paid, subject to withholding tax is recorded. Any other compensation not subject to withholding tax is also recorded. An example of this might be money paid to an employee for travel expenses.

- The amount of FICA tax withheld must be listed as well as the total amount of wages paid subject to FICA tax during the year.

- Space is also provided on the form to record the amount of state or city tax withheld.

- The gross state or local wages and the name of the state are entered in boxes 9 and 10 respectively.

If an employee has left the dental practice without leaving a forwarding address, an attempt should be made to locate him. A first step would be to contact his old address; a family member may be able to provide the

		Wage and Tax Statement		**1975**
X Corrected By Employer 64-0000000 John Melvin Doe, D.D.S. 300 Dental Drive Anywhere, USA 39000		Type or print EMPLOYER'S name, address, ZIP code and Federal identifying number.	**Copy D** For employer	
			Employer's State identifying number 64-0000000	

Employee's social security number	1 Federal income tax withheld	2 Wages, tips, and other compensation	3 FICA employee tax withheld	4 Total FICA wages
427-73-8766	$832.00	$7200.00	$402.99	$7200.00

Type or print Employee's name, address, and ZIP code below.	5 Was employee covered by a qualified pension plan, etc.?	6	7
Jane Ellen Doe 901 Nowhere Street Anywhere, USA 39000	8 State or local tax withheld $119.00	9 State or local wages $7200.00	10 State or locality USA
	11 State or local tax withheld	12 State or local wages	13 State or locality

Form **W-2**   Department of the Treasury—Internal Revenue Service

Fig. 18-2   A corrected copy of a Wage and Tax Statement.   Notice the X and the notation in the upper left-hand corner denoting the form was corrected by the employer.

new address.   If after reasonable attempts, the former employee cannot be located, his or her W-2 forms along with Form 941 should be mailed to the Internal Revenue Service.

Occasionally, a mistake will be made on a W-2 form.   The mistake may not be noticed until after the forms are delivered to the employees.   A corrected copy must then be made and given to the employee. The corrected W-2 form must be clearly identified as a corrected copy.   A large X and the words *corrected by employer* should appear on the corrected copy in the upper left-hand corner, figure 18-2.   If an employee loses a W-2 form, an additional form may be issued by the employer.   It must be marked

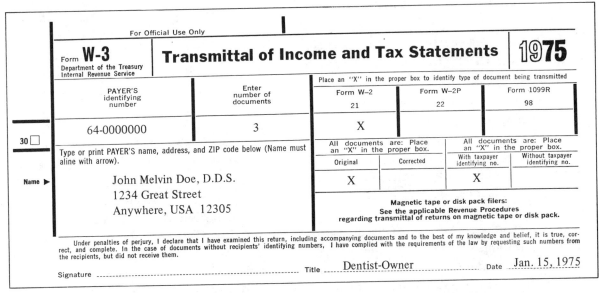

Fig. 18-3 A Transmittal of Income and Tax Statements. Form W-3.

as a substitute copy and should show the words, *reissued by employer.*

TRANSMITTAL OF WAGE AND TAX STATEMENTS (FORM W-3)

The W-3 form is a reconciliation of income tax withheld and the transmittal of tax statements, figure 18-3. The form is due on or before February 28 each year. The W-3 comes in duplicate. One copy is for the Internal Revenue Service and the second copy marked *your copy* is retained by the dental office.

This form must be filed by employers and other payers as a transmittal for the W-2, W-2P, or 1099R forms. On the right of the form, boxes are provided to indicate which type of documents are being transmitted. The W-2, Wage and Tax Statement, was discussed earlier in this unit. The W-2P is a Statement for Recipients of Annuities, Pensions, or Retired Pay. Form 1099R is a Statement for Recipients of Lump-Sum Distributions from Profit-Sharing and Retirement Plans. The IRS provides detailed instructions and explanations of the W-2P and the 1099R on the sheet attached to the W-3 form. Figure 18-3, page 165 shows only that portion of Form W-3 which is to be mailed to the IRS Service Center.

EMPLOYER'S ANNUAL FEDERAL UNEMPLOYMENT TAX RETURN (FORM 940)

Form 940 is another form that may be required for the dental office. This form is the unemployment tax return. Any employer or organization that employs one or more employees at least one day for 20 calendar weeks is required to file Form 940. Unemployment tax is a certain percentage of wages paid to employees. The percentage of federal unemployment tax may be changed by the federal government. In 1973, the amount was 3.28 percent of wages paid. However, the percentage rate may be different for an office whose employees have not filed for unem-

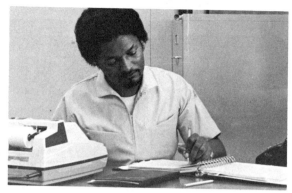

Fig. 18-4   Auditor working on annual federal tax returns.

ployment. Again, Circular E should be consulted for the proper amount. This tax is paid by the *employer;* it may not be deducted from the salary of the employee.

If the dental office filed an unemployment form for the previous year, a preaddressed form will be sent to the office. If forms are needed for the first time, they can be requested from the Internal Revenue Service. Form 940 will usually be prepared by the office accountant.

STATE AND FEDERAL INCOME TAX RETURNS

Most dental offices employ the services of a certified public accountant (CPA) or auditor to complete the final preparation of the state and federal income tax returns. It is more economical for the dentist to employ a certified public accountant than to risk costly errors. This accountant may be employed to visit the office on a monthly, quarterly, or yearly basis, depending upon the needs of the practice. Many offices require the secretarial dental assistant to complete all of the monthly and quarterly tax requirements. Then the accountant visits the office yearly; this visit is made after January 1 and before April 15 of each year. April 15 is the deadline for the federal and state income tax returns.

A telephone call should be made to the accountant to set up an appointment for the yearly visit to the dental office. The accountant may desire to work in the dental office for a few days. This may be more convenient than carrying all the records to his office. A working space should be made available near an adding machine or calculator. Having everything ready will simplify the task. If the accountant is employed on an hourly basis, both time and money will be saved.

The secretarial dental assistant should have all of the files ready for the accountant. All records for the previous year must be in order. The daily log should be ready and the daily pages added into monthly, quarterly, and yearly totals. Expense sheets should be summarized as well as the employee's earning records. All files pertaining to financial matters of the office should be properly labeled and placed on the working space near the accountant. Copies of all the federal forms which have previously been prepared and filed by the secretarial dental assistant should be in proper order, and the current forms to be prepared should be placed with the other materials.

The dental office must keep any records pertaining to federal income taxes readily available for the Internal Revenue Service to inspect if the need arises. Duplicate copies of all the forms submitted must be kept in the office tax file. The records should be kept for at least four years. However, most offices will probably keep the records longer unless filing space is a real problem.

SUMMARY

Usually the secretarial dental assistant is responsible for completing several federal forms at the close of each year. The W-2 and W-3 forms are prepared after December 31. They must be completed and mailed before February 28 of the current year. The W-2 form is a wage and tax statement prepared for each employee who was on the payroll during the year. This form verifies the amount of wages paid and deductions made on each employee who was employed during any portion of the year. The W-3 form is used for the transmittal of income and tax statements.

The dental office usually employs an accountant to prepare the Employer's Annual Federal Unemployment Tax Return, and the state and federal annual income tax returns. Someone with expertise in taxes is needed to complete these annual forms. The secretarial dental assistant can help the accountant by having all the necessary items ready. All financial records should be up-to-date before the accountant arrives; having all the files and records ready saves time and money for the dental office.

SUGGESTED ACTIVITIES

- Make arrangements with the instructor to invite a certified public accountant to visit the class and talk to the group on ways the secretarial dental assistant can help accountants complete their annual federal tax forms.

- Prepare a small chart on all federal and state forms required in dental office management. The chart should show the number of the form, the deadline date, and any other pertinent information.

REVIEW

A. Match the form number with the name of the form.

    ____ 1. W-2 Form   a. Employer's Annual Federal Unemploy-
    ____ .2. W-3 Form   ment Tax Return.
    ____ 3. 940 Form   b. Wage and Tax Statement.
                                  c. Transmittal of Income and Tax State-
                                    ments.

B. Match the following copies of the W-2 Form:

    ____ 1. Copy A   a. for the employee's federal return.
    ____ 2. Copy 1   b. for the employee to file with the state or
    ____ 3. Copy B   city return. .
    ____ 4. Copy C   c. for the state or city tax department.
    ____ 5. Copy 2   d. for the employer to retain in his file.
    ____ 6. Copy D   e. for the Internal Revenue Service.
                                    f. for the employee's records.

C. Select the best answer.

1. A Wage and Tax statement (W-2) is completed

    a. for the employer and by his partners.
    b. for any person employed during any portion of the year.
    c. only for the employed person who works at least 30 days.
    d. only for any employee who leaves the practice before January 1.

2. The W-2 form must be prepared and given to the currently employed person

    a. on or before January 31 each year.
    b. on or before December 31 each year.
    c. at the end of each quarter.
    d. 30 days after the end of each quarter.

3. The W-2 form is prepared and given to the employee who has permanently left the dental practice

    a. on or before January 31 each year.
    b. when the final paycheck is written.
    c. within 30 days after the final paycheck was received.
    d. 30 days after the end of the last quarter the employee worked.

4. The Transmittal of Income and Tax Statements (W-3) is due

    a. on or before February 28 each year.
    b. on or before April 30 each year.
    c. on or before April 15 each year.
    d. on or before January 1 each year.

5. Federal unemployment tax is paid

    a. by the employer.
    b. by the employee.
    c. by the employee and matched by the employer.
    d. by the employee and matched by the federal government.

6. Most dental offices employ the services of a certified public accountant to complete the state and federal annual income tax returns because

   a. it is a federal regulation that a certified public accountant complete these forms.
   b. these forms involve financial records of the office and call for expert tax knowledge.
   c. the state board of dental examiners urges the dentist to employ an accountant.
   d. the state tax commission requires all businesses to employ a certified public accountant.

7. The deadline for the federal and state income tax returns is

   a. January 31.   c. April 15.
   b. April 30.   d. January 15.

D. 1. After examining the employee's earning records for the year, correctly complete the three W-2 forms.

Payroll December

NAME: *Mary Jane Smith*   SOC. SEC. NO. *427-81-5738*   NUMBER OF EXEMPTIONS *1*

DATE	HOURS	RATE	GROSS PAY	FED. I.T.	F.I.C.A.	STATE I.T.				NET PAY
12-15			300 00	47 60	17 55					234 85
12-30			300 00	47 60	17 55					234 85
		TOTALS	600 00	95 20	35 10					469 70
QUARTER		BROUGHT FWD.	1200 00	190 40	70 20					939 40
		TO DATE	1800 00	285 60	105 30					1409 10
YEAR		BROUGHT FWD.	5400 00	856 80	315 90					4237 30
		TO DATE	7200 00	1142 40	421 20					5646 40

NAME: *Beverly Power*   SOC. SEC. NO. *537-83-8421*   NUMBER OF EXEMPTIONS *2*

DATE	HOURS	RATE	GROSS PAY	FED. I.T.	F.I.C.A.	STATE I.T.				NET PAY
12-15			250 00	29 50	14 63					205 87
12-30			250 00	29 50	14 63					205 87
		TOTALS	500 00	59 00	29 26					411 74
QUARTER		BROUGHT FWD.	1000 00	118 00	58 52					823 48
		TO DATE	1500 00	177 00	87 78					1235 22
YEAR		BROUGHT FWD.	4500 00	531 00	263 34					3705 66
		TO DATE	6000 00	708 00	351 12					4940 88

NAME: *William C. Croft*   SOC. SEC. NO. *427-73-5739*   NUMBER OF EXEMPTIONS *3*

DATE	HOURS	RATE	GROSS PAY	FED. I.T.	F.I.C.A.	STATE I.T.				NET PAY
12-15			300 00	29 70	17 55					252 75
12-30			300 00	29 70	17 55					252 75
		TOTALS	600 00	59 40	35 10					505 50
QUARTER		BROUGHT FWD.	1200 00	118 80	70 20					1011 00
		TO DATE	1800 00	178 20	105 30					1516 50
YEAR		BROUGHT FWD.	5400 00	534 60	315 90					4549 50
		TO DATE	7200 00	712 80	421 20					6066 00

Wage and Tax Statement 1975

64-0000000
John Melvin Doe, D.D.S.
300 Dental Drive
Anywhere, USA 39000

Type or print EMPLOYER'S name, address, ZIP code and Federal identifying number.

Copy D
For employer

Employer's State identifying number
64-0000000

Employee's social security number	1 Federal income tax withheld	2 Wages, tips, and other compensation	3 FICA employee tax withheld	4 Total FICA wages
Type or print Employee's name, address, and ZIP code below.		5 Was employee covered by a qualified pension plan, etc.?	6	7
		8 State or local tax withheld	9 State or local wages	10 State or locality
		11 State or local tax withheld	12 State or local wages	13 State or locality

Form W-2   Department of the Treasury—Internal Revenue Service

---

Wage and Tax Statement 1975

64-0000000
John Melvin Doe, D.D.S.
300 Dental Drive
Anywhere, USA 39000

Type or print EMPLOYER'S name, address, ZIP code and Federal identifying number.

Copy D
For employer

Employer's State identifying number
64-0000000

Employee's social security number	1 Federal income tax withheld	2 Wages, tips, and other compensation	3 FICA employee tax withheld	4 Total FICA wages
Type or print Employee's name, address, and ZIP code below.		5 Was employee covered by a qualified pension plan, etc.?	6	7
		8 State or local tax withheld	9 State or local wages	10 State or locality
		11 State or local tax withheld	12 State or local wages	13 State or locality

Form W-2   Department of the Treasury—Internal Revenue Service

---

Wage and Tax Statement 1975

64-0000000
John Melvin Doe, D.D.S.
300 Dental Drive
Anywhere, USA 39000

Type or print EMPLOYER'S name, address, ZIP code and Federal identifying number.

Copy D
For employer

Employer's State identifying number
64-0000000

Employee's social security number	1 Federal income tax withheld	2 Wages, tips, and other compensation	3 FICA employee tax withheld	4 Total FICA wages
Type or print Employee's name, address, and ZIP code below.		5 Was employee covered by a qualified pension plan, etc.?	6	7
		8 State or local tax withheld	9 State or local wages	10 State or locality
		11 State or local tax withheld	12 State or local wages	13 State or locality

Form W-2   Department of the Treasury—Internal Revenue Service

170

2. Complete the W-3 form below, using the earnings record and W-2 forms in the preceding question.

For Official Use Only			

Form W-3 — Department of the Treasury, Internal Revenue Service — **Transmittal of Income and Tax Statements** — **1975**

Place an "X" in the proper box to identify type of document being transmitted

Form W-2 21	Form W-2P 22	Form 1099R 98

PAYER'S identifying number | Enter number of documents

30 ☐

Type or print PAYER'S name, address, and ZIP code below (Name must aline with arrow).

Name ▶

All documents are: Place an "X" in the proper box.

Original	Corrected

All documents are: Place an "X" in the proper box.

With taxpayer identifying no.	Without taxpayer identifying no.

Magnetic tape or disk pack filers:
See the applicable Revenue Procedures
regarding transmittal of returns on magnetic tape or disk pack.

Under penalties of perjury, I declare that I have examined this return, including accompanying documents and to the best of my knowledge and belief, it is true, correct, and complete. In the case of documents without recipients' identifying numbers, I have complied with the requirements of the law by requesting such numbers from the recipients, but did not receive them.

Signature _____ Title _____ Date _____

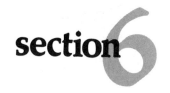

section 6

Written Communications

Unit 19 The Business Letter

OBJECTIVES

After studying this unit, the student should be able to

- Identify the parts of a letter and their proper location within the letter.
- Describe six styles of business letters.
- Explain the three types of punctuation used in business letters.
- Address a business envelope using the correct format.

A business letter is a joint effort between the secretarial dental assistant and her employer. The employer provides knowledge and skill in composing the body of the letter, and the secretarial dental assistant demonstrates knowledge and skill in preparing the letter for mailing. There are a few points to keep in mind when writing and typing a business letter:

- The letter should be attractive — first impressions are lasting ones; the letter is arranged on the page as a picture is in a frame.

- All errors are neatly corrected so they are not obvious.

- The letter is correct in English usage, punctuation, and spelling.

- Dates and facts should be double checked for accuracy.

- The body of the letter is clear, concise, and sincere. A letter that is confusing or makes no sense is of little value.

- Modern terminology should be used rather than out-of-date phrases. The most effective business letter is written in the same language style as the spoken word.

PARTS OF A LETTER

There are eight major parts of a letter which are standard in most business letters.

Letterhead

Most dental offices use a printed letterhead. The letterhead should be typed if plain stationery is used.

Date Line

The date should be typed on one line; no abbreviations are used.

Inside Address

The inside address should be single spaced. If the addressee is a person, the title is included. There are currently two trends of thought as to the use of abbreviations in the inside address: the traditional method of using no abbreviations, and the modern method of using the Post Office Department's two-letter state abbreviations. Either usage is considered to be correct.

Salutation

The salutation should agree with the inside address. If the letter is addressed to a person, the salutation should read, "Dear Mr. . ." or "Dear Ms." If the letter is addressed to a company, the salutation should read, "Gentlemen." If the letter is addressed to a title (Personnel Manager, ABC Company), the salutation should read, "Dear Sir."

Body of the Letter

The body of the letter should consist of at least two single spaced paragraphs with a double space between the paragraphs.

Complimentary Close

Only the first word of a complimentary close is capitalized. The most frequently used closings are: Yours truly, Very truly yours, Sincerely, and Sincerely yours.

Signature Line

This is the name and/or title of the person writing the letter. It is customary to leave four blank lines for the handwritten signature. However, if the handwritten signature is extremely small or excessively large, the number of spaces allowed may be adjusted accordingly.

Reference Initials

The usage of reference initials is determined by company policy. A common procedure is to type the initials of the dictator and the initials of the secretarial dental assistant separated by either a colon or a diagonal mark. If the secretarial dental assistant composes the letter herself, only her initials appear on the letter. All initials of the dictator are usually typed in capital letters; the secretarial dental assistant's initials may be typed in either capital or lowercase letters (DOM: JH or DOM/jkh).

Others

There are a few parts of a business letter that are used occasionally.

Special Reminder. (Personal or Confidential) This is placed three spaces above the inside address, beginning at the left margin; each letter is capitalized.

Mailing Notation. (Special Delivery) This is placed two spaces below the date and ends at the right margin; it, too, is typed in capital letters.

Attention Line. The attention line may be used if the letter is addressed to a company. It indicates the name of the person or department to whom the letter is directed. The attention line is usually preceded by the word *attention,* followed by a colon (Attention: Mr. D.A. Smith). It is typed two spaces below the inside address.

Subject Line. The subject line is frequently found in business letters today. It is typed two spaces below the inside address or, if an attention line is used, two spaces below the attention line; it is placed two spaces above the salutation of the letter. The subject line is usually preceded by the word *subject,* followed by a colon (Subject: Dental Conference). The subject line may be typed in capital letters if desired; this is optional. Also, it may or may not be preceded by the word *subject.* However, it stands to reason that if the letter contains the aforementioned attention line in capitals, the subject line should also be in capitals when used; this adds to the uniformity and attractiveness of the letter.

Company or Clinic Name. The name of the company or clinic is sometimes included in a business letter when the writer acts as its representative. When it is used, the company name is typed in capital letters two spaces below the complimentary close. The name and title of the person writing the letter will be used for the signature line.

Enclosure Notation. When an enclosure is sent with the letter, the word *Enclosure* or the abbreviation, Encl., is typed below the reference initials.

Carbon Copy Notation. This is typed on a business letter when a third person is to receive a copy of the letter — file copies are not indicated with carbon copy notations. The carbon copy notation is typed below the enclosure notation and may be indicated by *cc, CC,* or *CC: Mr. John Smith.* A notation may be made on a carbon copy when the writer does not wish the notation to appear on the original; this is referred to as a *blind carbon copy notation.* After the letter is completed, remove the original and type only on the carbon copies. The blind carbon copy notation is typed in the top left-hand corner as *bcc: Mr. John Smith.*

Postscript. A postscript sometimes appears in a business letter. It is always the last item to be typed. It may be introduced by the abbreviation *P.S.* or by the word *Postscript.* The message may also be typed without an introduction.

TYPING THE BUSINESS LETTER

Before a letter is to be typed, several factors must be determined:

- The kind of punctuation to be used.
- The style of business letter.
- The length of the letter and its margins.
- The format and placement of items.

Punctuation

When typing a business letter, there are three different styles of punctuation that may be used:

Mixed Punctuation. A colon appears after the salutation and a comma after the complimentary close. This is the most frequently used style of punctuation. (See figures 19-1 and 19-2).

Open Punctuation. No punctuation appears in the letter except routine punctuation within the body. (See figures 19-3 and 19-4).

Closed Punctuation. A colon, a comma, or a period appears at the end of each line in the letter except the body. This style is considered very formal and is seldom used today. See figures 19-5 and 19-6.

Letter Styles

There are several arrangements of business letters — some are considered formal, some streamlined, and others traditional. Probably the most frequently used and the most flexible to use is the Modified Block style. However, other styles will also be briefly described in this unit.

Modified Block Style. The date line may be centered, may begin at the horizontal center, or may end flush with the right margin. The complimentary close, the company name (if used), and the signature line are typed beginning at the horizontal center, figure 19-1. All other parts of the letter begin at the left margin.

Semi-block Style. This style is arranged similar to the Modified Block; however, paragraphs are indented either five or ten spaces, figure 19-2.

Full-Block Style. This is a fast, easy style to type. All parts of the letter begin at the left margin, figure 19-3.

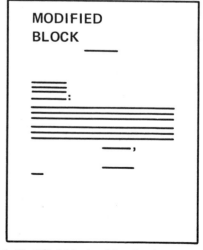

Fig. 19-1 Modified block with mixed punctuation.

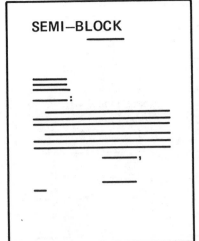

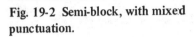

Fig. 19-2 Semi-block, with mixed punctuation.

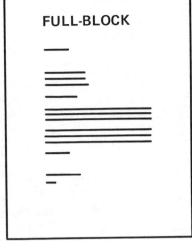

Fig. 19-3 Full-block, with open punctuation.

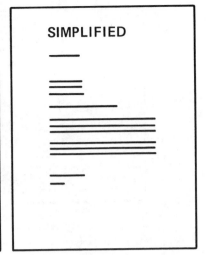

Fig. 19-4 Simplified, with open punctuation.

Simplified Style This is recommended by the American Management Association. It is concise and direct in both arrangement and content. All parts of the letter begin at the left margin. The salutation and the complimentary close are omitted, and a subject line is included, figure 19-4. All of the letters in the subject line and the signature line are capitalized.

Indented Style. This is considered extremely formal and is seldom used for business letters today, figure 19-5.

Hanging Indented Style. This is used as an eye-catcher, usually a sales letter, figure 19-6. The first line of each paragraph is blocked and the succeeding lines are indented.

It should be mentioned that a new letter style is becoming popular but it is rather direct and impersonal. However, the secretarial dental assistant should be aware of this style. In place of the salutation "Dear Mr. Smith," the letter begins with a sentence such as, "There seems to be a mistake, Mr. Smith . . .;" double space and then begin the body of the letter.

Format and Placement

Letters are classified as short, average, long, and two-page. When determining the

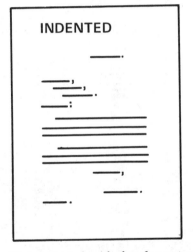

Fig. 19-5 Indented, with closed punctuation.

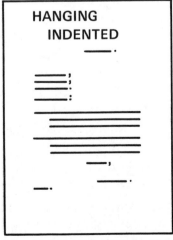

Fig. 19-6 Hanging indented, with closed punctuation.

			TRADITIONAL	FLOATING DATE
Letter Length	Number of words	*Line-Length	Spaces between date and inside address	Location of date line
Short	0-100	4 inch	7-11 spaces	Line 18-20
Average	100-200	5 inch	5-7 spaces	Line 14-16
Long	200-300	6 inch	3-5 spaces	Line 12
Two-Page	Over 300	6 inch	3-5 spaces	Line 12

*A vertical inch equals 6 line spaces.
A horizontal inch equals 10 spaces on Pica type size, 12 spaces on Elite type size.

Fig. 19-7 Determining Letter Length and Format.

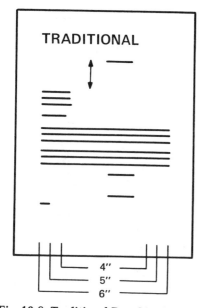

Fig. 19-8 Traditional Date Line Method.

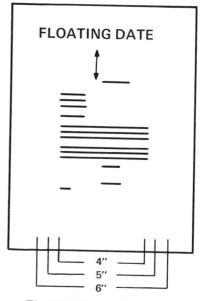

Fig. 19-9 Floating Date Line.

length and margins needed, other factors are also taken into consideration such as whether a subject line, attention line, or other optional parts of a business letter are to be included.

After the length of the letter and the margins have been determined (see figure 19-7), the format of the letter is decided. Two commonly used methods are the Traditional and the Floating Date Line method. The second page of a letter may be typed in a *block* or *spread* method.

Traditional. The date is located two spaces below the letterhead. A variation from 3 to 11 spaces is allowed between the date and the

inside address, depending on the length of the letter, figure 19-8.

Floating Date Line. The date line fluctuates between Line 12 and Line 20, depending on the length of the letter. There are always three blank lines between the date and the inside address, figure 19-9.

Second Page Heading. When a letter contains more than 300 words, a second page will be necessary. The first line of type begins one inch from the top margin (type on Line 7). Either of the following methods may be used for the heading of the second page.

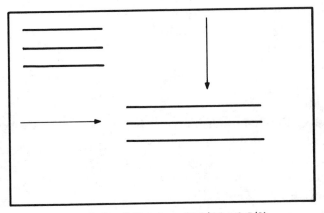

Fig. 19-10 Small Envelope (6 1/2 by 3 5/8).

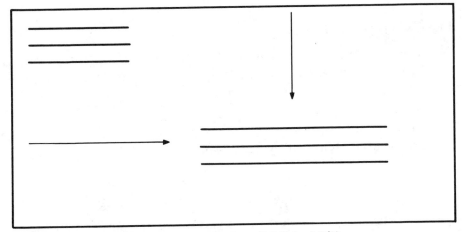

Fig. 19-11 Large Envelope (9 1/2 by 4 1/2).

• Blocked Method.   The name of the addressee, page 2, and the date are blocked at the left margin; double space before typing the body of the letter.

• Spread Method. The name of the addressee begins at the left margin and page 2 is centered on the same line. The date ends flush with the right margin on the same line; double space before typing the body of the letter.

ADDRESSING THE ENVELOPE

The Post Office Department has specific standards for handling envelopes. These standards must be met so that the envelope can be read by the optical scanning machines.

The return address should be typed on the second line of the envelope, three spaces from the left edge, block style, single spaced. The writer's name, street address, city, state, and ZIP Code number is included; his or her title does not usually precede the name.

Special reminders, such as the word, *Personal,* should be typed three spaces below the return address and three spaces from the left edge of the envelope. It may be underlined or typed in capital letters.

Special mailing notation, such as SPECIAL DELIVERY, should be typed in capital letters below the stamp but at least three lines above the envelope address

The envelope address should include the name, street address, city, state, and ZIP Code of the addressee. If the addressee is an individual, a title should precede the name. The city, state, and ZIP Code should always appear on one line. The envelope address should always be single spaced and nothing should be typed below the envelope address.

State abbreviations published by the Post Office Department should be typed in all capital letters, no periods, no spaces. The ZIP code number may be typed one, two, or three spaces after the state abbreviation. (One or two spaces is preferred by most business offices.)

Small Envelope Arrangement

The envelope address should be typed 2 inches (12 line spaces) from the top edge and 2 1/2 inches (25 spaces Pica, 30 spaces Elite) from the left edge, figure 19-10, page 177.

Large Envelope Arrangement

The envelope address should be typed 2 1/2 inches (15 line spaces) from the top edge and 4 inches (40 spaces Pica, 38 spaces Elite) from the left edge, figure 19-11, page 177.

SUGGESTED ACTIVITIES

- Collect five examples of business letters that have been received through the mail; evaluate each one as to appearance, correctness, placement, and style.

- With other members of the class, prepare a bulletin board display, using various letter styles which have been received through the mail from businesses.

- Survey three dental offices to determine if a standard procedure has been established in that office as to style of letter, kind of punctuation, and other factors regarding format.

REVIEW

A.   Label the 8 major parts of a business letter:

1. _____

2. _____

3. _____

4. _____

5. _____

6. _____

7. _____

8. _____

B.   Using the letters, *O* for open punctuation, *C* for closed punctuation, and *M* for mixed punctuation, identify the examples given in the first column.   Some examples may have more than one answer.

1. Dear Mrs. Jones   1. _____
2. Mr. James Brown,   2. _____
    143 South Street,
    Jackson, MS 39201
3. Sincerely yours,   3. _____
4. January 12, 1973   4. _____
5. DOM:jh   5. _____

C.   Complete the following statements.

1. The most frequently used letter style is the_____ .

2. The most frequently used punctuation style is _____ .

3. The most widely used and the most flexible business letter style is the _____ .

4. A _____ must appear on all business letters.

5. The _____ of the complimentary close should be capitalized.

6. Most business letters are _____ spaced with_____ _____ between paragraphs.

7. The Post Office Department's abbreviations for the various states consist of _____ letters.

8. The _____ style is a fast, streamlined style to type.

9. The Post Office Department requests that all envelope addresses be _____ spaced.

10. The enclosure notation is typed _____ the reference initials.

Unit 20 Incoming and Outgoing Mail

OBJECTIVES

After studying this unit, the student should be able to

- List categories for incoming mail and explain how each is handled.
- Describe the four classes of mail.
- State the advantages of a postage meter.
- Correctly prepare a telegram message.

Incoming and outgoing mail are forms of written communications and should be handled properly. The secretarial dental assistant is usually responsible for taking care of all the mail in the dental office. Unfortunately, mailing procedures in the dental office are often taken for granted; rarely does the dental office manual outline proper mailing procedures. This is a mistake as persons may judge office efficiency by the way incoming mail is handled and/or by the appearance of outgoing mail.

INCOMING MAIL

Incoming mail should be sorted and distributed as soon as possible. The mail may contain an urgent message either from patients regarding a treatment or appointment or from professional organizations regarding an announcement. In other words, certain letters may contain items that need immediate attention from the dentist or the secretarial dental assistant. This type of mail is called *priority mail.*

The dentist should inform the secretarial dental assistant as to his policy regarding the opening of mail. This information is given at the beginning of employment. Some dentists prefer to open much of the office mail personally. Other dentists prefer that the secretarial dental assistant open and sort all the mail. It is then distributed to the person

for whom it is intended. It may be difficult to differentiate between business office mail and private office mail as many offices do not use statement return envelopes. However, mail marked Personal should never be opened by anyone other than the person to whom it is addressed.

Incoming mail may be divided into several categories:

- Personal mail to the dentist.
- Mail containing payments (accounts receivable).
- General office correspondence.

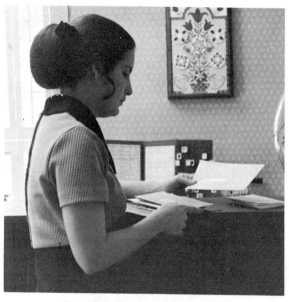

Fig. 20-1 Sorting Incoming Mail.

- Statements and invoices from firms with whom the office does business.
- Magazines, journals, and newspapers (periodicals).
- Advertisements.
- "Junk" mail.
- Dental laboratory cases.

Personal Mail

Personal mail directed to the dentist is any correspondence that requires the dentist's attention whether or not it is marked Personal. An opened letter which is of a personal nature but was unmarked may be attached to its envelope by a paper clip.

Personal mail is placed in a conspicuous place on the dentist's private desk. If not placed in a conspicuous place, the letter or letters may get lost and not receive the needed attention. The results could be unpleasant if the message was urgent.

Incoming mail may come from doctors to whom patients have been referred. If this should be the case, the patient's treatment chart should be taken from the files and clipped to the letter before placing it on the dentist's desk. Performing simple tasks like this will save time. The secretarial dental assistant who thinks ahead and performs her duties thoughtfully becomes a valuable asset to the dentist.

Payments

All mail containing payments should be stacked together and secured with a rubber band until the secretarial dental assistant is ready to start posting accounts. NEVER remove the check or money order from the envelope prior to posting. The name of the account for whom payment is being made does not always appear on the remittance. Many times a wife may have a separate checking account in her given name (Mary Smith), but her

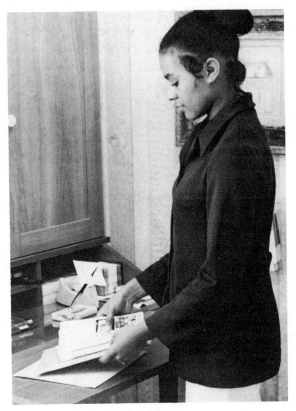

Fig. 20-2 **Personal mail should be placed on the dentist's private desk.**

record may be listed in her husband's name (Mrs. John Smith). Also, some married women keep their maiden name for professional purposes. Therefore, the envelope with the return address may be helpful in locating the correct record. For this reason the envelope should not be discarded until the account has been posted. Also, the envelope portion of the statement returned with the check may have needed information. Payments received by mail from patients should be posted daily. This will keep bookkeeping records up-to-date. Receiving payments by incoming mail is certainly a vital part of the dental practice. Absolute accuracy is essential in handling this portion of incoming mail.

General Office Correspondence

Much of the incoming general office correspondence can be handled by the secretarial dental assistant without referring to the dentist. For example, the writer may ask for a change in appointment. The secretarial dental assistant should be able to compose letters that answer simple incoming requests such as appointment changes and payment of accounts. Near the end of the year, patients often request yearly itemized statements. This type of incoming request should be answered promptly in order for the patient to use the statement for income tax preparation.

Statements and Invoices

Statements and invoices are important pieces of incoming mail. These are statements and invoices from firms with whom the dental office does business. The statements should be opened and checked against the invoice file for verification. The statements should then be placed in the proper file for monthly payment. Invoices should be placed in the file under the heading of the company.

Periodicals

The bulk of the mail may be periodicals in the form of magazines, journals, and newspapers. The magazines and newspapers received for the reception area should be placed in the proper rack or cover. Magazines or newspapers which are out-of-date should be removed. The magazines may be disposed of by donating them to a charity organization.

More than likely, the dentist receives several professional journals. Most dentists belong to the American Dental Association and receive the Journal of the American Dental Association monthly. All professional journals should be placed on the dentist's desk. He may wish to take them home.

Advertisements

Advertisements should be looked over carefully. The dentist, in most cases, will want to examine the advertisements pertinent to dental supplies and dental equipment. There

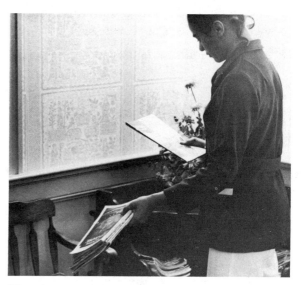

Fig. 20-3   Incoming mail may include current magazines for placement in the reception area.

may be "specials" he may be interested in purchasing. The secretarial dental assistant may be instructed to throw away other advertisement mail after examining it.

So called *"junk mail"* may be received in the dental office. This is mail that has no value to the dental practice and may be discarded by the secretarial dental assistant after careful examination.

Laboratory Cases

Laboratory cases that have been completed may be sent to the dental office by first class mail or parcel post. When sent by parcel post they should be marked SPECIAL HANDLING. The laboratory case will be sent in a carefully packaged laboratory box. The secretarial dental assistant should carefully open the package, remove the contents and place them in the dental laboratory. A note informing the dentist of the arrival of the case is immediately written and placed on his desk.

OUTGOING MAIL

Attractive and professional looking outgoing mail is an essential to a dental office.

REGISTERED:	First class mail that is valuable enough to be insured. A return receipt may be obtained. Rates depend on the value of the contents.
CERTIFIED:	First class mail that is less valuable than Registered and may not be insured. A return receipt may be obtained.
INSURED:	Third and Fourth class mail that is insured. Fee is according to the value of the contents.
SPECIAL DELIVERY:	First, Second, Third, or Fourth class mail that is delivered as it reaches the post office. This service is available only in towns and cities.
SPECIAL HANDLING:	Third and Fourth class mail that is delivered with other mail but receives quicker handling than other Third and Fourth class mail.

Fig. 20-4 Special Classifications of Mail.

The person or firm to whom the dentist is writing may never have occasion to see the dental office. Therefore, they may judge the dental practice by the quality of the outgoing mail. A letter mailed with errors, untidy corrections, or in an envelope with smudged fingerprints gives a poor image of the dental office. Appearance of both the letter and the envelope is important. Most outgoing mail from the dental office is in the form of statements to patients or general office correspondence. These topics will be covered more fully in later units. At this time, suggestions for improving procedures involved with the outgoing mail are given as guidelines.

Classification of Mail

There are several classifications of outgoing mail, the most common being first class mail. *First class mail* consists of sealed letters and postcards. Outgoing statements and business letters from the dental office are classified as first class mail. *Second class mail* consists of newspapers and periodical publications. *Third class mail* is bulk mail weighing less than 16 ounces such as circulars, books, catalogs. etc. *Fourth class mail* is commonly referred to as parcel post. Parcel post includes packages or printed materials that weigh more than 16 ounces. Parcel post rates will vary according to the distance mailed.

Formerly, air mail service was a classifi-

cation of a faster service at a higher postage rate per ounce. Effective October 10, 1975, the U.S. Postal Service eliminated air mail service as a classification. It was eliminated because *most* mail was already traveling by air.

If a letter or item requires special attention, it must be sent registered, certified, insured, special delivery, or special handling. See figure 20-4 for further explanation of these classifications. If special attention is not required, stamped envelopes may be purchased from the local post offices. These are envelopes with first class postage printed on them. They are sold by the post office for a small fee.

There are several ways to make mail move a little more rapidly. Mail at times *other than* 5:00 p.m. as there is usually an overload of mail to be processed at this time. Mailing large quantities of mail such as statements or monthly recall letters at this time may slow down service. If mail is not picked up at the office, visit the local post office and ask what is the best time to deliver outgoing mail to the post office.

Separating local and out-of-town items before mailing may greatly speed up service. The zip code must be added to all outgoing mail. Failure to use the zip code slows down service. A national zip code directory may be purchased from the post office; a local directory is also available.

THE ZIP CODE STORY

The zip code's purpose is to increase accuracy and speed in the delivery of mail. Each zip code consists of five digits. These digits identify the post office in the United States. The zip code also assists the larger post offices with routing the mail for delivery to its various units. The first three digits identify the major city or sectional center. The last two digits identify the various post offices or units within the city.

A national zip code directory may be purchased from the post office. This directory provides a list of all zip codes for all post office addresses.

The zip code should be placed immediately to the right of the city and state on an envelope or package. A comma is not to be placed between the state and the zip code. If space permits the zip code from being placed to the right of the city and state, it may be placed immediately beneath the city and state. No other digits should precede or follow the zip code if placed on a line by itself.

Mailing packages containing laboratory cases requires special attention. The zip code is very important on packages because the first three numbers of the zip code are used for figuring postal charges. It is not necessary to place address labels on all sides of the package. One correctly addressed label that includes a return address is sufficient. Packages must be securely wrapped to insure proper handling. If postage is not paid by the laboratory, a scale for weighing packages should be available in the office.

Mail that is larger than the average business envelope may require special attention. If large envelopes (such as a 5" x 7" or an 8" x 10") are to be frequently used for mailings, envelopes with a green diamond border should be used to quickly identify the mail as first class. Large envelopes with this green border and a FIRST CLASS imprint are available from the post office. Otherwise large envelopes may be handled as third class mail, which is less expensive but much slower than first class mail. It is not likely that the dental office will have much need for mailing items either second or third class.

Remember: Postage must be placed on envelopes. Currently, postage regulations prohibit delivery of unstamped mail.

Postage Meter

A postage meter increases the speed, convenience, and efficiency of outgoing mail. It

(Courtesy of Postal Service)

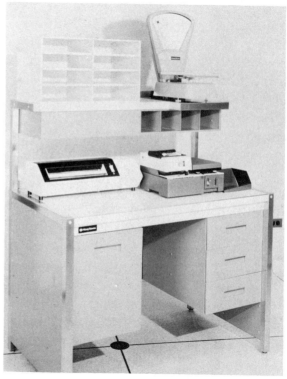

Fig. 20-5 A complete postage center.

actually prints the postage on the envelope. If a package is to be mailed, the postage meter prints the amount of postage on a piece of adhesive paper which can then be placed on the package. A postage meter faces, postmarks and cancels the mail. This eliminates the need for the post office to do these procedures, thus speeding the mail service. Machines may be purchased which, once the letter is inserted, seal the envelope and print

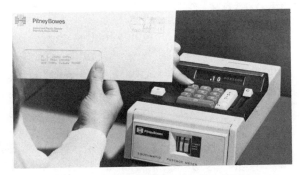

Fig. 20-6 A Touchmatic postage meter.
(Courtesy Pitney-Bowes)

the postage; it is not a pleasant task for the secretarial dental assistant to moisten stamps or envelopes, especially on heavy mailing days.

Many times stamps are misused in the dental office by the dental team members. A postage meter eliminates the misuse or borrowing of stamps and stamp money. Also, the secretarial dental assistant will not have to keep a check on loose stamps.

Postage meter equipment usually consists of two parts: a mailing machine and a removable postage meter. The postage meter must be licensed for use by the US Postal Service. Since these meters are printing United States postage, they cannot be sold. The meters must be rented from an authorized manufacturer who is responsible to the post office for proper operation and replacement.

The dental office purchases the office mailing machine and leases the postage meter; both units come together. The postage meter is simply detached and carried to the local post office where post office personnel will set the meter. The dental office pays for the postage in advance and the meter is set according to the amount paid.

There are several styles of postage meter equipment that may be purchased for use in the dental office. The Touchmatic postage meter is one example, figure 20-6. It is designed for use in small or medium size offices. The Touchmatic is an all-electric desk model that features a pushbutton keyboard. The keys are pressed according to the postage needed and the postage is automatically printed on the letter or tape. The postage is registered so that the secretarial dental assistant knows exactly how much postage has been used and how much postage is left in the machine.

It is not difficult to learn to operate a postage meter. The secretarial dental assistant may be taught to use the machine in just a few minutes. Gummed postage tape is available for packages or bulky material. A postage meter can save much time and money. The outgoing mail also looks more attractive and professional.

TELEGRAM TO BE SENT TO:

Dr. Kirby Davis
600 Medical Arts Building
Anytown, USA 39206
Telephone Number 362-1891

TELEGRAM MESSAGE

ACCEPT INVITATION SPEAKING TO CENTRAL DISTRICT
DENTAL SOCIETY, JANUARY 17.

ARRIVE JANUARY 16, 6:00 p.m., DELTA FLIGHT 641

Fig. 20-7 A brief telegram message.

TELEGRAMS

The secretarial dental assistant should know how to send a telegram as, occasionally, the dentist may want to send a telegram from the dental office. The number of a telegraph office can be found in the yellow pages of the local telephone directory. Western Union has offices listed in most cities of the United States.

The dentist will probably specify the type of telegram he desires to make. Most short telegrams are sent direct and are delivered by telephone. A lengthy telegram is usually sent overnight and received the following morning. All telegrams should be written as briefly as possible since the cost is determined by the number of words. The secretarial dental assistant should write out the message and have the correct name, address, and telephone number of the receiver ready before dialing the telegraph office.

SUMMARY

Incoming and outgoing mail in the dental office should be efficiently handled. Incoming mail should be sorted and distributed as soon as possible after it arrives. There may be items that need immediate attention from the dentist or the secretarial dental assistant. Outgoing mail should be correct, attractive and legible. Many times the dental office is judged by the appearance or the quality of the outgoing mail. Having a postage meter in the dental office may help to make the outgoing mail more professional looking as well as speed up the delivery of mail. Written communications should not be carelessly prepared and mailed. The secretarial dental assistant must be efficient in handling both incoming and outgoing mail. She should also know how to send a telegram. Telegrams are written as briefly as possible to save money.

SUGGESTED ACTIVITIES

- Visit the local post office. Obtain brochures on postage rates, how to address mail, and how to pack and wrap parcels for mailing.

- Invite a representative from a dental laboratory to speak to the class on the proper method of preparing laboratory cases for mailing.

- Prepare a poster on postage rates for all classifications of mail using current rates.

REVIEW

A. Select the best answer for the first five questions. The remaining questions require more than one answer.

1. Letters not marked Personal but requiring the personal attention of the dentist should be opened by the secretarial dental assistant and

   a. carefully placed back in the envelope.

   b. resealed so the dentist will not know the letter has been read.

   c. clipped to the envelope and placed in a conspicuous place on the dentist's private desk.

   d. the letter answered to the best of the assistant's ability.

2. Mail that has no value to the dental office is sometimes referred to as

    a. advertisement mail.

    b. junk mail.

    c. third class mail

    d. fourth class mail.

3. Zip codes are very important on letters and packages. They are essential for mailing packages parcel post because

    a. the last two digits are used to figure the correct postage rate.

    b. the third and fourth digits are used to route the mail.

    c. the first three digits are used to figure the correct postal charges.

    d. zip codes make the address look more professional.

4. A green diamond border as well as the class imprint readily identifies the large envelope as

    a. first class.

    b. second class.

    c. third class.

    d. fourth class.

5. All telegrams should be written as briefly as possible because

    a. the receiver has limited time to read telegrams.

    b. telegrams are written only for short letters.

    c. a lengthy telegram may not reach its destination any sooner than a letter.

    d. the cost is determined by the number of words.

6. Persons or firms may be influenced by the

    a. way the incoming mail is handled.

    b. appearance of the envelope.

    c. way corrections are made on the correspondence.

    d. way corrections are made on the envelope.

7. Mail marked Personal for the dentist should

    a. be opened by the secretarial dental assistant since the dentist is too busy to be bothered.

    b. never be opened by anyone other than the person to whom it is addressed.

    c. placed on the dentist's private desk in a conspicuous place.

    d. be given to the chairside dental assistant since she knows how to answer technical questions.

8. Envelopes containing payment checks or money orders should not be discarded until posting is completed because

   a. the return address may be helpful in locating the correct record.

   b. the envelope portion of the returned statement may have needed information.

   c. some of the envelopes may have uncancelled stamps that may be used again.

   d. the envelopes may be restamped and used again.

9. Letters or items that require special attention may be sent by

   a. registered mail.

   b. certified mail.

   c. insured mail.

   d. special delivery.

   e. special handling.

10. A postage meter in the dental office

    a. eliminates the use of a stamp box and stamp money.

    b. makes outgoing mail go at a cheaper rate.

    c. speeds up service through the post office.

    d. prevents the misuse of stamps.

    e. registers postage so that the office knows exactly how much postage has been used or is left in the machine.

    f. is loaned free of charge to the office by the post office.

B. Match the following according to the classifications of mail

Column I	Column II
1. First class	a. Circulars, books, catalogs or printed matter weighing less than 16 ounces.
2. Second class	
3. Third class	
4. Fourth class	b. Eliminated by the postal service October 10, 1975.
5. Air mail	
	c. Sealed letters or postcards.
	d. Packages or printed material weighing more than 16 ounces, called parcel post.
	e. Newspapers and periodical publications.

C.   Write the following message to be sent as a telegram.

Dr. Jack Fowler desires to send a telegram to Miss Regina Harper, 4542 Kirkley Drive, Baltimore, Maryland, telephone number 366-1405. Miss Harper is an out-of-town patient who has an appointment with Dr. Fowler tomorrow, July 2, at 3:00 p.m. Dr. Fowler regrets that he has been called away from his office due to a family emergency in another city. He will be unable to see her for her scheduled appointment; he has reserved time for her on July 10, at 3:30 p.m. Dr. Fowler is sorry about the delay but the postponement is unavoidable.

Telegram to be sent to:

Message:

Unit 21 General Office Correspondence

OBJECTIVES

After studying this unit, the student should be able to

- List examples of interoffice communication.

- Describe three methods of referring patients.

- Explain the use of dental certificates, school excuse cards, patient introduction-referral slips, and extraction notes.

Every dental office has a system of communications. Many small courtesies are omitted that could be very helpful because offices do not realize the importance of communications. These courtesies not only add to building a dental practice but are means of telling the patients about office policies. They also advise the patients of their responsibilities and what they may expect from the office.

There are many forms of written communications that are very important in the dental office. Each of these forms of communication helps produce a smooth-running dental office. Several forms of communication and examples of each will be discussed in this unit:

- Interoffice communication.

- Letters to new patients.

- Letters referring patients to other offices.

- Dental certificates.

- School excuse cards.

- Miscellaneous cards and letters.

Since an earlier unit dealt with the format, only contents will be discussed in this unit.

INTEROFFICE COMMUNICATION

Interoffice communications are a very important part of the office routine. There are times when decisions have to be made and policies changed between staff meetings. If changes are made and the staff is not informed, confusion and unhappiness will result. This could be eliminated by a simple memo to all the staff telling them of the change. The memo could be headed, ATTENTION – ALL STAFF.

ATTENTION: Staff   March 15, 1976

Monday, April 8, at 9:00 a.m., we will attend a dental seminar on advanced dental practice management at the University Medical Center. Everyone will be expected to arrive at 8:30 a.m. in Room 105 for registration. Your registration fee will be paid for by this office. Lunch is included in the fee.

Fig. 21-1 An example of an interoffice communication. Be sure to leave enough space for the members of the staff to initial.

Be sure that everyone has a chance to see the memo. Each member of the staff should initial the memo to indicate it was read, figure 21-1. If the entire staff is working that particular day, the notice can be removed at the end of the day, if all have indicated they have read the memo.

If the staff members alternate working days, a good form of interoffice communications would be for the secretarial dental assistant to make up a work chart for the staff. This way the staff could tell at a glance what days they are scheduled to work.

The bulletin board is an excellent place for these interoffice memos. It should be located in an area that is convenient and heavily used by the dental team, such as the auxiliary lounge or laboratory. The office runs smoother and the dental team is happier when everyone knows what is going on. Interoffice communications are not meant to take the place of staff meetings. However, they are a good means of keeping everyone aware of current events in the office.

LETTERS TO NEW PATIENTS

Space is not available in the appointment book for all information about new patients. A new-patient notebook can be used to record this information. There are several reasons for recording information about the patient before he arrives. For example, if the patient is new in the area, the dental office may send a letter welcoming the family to the neighborhood. If they need advice as to physicians, orthodontists, or other specialists, they should feel free to call the dental office and inquire.

A dentist who has a specialty practice, such as orthodontics or pedodontics, could have his secretarial assistant send a letter to the children welcoming them to the practice, figure 21-2. Parents are appreciative of any token of interest displayed. Enclose some

---

Dr. John Melvin Doe
300 Dental Drive
Anywhere, USA 29000

January 1, 1976

Dear Johnny,

We are looking forward to having you as a patient in our office. You have an appointment with us April 1, 1976 at 10:00 a.m.

Please have your parents read the enclosed pamphlets with you. They will answer some of the questions you may have about what we are going to do for you.

Ask your mother to call us if she has any questions before your first visit. Sincerely,

John Melvin Doe, D.D.S.

JMD/mcd
Enclosure

Fig. 21-2 An example of a letter written to a new child patient.

literature pertinent to the child's dental problem. A letter directed to the child gives him a feeling of importance. The letter does not have to be lengthy, but it does help the new patient feel welcome. The new-patient notebook should include the following:

- Name of the patient
- Age (if a child)
- Parents' initials (if a child)
- Address
- Telephone number
- Date
- Person who referred the patient
- Date of appointment
- Time of appointment
- Disposition of the patient (status of treatment)

An ordinary notebook could be used for this purpose as long as it is large enough to record the necessary information. It should be used each time a new patient calls to make an appointment. With this information in one notebook, the secretarial dental assistant can quickly write letters to the parents or the referring party. Also, valuable time will not be lost looking for the time of the appointment in a crowded appointment book. *Disposition of the patient* is a means of keeping the dentist up-to-date on what is happening. The dentist can tell at a glance whether treatment has been started elsewhere, what phase of treatment the patient is in, whether the patient was just shopping, or if the patient is a transfer patient. This can be initialed coding that the secretarial dental assistant has prearranged with the dentist. The status of the patient's dental treatment must be kept current as this is important information for the dentist.

Dr. John Melvin Doe
300 Dental Drive
Anywhere, USA 39000
Telephone 872–8017

Introducing ______________________ Age ____

Specific Area of Concern

__ Diastema	__ Space Deficiency
__ Overbite	__ Serial Extraction
__ Crossbite	__ Thumb Sucking
__ Open Bite	__ Tongue Thrusting
__ Crowding	__ Impaction
__ General Treatment	__ Congenitally missing teeth
__ Space Maintainer	__ Prosthetics

Remarks:

Stage of Dental Treatment

__ Examination
__ Prophylaxis
__ Treatment in Progress
__ Restorations Complete

Have FMX-Rays been taken recently?

__ Yes __ No

If Yes, give date ______________________

__ Please call patient for appointment. Phone no.__________

__ Please call me regarding patient.

Dr.__________________

Fig. 21-3 Introduction-referral slip.

REFERRING PATIENTS TO OTHER OFFICES

Diagnostic letters which refer patients to a specialist are an important part of communications. The dentist may write a letter to give a summary of the patient's dental condition and tell why the patient is being referred to the specialist. The specialist may outline his treatment plan so that both may work together for the patient, thereby providing a very necessary link between the dentist and the specialist.

Patient introduction-referral slips may be designed in all sizes, shapes, and colors. They are given to the patient to take with him when he goes to the dentist. In smaller cities, the doctor's name, address, phone number, and a space for the necessary treatment may be sufficient information, figure 21-3. Some slips include the specialty of the referring doctor. In larger cities, maps may be added to mark the various routes a person may take to locate the office.

Extraction notes are another form of written communication. They also may be designed in various sizes, shapes, and colors.

Proper identification and sufficient information is contained on the form so that the doctor has only to check certain items. The checkmarks indicate the work to be done by the dentist. One type of extraction note is done in triplicate, printed on paper that does not require carbon. A copy may be given to

---

RECORD OF ORTHODONTIC APPOINTMENT

To Principal or Teacher of School:

For your information and record,

_____
(Name of Pupil)

was in my office for professional services from _____
(hour)

to _____ on _____
(hour)   (date)

D.D.S.-P.A.
_____
Orthodontist

Fig. 21-4 A typical school excuse card.

**Dr. John Melvin Doe
300 Dental Drive
Anywhere, USA 39000**

March 1, 1975

Miss Rhonda Croft
Teacher, Johns Elementary School
4857 Sunset Road
Anywhere, USA 39000

Dear Miss Croft:

Michael John Smith has just had orthodontic appliances placed on his teeth. It is essential that he be allowed to brush his teeth after eating lunch each day.

We would appreciate your cooperation in this matter.

Sincerely,

John Melvin Doe, D.D.S.

Fig. 21-5 A letter written to the teacher of a child with an orthodontic appliance.

the parents or the patient, one copy may be mailed to the dentist, and one copy may go into the patient's folder for reference. This method is probably the most efficient type of extraction note.

DENTAL CERTIFICATES

Dental certificates may be obtained from the local health department. It is very important to have an ample supply in the general dentistry office or the pedodontic office, particularly in the late spring or summer. Some states require a dental certificate to enroll children in kindergarten or first grade. This dental certificate may be filled out and given to the parent when the child's work is completed.

SCHOOL EXCUSE CARDS AND LETTERS

Excuse cards for the child to give to school officials are available for children who must have appointments during school hours.

The patient's name, time of the appointment, and the dentist's name can be filled in prior to the time of the appointment. The time of departure would be filled in at the end of the dental treatment. A typed or printed card looks more professional than a hurriedly written note. It takes only a few minutes to fill out an excuse card but it is appreciated by the parent and the child. It also makes it easier for the school official to complete his records.

It may be necessary for the dentist or secretarial dental assistant to write a card or letter to the teachers of children with orthodontic appliances, figure 21-5, page 193. The orthodontist may feel it is necessary to explain to the teacher that the patient be allowed to brush after meals as the teacher may be hesitant to excuse the student for this purpose.

MISCELLANEOUS CARDS AND LETTERS

Sending sympathy cards to patients when a member of their family dies is a thoughtful

Dr. John Melvin Doe
300 Dental Drive
Anywhere, USA 39000

June 15, 1974

Mr. James P. Smith
987 Nowhere Street
Anywhere, USA 39000

Dear Mr. Smith:

We have received the final payment for Mary's orthodontic treatment. Thank you for being so prompt with your payments. It has been a privilege having Mary as a patient.

As you know orthodontic treatment extends many months beyond removal of the appliances and initial placement of the retainers. This retention phase of treatment has been prepaid as part of the total fee and therefore no charges will be made for these office visits. We do, however, want to stress the importance of the retention phase of treatment. We would appreciate the same diligence in making these appointments as was shown during active treatment.

Sincerely,

John Melvin Doe, D.D.S.
JMD/mcd

Fig. 21-6 A thank-you letter written on completion of extensive dental treatment for a child.

way of showing patients the office does care about them. This will require daily reading of the obituary columns and a knowledge of the names of the clientele of the dental practice. The card may be signed "Dr. Doe and staff" or may give the dentist's name only. Patients feel appreciative of this gesture by the dentist — this thoughtfulness in sending a personal card does not go unnoticed.

It is important to send a letter to the parents on completion of extensive dental treatment for their child; this letter is especially important for the orthodontist or pedodontist. The letter should thank the parents for having given the office the privilege of having the child as a patient. It may also stress the importance of continued dental appointments and regular prophylaxis, figure 21-6.

Another way of showing appreciation to the patient is to send a thank-you letter when the account has been paid in full. This type of letter always brings pleasant comments from the recipient. Also, thanking the patient who has referred other patients to the office is a thoughtful act.

Deficiency cards are sometimes used to notify parents of problems, especially those which arise during orthodontic treatment. Children and young people are familiar with the meaning of deficiency marks in school so they relate well to deficiency marks from their dentist, hygienist, pedodontist, or orthodontist. Deficiency cards may have all the necessary remarks printed on them, figure 21-7. The dentist or hygienist checks the appropriate blocks. The card is dated and addressed for mailing. The parents should sign and return the card to indicate they are aware of the infraction. The reason why the deficiency card is being sent should be stated clearly so that both the patient and the parents understand. The card is perforated so that one portion can

---

Date _____

Name _____

☐ HG
☐ Chart
☐ Elastics
☐ Appliance
☐ Hygiene
☐ Diet
☐ Late Appt.
☐ Broken Appt.
☐ Retainer
☐ Attitude
☐ Other
☐ $ _____

☐ Returned
Date _____

Name _____ Date _____

Dear Parent: _____

A first-time infraction of an important aspect of your child's cooperation is noted below. Your help in correcting this problem is essential. Would you please sign and return this card immediately to the office. Please call if you have any questions.

☐ Poor headgear wear   ☐ Not filiing in time chart

☐ Inadequate use of elastics   ☐ Abuse of Appliances

☐ Failure to keep appliance clean and   ☐ Late for appointment
   tissues healthy
                                         ☐ Broken or lost retainer
☐ Not following diet restrictions
                                         ☐ $_____ extra charge
☐ Broken appointment or failure to notify
   office 24 hours in advance of cancellation   ☐ Attitude not conducive
                                                   toward good results

☐ Other _____

☐ Remarks _____

Parent's signature _____

Fig. 21-7 An orthodontic deficiency card.

be detached and kept in the patient's file. A notation is made on this portion in order to keep the records current.

The need may arise in the dental office for many other letters to be composed. Recall letters were explained in unit 8. Collection letters are explained in unit 23.

SUMMARY

Many times, dental offices do not realize the importance of word communication with the patient. All forms of communication help to produce a smooth-running dental office.

Many courtesies may be extended to the patient by written communications. Interoffice communications can keep the dental team aware of current events in the office. Letters to new patients are informative and appreciated by the patient. Letters of referral provide a method of coordinating dental treatment. Dental certificates and school excuse cards are important to the school-age patient. There are many miscellaneous cards and letters that can be sent to patients which show that the dental office is interested in them.

SUGGESTED ACTIVITIES

- Write a letter to

    a. a new patient welcoming the family to the neighborhood.

    b. a referring dentist.

    c. a patient thanking him for the way he paid his account.

    d. a teacher explaining the necessity of allowing the child patient the time to brush after lunch.

- Using 4 x 6 index cards, sketch a sample of a

    a. dental certificate.

    b. school excuse card.

    c. deficiency card.

    d. patient introduction-referral slip.

    e. extraction note.

REVIEW

A. Select the best answer for the first six questions. The remaining questions require more than one answer.

   1. One way to improve and keep a pleasant relationship with patients is to

       a. send a letter of appreciation upon completion of dental treatment.

       b. send a letter of deficiency.

       c. advise them of regular staff meetings.

       d. alert them to current interoffice events.

2. A new-patient notebook accelerates writing letters to new patients because

   a. the notebook outlines form letters to be written.

   b. it is a method of welcoming new patients to the office.

   c. information like name and address is readily available in the notebook.

   d. it may be given to the new patient to study the office policies.

3. Diagnostic letters written to referring dentists

   a. provide a necessary link between two dentists so that treatment plans may be coordinated.

   b. enable the referring dentist to know the disposition of the patient by initialed coding.

   c. enables the patient to select a referring dentist of his choice.

   d. may make the patient feel a special closeness to the doctor.

4. Ideally, extraction notes should be done in triplicate because

   a. the patient, the referring doctor, and the referring patient receive copies.

   b. the patient, referring dentist, and the patient's file receive copies.

   c. the referring dentist, the secretarial dental assistant, and the dentist receive the copies.

   d. the patient, the hygienist, and the orthodontist receive the copies.

5. A card written for school officials showing the patient's name, time of the appointment, dentist's name, and time of departure from the office is a

   a. deficiency card.

   b. dental certificate.

   c. referral card.

   d. school excuse card.

6. A letter written to parents on completion of extensive dental treatment for a child may thank the parents and

   a. enable the parent to refer others to the office.

   b. stress the importance of continued dental appointments and regular prophylaxis.

   c. also serve as a deficiency reminder to the child.

   d. save postage by enclosing a copy of the bill.

7. A bulletin board in the dental office may

    a. serve to alert the dental team to any change made in the office routine.

    b. take the place of regular staff meetings.

    c. serve as a method of keeping everyone aware of current events in the office.

    d. provide a visible means of letting patients know the office is interested in their activities.

8. Letters written to new children patients

    a. give the child a feeling of importance.

    b. provide the child with advice as to physicians in the area.

    c. provide a way to send the child some literature that may be helpful on the day of the appointment.

    d. show the parents the office is interested in the child.

9. Dental certificates are needed more often in the

    a. winter.

    b. spring.

    c. summer.

    d. fall.

10. Three methods of referring patients to other offices are

    a. introduction-referral slips.

    b. dental certificates.

    c. diagnostic letters.

    d. extraction notes.

11. Written communication with patients

    a. helps build up the dental practice.

    b. informs patients about the office policies.

    c. informs the patient about his responsibilities to the office.

    d. is wasteful because it takes up time which could be used more effectively.

Unit 22 Monthly Statement Preparation

OBJECTIVES

After studying this unit, the student should be able to

- Define a treatment plan.
- List the payment methods used in many dental offices.
- Differentiate between a contract plan and a bank plan.
- Describe seven ways to prepare monthly statements.

Collecting fees is a very important and necessary part of the dental practice that is usually delegated to the secretarial dental assistant. Most dentists do not care to be involved with this task and prefer to have an efficient secretarial dental assistant handle fee collection. The dentist usually relies very heavily on the person assigned to the business desk to take complete charge of this task.

Collecting fees is not difficult if the method of collecting is planned. The collection plan must be thoroughly explained to the patient before dental treatment begins. If the patient understands the plan, collection is easier. It is usually a lack of understanding on the patient's part that creates problems in collecting fees. When a new patient enters the dental practice, the secretarial dental assistant should explain office policy regarding fees. This can be done either when the patient calls the office for an appointment or on the patient's first visit to the office. Some offices send the new patient a written statement.

If extensive dental work is to be done, a treatment plan should be presented to the patient. A treatment plan explains exactly what dental work is recommended by the dentist and its approximate cost. Many times, two treatment plans are presented — an optimum plan as the ideal method of treatment and an alternate plan in the event the patient

is unable to accept the optimum plan. Usually the dentist presents the treatment plan to the patient, however, he may ask the secretarial dental assistant to present the plan. The secretarial dental assistant must be very knowledgeable about dentistry if she is to discuss treatment with the patient. She should be able to answer questions concerning the recommended dental treatment; however, she must not hesitate to contact the dentist if she is not sure of her answer.

METHODS OF PAYMENT

Methods of payment vary with each dental office. The method that works well for one office may not suit the needs of another. The dentist will be the one to decide what method will be workable for the practice.

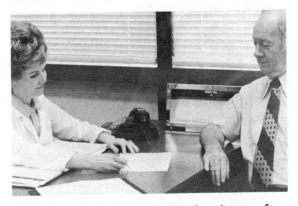

Fig. 22-1 The secretarial dental assistant often explains the treatment plan.

Dr. John Melvin Doe
300 Dental Drive
Anywhere, USA   39206

December 16, 1975

Mrs. Jack Williams
255 Fairfield Drive
Anywhere, USA   39206

Dear Mrs. Williams:

Thank you for the confidence you have shown in me by allowing me to be your family dentist. It is a pleasure to have patients like you and your family. May I also thank you for the way you have handled your account with my office over the past six years.

It has become necessary for my office to eliminate the monthly statement method of payment. In an effort to maintain our office efficiency and to avoid an increase in fees, we are going to initiate a "cash" policy for dental treatment. As much time is used each month by our staff to prepare monthly statements, we feel that we may increase our office efficiency if we change methods of payment.

We trust that you will understand our reasons for this change. If you should have any questions concerning our new policy, please call our office.

Thank you, again, for your cooperative manner in handling all of the financial transactions with our office.

Sincerely,

John Melvin Doe, D.D.S.

JMD/mcc

Fig. 22-2 A sample letter explaining the necessity of going to an all-cash policy.

There are usually several methods used by each dental office due to the varying financial needs of the patients. It is rare to find an office that uses only one method of payment. The following payment methods are commonly used in dental offices:

- Patient pays cash as the treatment is rendered.

- Patient is sent a monthly statement.

- Patient pays an agreed amount each month.

- Patient participates in a contract plan or a bank plan.

Some dental offices operate on an all-cash basis. They expect to be paid in full for the treatment as soon as the patient is dismissed. If this is the policy, a small placard can be placed in the reception area or in the business area to remind the patients. Occasionally, a dentist may decide to change to an all-cash policy after years of practice. A letter should be written to all the active patients informing them of this new policy, figure 22-2. The letter may be a combination thank-you and information letter. Thanking the patient for the way he or she has always handled the account may prepare the patient for the information to follow. The all-cash policy is better received if the explanation is presented in a way that shows this is an effort to maintain efficiency so that fees will not have to be raised. Most people are receptive to ideas when they feel the dentist is being considerate of his patients.

It is a fact that an all-cash policy is less expensive to the dental office. Much time and money is saved by eliminating monthly statement preparation, postage, and record keeping of accounts receivable. The patient pays as he is dismissed, a receipt is made, and the entry is recorded on the patient's chart. After recording on the daily page, the patient's chart is filed in the active file. Record keeping is complete for the patient in a few minutes.

Within the last few years, it has become popular for dental offices to accept credit cards such as Master Charge or BankAmericard. This type of payment is permissible. The local bank may need to be consulted for information regarding credit card payments.

MONTHLY STATEMENTS

Many dental offices bill the patient monthly for services rendered. The monthly statement may be sent at the end of the month. It is also permissible to send the statement immediately after the patient has visited the office. Another method may be to *cycle* the statements. Cycling involves dividing the alphabet into the working days of the month. Statements for patients whose names begin with certain letters are billed on certain days. The advantage of this method is that it evenly divides the statement preparation over a month's time. This method eliminates those hectic days at the end of the month which are spent preparing all the statements in a limited time period. If the statements are sent at the end of the month, a definite time should be designated as the monthly closing time. It is suggested that the statements be prepared for mailing on the 25th of each month. This places the statement in the home several days before the first of the month. As many people pay bills on a first come basis, it is probable that prompt payment will be made.

Statement preparation may be a chore for the dental office unless effective planning is made. The dentist should take a good look at the present method of collecting fees. If time is being taken from appointment control for the purpose of preparing statements, it is time to change methods. The dental office may use one of the following methods in preparing monthly statements. After observing the various methods and comparing costs, the most effective method can be selected.

- Send a photocopy of the patient's financial record.

- Prepare a statement on a printed statement form.

- Use a special printed self-mailer.

- Mail a pegboard "write it once" copy.

- Employ a duplicating firm to come to the office on a certain day and prepare the statements.

- Employ a special billing company to render this service.

- In a large modern group practice, use a computer.

Photocopies of Record

A photocopy of the patient's financial record, commonly referred to as the ledger card, may be copied in the office, figure 22-3. This requires the purchase of duplicating equipment for the office. If more than 150 statements are sent monthly, the time saved in statement preparation may be worth the cost of the equipment. The yellow pages of the local telephone directory may be consulted for the names of companies offering this equipment. Duplicating equipment will be discussed in a later unit.

Printed Statements

Writing statements on a printed statement form may be advisable for the office

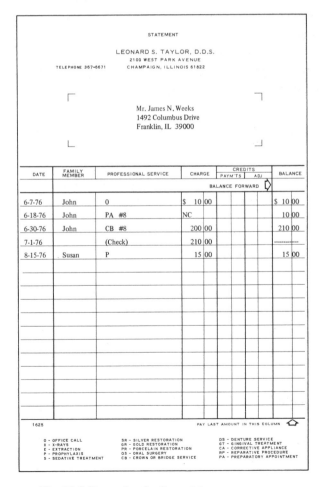

Fig. 22-3 Example of a financial statement.

STATEMENT

LEONARD S. TAYLOR, D.D.S.
2100 WEST PARK AVENUE
CHAMPAIGN, ILLINOIS 61820

TELEPHONE 367-6671

Mr. David W. Weeks
3876 Nowhere Street
Anywhere, USA 39000

DATE	PROFESSIONAL SERVICE	CHARGE	PAID	BALANCE
2-3-74	Cleaning, Radiographs	$16.		$16.
2-9-74	One two-surface silver	14.		30.
	restoration			

PAY LAST AMOUNT IN THIS COLUMN

O — OFFICE CALL
X — X-RAYS
E — EXTRACTION
P — PROPHYLAXIS
S — SEDATIVE TREATMENT

SR — SILVER RESTORATION
GR — GOLD RESTORATION
PR — PORCELAIN RESTORATION
OS — ORAL SURGERY
CB — CROWN OR BRIDGE SERVICE

DS — DENTURE SERVICE
GT — GINGIVAL TREATMENT
CA — CORRECTIVE APPLIANCE
RP — REPARATIVE PROCEDURE
PA — PREPARATORY APPOINTMENT

THIS IS AN EXACT COPY OF YOUR ACCOUNT PREPARED ON 3M ''JIFFMASTER'' COPY PAPER

Fig. 22-4 Sample of an itemized statement.

where a limited number of statements are sent monthly. The statement should show the date or dates of the visits and the amount of the fee for each visit. If the patient was given a charge slip or was told the amount of the fee, it will not be necessary to itemize the statement. Otherwise, it may be necessary to itemize all services rendered, figure 22-4.

Dental abbreviations should not be used unless they are explained at the bottom of the statement. Neither should unexplained technical terms be used. The average patient may not understand the unexplained abbreviation or technical term. If the service rendered was a #2 MOD Amalgam, it could be written as a three surface amalgam restoration. Stating the number of the surfaces may eliminate questions as to the variation of fees for restorations. When writing the amount, leave off the zeros if all the fees are in even amounts. When a patient sees the figure $20, it does not seem as much as $20.00. This may facilitate payment. The statements should be typed if at all possible. The need for addressing envelopes will be eliminated if a window envelope is used for mailing. The statement is folded so that the patient's name and address will appear in the window. When plain envelopes are used, it will save time to type the name and address of the patients on self-adhesive labels. The labels can then be quickly placed on the envelopes. Packages of these labels are available at stationery stores.

Self-Mailer

A self-mailer envelope may be referred to as a three-in-one statement, figure 22-5. It is a mailing envelope, a statement, and a return envelope. The statement portion of the self-mailer may be removed at the perforation by the patient and kept for his record. The remaining portion is an addressed return envelope with a gummed flap for the patient to mail the payment to the dental office. Using the self-mailer saves time and money for both the dental office and the patient. Time is not wasted in stuffing envelopes; nor is money spent for additional printing of envelopes.

Pegboard System

If the *pegboard "write-it-once" system* is used in the office, monthly statement preparation may be made even easier. Special ledger cards which provide ease in photocopying can be purchased for the pegboard. A set may be purchased that includes the patient's ledger card and a series of three monthly statements. This new approach to billing has proven satisfactory to dental offices which have been using the write-it-once system. The statement, ledger card, receipt, and daily journal are prepared at one writing. The statement portion is then detached and mailed to the patient. By using this method, an itemized statement is prepared without extra effort on the part of the secretarial dental assistant.

Duplicating Firms

Some duplicating firms contract with dental offices to prepare statements. These companies bring duplicating equipment to the dental office in a van-type vehicle. Patient ledger cards are carried to the vehicle and the information is duplicated into a statement. For the office that sends more than 200 statements monthly, this can be a valuable aid. This method of statement preparation may also be advisable for the office with limited personnel. It is very difficult for an office staff of one or two employees to find time for statement preparation in a busy practice. The expense of a duplicating firm may be justified when the dentist considers the lack of efficiency in his office during statement preparation.

Billing Services

Electronic equipment may be used in large city practices for statement preparation.

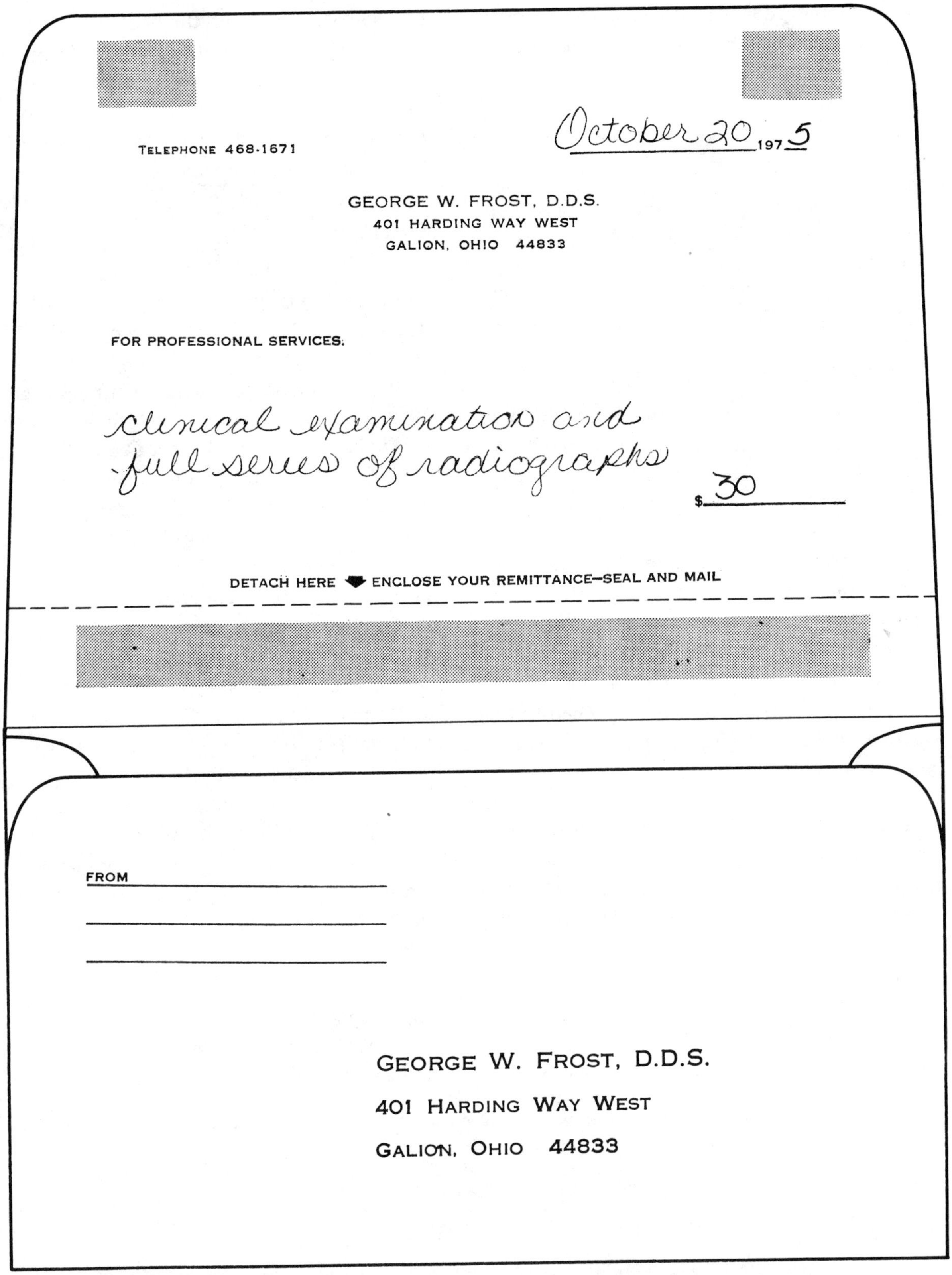

TELEPHONE 468-1671

October 20, 197*5*

GEORGE W. FROST, D.D.S.
401 HARDING WAY WEST
GALION, OHIO 44833

FOR PROFESSIONAL SERVICES:

*clinical examination and
full series of radiographs*

$ *30*

DETACH HERE ⬇ ENCLOSE YOUR REMITTANCE—SEAL AND MAIL

FROM _____

_____

_____

GEORGE W. FROST, D.D.S.

401 HARDING WAY WEST

GALION, OHIO 44833

Fig. 22-5 A self-mailer statement. The patient's name and address are on the reverse side of the top portion.

The secretarial dental assistant sends statement information to a billing service which electronically prepares the statements. The statements are also mailed by the billing service. Most companies will provide a free demonstration.

Computer Usage

In a large, modern group practice, computer billing may be possible. Computers are fast becoming popular in all types of professional offices. However, the cost is usually too high for the average dental office.

CONTRACT AND BANK PLANS

If extensive dental work is to be done, the dental office may suggest a contract plan or a bank plan. These plans can make extensive dental care available to persons who could not otherwise afford it.

The contract plan is an agreement between the patient and the dental office. An agreed amount is paid each month to the dental office. The dental office may add a small monthly finance charge to the unpaid balance. Details of the plan should be explained to the patient at the time the treatment plan is presented.

A bank plan is offered in some cities. A bank loan application for the patient is completed by the secretarial dental assistant. The information is telephoned to the credit department of the bank. After several days of checking the patient's credit, the bank will report to the dental office their decision concerning the loan to the patient. If the decision is favorable, the bank mails a coupon payment book to the patient and a check to the dental office for the amount of the loan.

SUMMARY

Collecting fees is an important part of any dental practice. This task is not difficult if the method of collecting is planned. The collection plan must be thoroughly explained to the patient before dental treatment begins. Most dentists prefer the secretarial dental assistant to have complete charge of collecting fees.

Payment methods vary from one dental office to another due to the varying financial needs of patients. Payment methods commonly used in dental offices are: patient pays cash as the treatment is rendered; patient is sent a monthly statement; patient pays an agreed amount each month; patient participates in a contract plan or a bank plan. Collection will be made easier if the patient understands the payment plan.

Many dental offices bill the patient monthly for services rendered. Statement preparation may be a chore for the dental office unless effective planning is made. There are various methods for preparing statements available to the dental office.

SUGGESTED ACTIVITIES

- Consult the yellow pages of the local telephone directory for a professional billing company. Make arrangements to have a representative of the company demonstrate statement preparation to the class.

- Write a sample letter informing an active patient that the dental office plans to change to an all-cash method of payment.

- Ask a secretarial dental assistant to explain the collection method used in her office. Report your findings to the class for discussion.

- Role play a secretarial dental assistant. Present a treatment plan to a class member who is role playing a patient.

REVIEW

A. Define the following:

1. Treatment plan.

2. Optimum treatment plan.

3. Alternate treatment plan.

4. Cycle billing.

5. A self-mailer.

B. Answer the following questions.

1. What are the four payment methods used in many dental offices?

2. Name seven methods of preparing monthly statements.

C. Select the best answer.

1. Cycle billing
    a. eliminates preparing monthly statements.
    b. hires a duplicating firm to come to the office only once during the month.
    c. evenly divides statement preparation over a month's time.
    d. utilizes computer billing.

2. A photocopy statement is a copy of the

   a. patient's treatment plan.

   b. patient's financial record.

   c. fees in the dental office.

   d. payment method agreement between the patient and the dental office.

3. If dental office abbreviations and technical terms are not explained, they should not be written on an itemized statement because

   a. it is more time consuming to copy from the record.

   b. it is in violation of the Principles of Ethics of the ADA.

   c. it is not very professional looking.

   d. the average patient may not understand the terminology.

4. Leaving off the zeros if fees are in even amounts seems to

   a. give the patient a false sense of security.

   b. confuse the patient as to the correct amount.

   c. appear less to the patient, therefore, may facilitate payment.

   d. slow down payment to the office.

5. An all-cash policy is preferred by many dentists because

   a. the cost of monthly statement preparation and postage is eliminated.

   b. record keeping is more detailed.

   c. the secretarial dental assistant will have less work to do.

   d. the patient receives a large discount for paying after treatment.

6. A contract method of payment is

   a. an agreement between the dentist and the billing company.

   b. an agreement between the dental office and a duplicating firm.

   c. an agreement that the patient will pay in full at the end of each month.

   d. an agreement between the patient and the dental office for the patient to pay a certain amount each month.

7. A contract plan or a bank plan may

   a. increase the fees of the offices in a regional area.

   b. make extensive dental care available to persons who could not otherwise afford it.

   c. only be initiated in major cities of the United States.

   d. be detrimental to a group dental practice.

8. A duplicating company may contract with the dental office to prepare statements by

   a. bringing the duplicating equipment to the office to mechanically prepare monthly statements.

   b. selling the dental office expensive duplicating equipment.

   c. sending a representative to the dental office for one week each month.

   d. demonstrating to the dental staff how monthly statements should be prepared.

9. Two reasons why a self-mailer is widely used is

   a. time is not wasted in stuffing envelopes.

   b. it provides the patient with a stamped return envelope.

   c. it provides the patient with a statement he can keep for his records.

   d. it is attractive in appearance.

D. Prepare an itemized printed form statement for the following:

   1. Mr. D.W. Jones of 255 Fairfield Drive, Anywhere, USA is responsible for the following account. His telephone number is 459-3993.

Dates	Patients	Treatment	Fee
a. Sept. 3	David	#3 MOD Amalgam	$18.00
b. Sept 10	Mary	Pro, BWXR	16.00
c. Sept. 23	Mr. D.W.	#14 DO Amalgam	
		#15 MO Amalgam	25.00

STATEMENT

LEONARD S. TAYLOR, D.D.S.
2100 WEST PARK AVENUE
CHAMPAIGN, ILLINOIS 61820

TELEPHONE 367-6671

DATE	FAMILY MEMBER	PROFESSIONAL SERVICE	CHARGE	CREDITS		BALANCE
				PAYM'TS	ADJ	

Unit 23 Collection Letters

OBJECTIVES

After studying this unit, the student should be able to

- Identify procedures that will keep overdue accounts to a minimum.
- Compose a series of four collection letters.
- Explain how a collection agency should be selected.

Writing collection letters may not be necessary if an efficient secretarial dental assistant is employed in the dental office. The efficient person will see that an understanding exists between the patient and the office concerning payment of fees. As stated in the preceding unit, it is often a lack of understanding on the patient's part that creates problems in collecting fees. Accounts usually do not become delinquent if the patient thoroughly understands the office policy. The efficient secretarial dental assistant will also watch each account closely. It is much easier to collect a three-month overdue account than a six-month overdue account.

There will usually be some delinquent accounts regardless of the office policy concerning payment of fees. At times, due to family crisis, patients are unable to follow office policy or agreements made. Sudden illnesses or deaths may result in critical financial problems for patients. The dentist and the secretarial dental assistant are usually very cooperative if the problems are known. A phone call or a letter written by the patient explaining a change in the ability to meet financial obligations should be noted immediately on the patient's financial record. It should be emphasized to the patient that *any* payment made on the account keeps the account from becoming delinquent. Many times patients feel that it is better not to send a payment if they cannot send it in full.

Stress to the patient that some payment should be made monthly even if it does not cover the full amount.

REMINDERS

Tact must be employed in collecting whether by telephone or by written communication. Insulting the patient may result in an even longer overdue account.

If no payment has been received since the last statement, a notation should be made on the next statement; the notation (reminder) may simply be a red check mark placed to the left of the balance, figure 23-1. If the statement has been overlooked by the patient, the red check mark may cause prompt payment. Others may be concerned about the appearance of the mark and send payment before other action occurs. It is amazing at the results this red check mark may bring. Another notification could be, *Payment has not been received since the last statement,* written on the statement or on a slip of paper enclosed with the statement. Management consultants of dental practices differ on how these notations should be made. Some feel that notations or phrases should not be written on the statement; they feel the patient would be embarrassed to send the payment. They prefer the notation to be written on a small piece of paper and included with the statement.

Printing companies provide stickers, usually in a series of three, for aid in collecting accounts, figure 23-2. The first sticker is a friendly reminder, the second a little more demanding, and the third is a firm demand for the payment. The dentist will decide if these stickers are to be used.

COLLECTION LETTERS

When writing a letter keep in mind that the appearance of any letter is important, especially the collection letter. The guidelines explained in the previous unit on letter format should be used in writing any collection letter.

The Mild Letter

If payment has not been received in two months, more attention should be given to the account. It is suggested that a mild, friendly letter be written to the patient, figure 23-3. This letter should be signed by the secretarial dental assistant. Many times the patients will pay after this letter. The patients may feel that since the letter was signed by the secretarial dental assistant, perhaps the dentist does

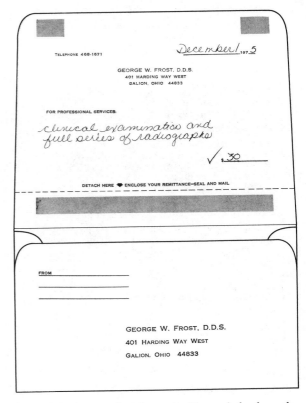

Fig. 23-1 A second statement with a red check mark reminds the patient of the balance due.

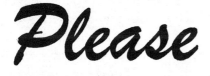

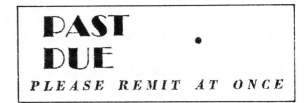

Your Remittance WILL BE VERY MUCH APPRECIATED

JUST A FRIENDLY REMINDER *... that your account is overdue. Won't you please mail remittance?*

FINAL NOTICE *Unless this account is paid in full within 10 days, it must be turned over for collection as provided by the laws of this state.*

Fig. 23-2 Stickers for use on statements to aid in collecting accounts.

211

Dr. John Melvin Doe
300 Dental Drive
Anywhere, USA 39206

January 5, 1975

Mr. William A. Jones
2558 Somewhere Street
Anywhere, USA 39201

Dear Mr. Jones:

We feel certain that you forgot to mail our office a check last month for dental services. Very often we write a good patient like yourself, only to have payment arrive in the next mail. Please disregard this letter if payment has been mailed within the last few days.

However, if you have forgotten to send our office a check, please try to do so before the next billing date.

If there are personal considerations that we should know about, please telephone our office. Problems may be worked out when good faith exists.

Sincerely,

Rhonda Douglas
Secretarial Dental Assistant

RD/chr

Fig. 23-3 An example of a mild collection letter. (#1)

Dr. John Melvin Doe
300 Dental Drive
Anywhere, USA 39206

February 5, 1975

Mr. William A. Jones
2558 Somewhere Street
Anywhere, USA 39206

Dear Mr. Jones:

Our office regrets having to write you the second time concerning your account. The amount of the account is $45.00. The last payment that we received was dated November 1, 1974.

If full payment can not be made, a partial payment will protect your credit standing. If there is some misunderstanding about the account, please call our office at 980-8017. We will be happy to discuss the account with you in detail. If you prefer, we will be happy to make an appointment for you to discuss this matter with Doctor Doe.

We urge you to give this account your immediate attention. Hopefully, we will hear from you within the next two weeks.

Sincerely,

Rhonda Douglas
Secretarial Dental Assistant

RD/chr

Fig. 23-4 Example of a firm collection letter. (#2)

not know about the overdue account. This may encourage payment because the patient does not want the dentist to know he is a slow payer. This type of collection letter is advisable for social friends of the dentist. It might be a touchy situation for the dentist's signature to appear on a collection letter to a friend or social acquaintance.

A notation should appear on the patient's financial record or treatment card that a letter was sent. The type of letter sent should also be noted. Each time an additional step is taken in the collection process, a notation must be made on the patient's record. It is very important that all steps taken be written and dated on the office records. These notations on the records serve a two-fold purpose. First, an accurate record is being kept of the progress of the collection. Second, a new employee or anyone in the dental office, may at a glance know the collection status of the patient.

The Firm Letter

A reminder letter may be sent if results did not occur from the mild, friendly letter, figure 23-4. This reminder letter should be a little more firm and specific but with a friendly tone. It is recommended that this letter include the amount of the account and the date of the last payment. Suggesting that the patient make an appointment to discuss the account tactfully emphasizes the importance of payment. This letter may be signed by the secretarial dental assistant or the dentist. If the account is a sizable figure, the dentist probably should sign it.

The Serious Letter

If a third letter is necessary, the account is seriously overdue. The fact that it is seriously overdue must be conveyed to the patient, figure 23-5. This letter should be signed by the dentist. The content and tone of the letter stresses the importance of prompt payment

Dr. John Melvin Doe
300 Dental Drive
Anywhere, USA 39206

March 5, 1975

Mr. William A. Jones
2558 Somewhere Street
Anywhere, USA 39201

Dear Mr. Jones:

It is with regret that we must write to you the third time about your overdue account. We do not understand why four statements and two letters have been ignored. Your account for professional services is $45.00. It is now four months past due.

We feel that we have been as lenient as we can be about your account. It is necessary that you send full payment immediately or contact our office for a definite settlement within the next few days.

Hopefully, you value your credit rating and will not permit our office to contact our collection agency for help with your account. However, we will have no choice unless we hear from you immediately.

Sincerely,

John Melvin Doe, D.D.S.

JMD/rd

Fig. 23-5 Example of a serious collection letter. (#3)

Dr. John Melvin Doe
300 Dental Drive
Anywhere, USA 39206

April 5, 1975

Mr. William A. Jones
2558 Somewhere Street
Anywhere, USA 39201

Dear Mr. Jones:

Again, we regret having to inform you that your seriously overdue account remains unpaid. We feel certain that you are aware that the account has been allowed to run much longer than normal credit practices permit. Ample time has been given for a definite arrangement to be worked out.

Unfortunately, we must seek legal help in collecting your account of $45.00. If payment is not received by April 10, 1975, our collections agency will be in touch with you.

Sincerely,

John Melvin Doe, D.D.S.

JMD/rd

Fig. 23-6 Example of a warning letter. (#4)

or prompt contact with the dental office. The specific information about the account should also be restated in this third collection letter. Firmness can be shown in a way that will not insult the patient. Never should the serious letter be written in the second person; for example, "You must pay this . . ." A poorly constructed collection letter results in poor relations; a written demand addressing the person directly only serves to irritate the patient, making collection even more difficult.

The Warning Letter

The fourth letter is a very serious letter to the patient; it is written because all other communication attempts have failed. The statement and notations were ignored, no action was received from the mild, the firm, and the serious letters. It is now time to let the patient know that other action is considered to be necessary. However, do not state that "other action will be necessary."

Tell the patient exactly what the office plans to do. If the patient is warned that the account will be turned over to a collection agency within ten days, the account should be given to a collection agency after ten days. Many offices have difficulty collecting overdue accounts because the actions stated in the oral and written communications are not carried out. Figure 23-6 shows an example of a warning letter to a patient. Notice that although the letter is very firm and serious it is still very professional.

COLLECTION AGENCIES

Close attention should be given to the selection of a collection agency. It is absolutely necessary that a reputable agency be selected. A nonreputable agency could be damaging to the dental practice. It is recommended that an agency be consulted which deals only with medical and dental accounts. If the agency representatives deal only with professional accounts, they are already familiar with professional ethics. This is a most important factor for the dental office to consider.

SUMMARY

Collection letters may be kept to a minimum if the secretarial dental assistant is efficient. Each patient's account should be watched closely each month; the longer the account remains unpaid, the harder it is to collect the fees. Tact must be used in all communications (oral and written) regarding fee collection. A poorly constructed collection letter may insult the patient so that payment is prolonged even longer.

If payment is not received a month after the first statement has been sent, the next statement is sent with a red check mark placed to the left of the amount. A written notation or a sticker may appear either on the statement or attached to it. If this fails, a mild, friendly letter is written to the patient. A second letter which is firm and specific is sent if no response is received from the first letter. A third letter indicates that the account is seriously overdue. A fourth letter may be the final communication with the patient before seeking legal aid in collecting the account. If the patient is told that legal aid will be sought in collecting the account within a certain period of time, then the aid should be sought within the stated time limit. If collection agencies are used, a reputable one which deals mostly with professional accounts should be selected.

SUGGESTED ACTIVITIES

- Invite a representative from a collection agency to speak to the class on methods of collecting professional accounts.
- Prepare a series of four 5 x 8 index cards with writing hints for collection letters.
- Type sample form letters which may be attached to 5 x 8 file cards for reference.

REVIEW

A.   Select the most appropriate response.

1. A red check mark placed to the left of the patient's balance on his statement may

    a. encourage prompt payment.

    b. slow down the collection process.

    c. signal the secretarial dental assistant to watch the account closely.

    d. Caution the dentist not to perform any treatment on the patient.

2. Some management consultants recommend that friendly, reminder messages be written on a separate slip of paper because

    a. it is less time-consuming for the office to prepare.

    b. the dentist needs a carbon copy of the written message.

    c. patients may find it embarrassing to mail payment with the reminder on the statement itself.

    d. the noted statement may be confusing to the patient.

3. A collection letter signed by the secretarial dental assistant may encourage prompt payment because

   a. the patient always has a more pleasant relationship with the secretarial dental assistant.

   b. the patient wants to pay the amount before the dentist is told about the delinquency.

   c. the patient wonders why the dentist's signature did not appear.

   d. the secretarial dental assistant is usually firmer than the dentist.

4. Two reasons why dated notations of any reminders and collection letters sent to the patient should always be made on his financial records are

   a. an accurate, up-to-date record is being kept of the collection process.

   b. the collection status of the patient will be available to anyone in the dental office who may need to refer to it.

   c. the Internal Revenue Service requires these notations to be written on all financial records.

   d. the patient may accidentally see the record.

B.   Name two factors to consider in selecting a collection agency.

C.   Write four collection letters. Contents of the letters must be different than that of the unit illustrations. Letters written for unit illustrations are guidelines.

   1. Letter which is mild and friendly.

   2. Letter which is a little more firm and specific.

   3. Letter for the seriously overdue account.

   4. A warning letter before possible legal action.

Letter 1 (Mild Collection Letter)

Dr. John Melvin Doe
300 Dental Drive
Anywhere, USA 39206

Letter 2 (Firm Collection Letter)

Dr. John Melvin Doe
300 Dental Drive
Anywhere, USA 39206

Letter 3 (Serious Collection Letter)

Dr. John Melvin Doe
300 Dental Drive
Anywhere, USA 39206

Letter 4 (Warning Collection Letter)

Dr. John Melvin Doe
300 Dental Drive
Anywhere, USA 39206

Unit 24 Manuscripts and Reports

OBJECTIVES

After studying this unit, the student should be able to

- Identify the items contained in manuscripts, formal reports, and informal reports.
- Prepare a final copy of a report or manuscript from an edited rough draft copy.
- Prepare the minutes of a meeting in an acceptable format.

The dentist who conducts research, participates in professional organizations, or writes articles, books, or speeches will expect the secretarial dental assistant to assist him in the preparation of these papers.

REPORTS AND MANUSCRIPTS

Reports may range from informal office memos to formal reports on research projects. *Manuscripts* (books or articles) are usually prepared for publication. Both reports and manuscripts should be written in Standard English; no slang or abbreviations are used. The material should be presented in a clear, straightforward manner and is written using the impersonal third person.

Rough Drafts

All reports and manuscripts are typed in rough draft form first, double or triple spaced so that corrections or changes can be easily made. If footnotes are present in the report, they may be typed in the body of the rough draft (immediately following the numbered reference) so that they are easily located when typing the final copy. The rough draft is edited for accuracy of facts, grammar and spelling, and for clear, concise presentation. If numerous changes have been made in the copy, a second or third rough draft may be

necessary to be sure that all changes are correct before typing the report in final form. All rough draft copies are saved for reference until the final copy has been typed.

When editing a rough draft copy, standard proofreading marks are normally used. These can be found in most dictionaries, but some of the more common marks are listed below:

Mark	Meaning
word or ℓ	delete or omit word
stet word or word	do not omit word
word or ∧	insert word or punctuation
＝	straighten up line
‖	straighten up margin
word	capitalize letter
word	put entire word in caps
⌐	move to left
¬	move to right
⊓	move up
⊔	move down
(sp)	spell out or do not abbreviate
#	add space
⌣	close up the space
¶	paragraph
word	underline word
ss ⌐	single space
ds ⌐	double space
wrogd	transpose letters

TEMPOROMANDIBULAR JOINT DIAGNOSIS

INTRODUCTION

During the past three decades, "temporomandibular joint problems have rested in a kind of medical no-man's land in that physicians have been generally handicapped by their limited understanding of oral and T-M joint function while the dentists have been handicapped by their lack of understanding of joints and joint problems."[1] Although it has been estimated that more than twenty percent of the population is afflicted with some form of TMJ dysfunction, the condition is misdiagnosed in a majority of cases. These patients belong to that segment of society who go from specialist to specialist, seeking relief from nagging head and neck pain.

It is the purpose of this paper to present currently accurate information concerning the differential diagnosis of the T-M joint pain and pains of the head and neck that may be diagnosed as relating to the T-M joint.

Unquestionably, no simple factor can be responsible for all of the varied symptoms. It is the interaction of the nervous muscular and vascular systems--at least in the affection region--which requires our attention.

---

[1] W. E. Bell, *Synopsis: Oral and Facial Pain and the Temporomandibular Joint*, (Dallas, 1967), p. 81

Fig. 24-1 Final copy with heading, side heading, and footnote superimposed on guide sheet with right-hand margin and numbers.

Final Copy

There are several formats for preparing reports or manuscripts which may be followed. If the publisher or agency submits specific instructions for the preparation of the report, follow the instructions closely and accurately. If no instructions are given, the following arrangement may be used, figure 24-1.

Paper. When typing the final copy of a report or manuscript, use a good quality, plain white paper, 8 1/2 inches by 11 inches. One or two carbon copies of the report should be made on a good quality onionskin paper.

Margins. All margins should be uniform. Use either a 1-inch or a 1 1/2-inch margin at the top, at the bottom, and on each side. If the report or manuscript is to be bound at the top or at the left, add an additional 1/2 inch to that particular margin. The first page of the report should have a 2-inch top margin.

Guide Sheet. A guide sheet can help in keeping the right-hand margin even and in determining spacing for footnotes. A guide sheet can be prepared on a piece of onionskin paper or other lightweight copy paper. Down the right edge of the paper, type numbers 1 through 66 so that each line on the sheet has been numbered. This numbering guide will indicate at a glance on what line you are typing and how many lines you have left. Then with a black felt-tip pen draw a line down the guide sheet just inside the numbers. A second line should be drawn down the guide sheet to indicate where the right-hand margin should end (either 1 inch or 1 1/2 inches to the left of the first line). Insert the guide sheet directly behind the original. Align the original with the first black line drawn so that the numbers on the guide sheet appear beside the edge of the original copy.

Spacing and Indentations. Double space the copy. Paragraphs may be indented either five

or ten spaces. Short quotations (no more than four lines) may be typed in the body of the report; longer quotations should be typed as a separate paragraph, single spaced and indented five or more spaces from each margin.

Headings. A main heading should be centered and typed in all capital letters. It is preceded and followed by a triple space. A side heading is placed against the left margin and is underlined or typed in capital letters. It is preceded by a triple space and followed by a double space. Paragraph headings are indented, underlined or typed in capital letters, and followed by a period. The first sentence of the paragraph should begin on the same line as the paragraph heading.

Page Numbers. The first page of the report is not numbered. All other pages should be numbered in the upper right-hand corner, aligned with the right margin. The page numbers are typed 1/2 inch above the top margin. If the report is to be bound at the top, the page numbers are centered at the bottom of the page 1/2 inch below the margin.

Footnotes. When footnotes are typed at the bottom of the page, they are separated from the body of the report by a single space, a 1 1/2-inch horizontal line beginning at the left margin, and a double space. Footnotes are single spaced with a double space between them. The first line is indented five spaces. The footnote number is raised 1/2 of a line space at the point of reference and at the beginning of the footnote. Footnotes may be numbered consecutively throughout the report, numbered anew for each chapter, or numbered anew on each page. Footnotes contain the author's name typed in normal sequence, the title of the chapter or article in quotation marks (if needed), the title of the book or magazine underlined, the edition, the volume number, the place and date of publication in parenthesis, and the page number. The abbreviation Ed. for edition, Vol. for volume, p. for page, and pp. for pages may be used in the footnotes.

Another method of handling footnotes, which is becoming more popular, requires that all reference material (regardless of classification) be alphabetized in the Bibliography and each reference is numbered in sequence. At the point of reference in the body of the report, the reference number and the page number are placed in parentheses; for example, (8, p. 221). This eliminates the need for footnotes at the bottom of the page and makes typing the report much faster.

Contents of Reports and Manuscripts

Preliminary material (all pages appearing before the actual report) and supplementary material (all pages appearing after the actual report) are prepared using the same margins and spacing as the body of the report. On the first sheet of the material, a 2-inch top margin is used, and the title is centered and typed in all capital letters. A short informal report or an article may have the title and the dentist's name typed at the top of the first page. Figure 24-2 outlines what should be included in manuscripts, formal and informal reports.

Title Fly. A title fly may be included if desired. The *title fly* is treated as the front cover and contains only the title of the report.

Title Page. The title page contains the title of the report, the name of the dentist, and the date.

Preface. A preface or introduction to establish the setting or circumstances may be included if desired.

Acknowledgment. An acknowledgment of help received or permission to quote another may be included if necessary or desired.

Table of Contents. Only the main headings of the report are usually listed in the table of contents along with all preliminary materials and supplementary materials. Preliminary pages are numbered in small roman numerals. Main headings and supplementary pages are numbered in arabic numerals. The table of contents is *leadered* (periods are double spaced, beginning at least one space beyond the head-

Manuscript	Formal Report	Informal Report
Title Fly	Title Fly	
Title Page	Title Page	Title Page
Preface	Preface	
Acknowledgments	Acknowledgments	
Table of Contents	Table of Contents	
Other Tables	Other Tables	
	Synopsis	
The Manuscript	The Report	The Report
Appendix	Appendix	
Bibliography	Bibliography	Bibliography
Index		

Fig. 24-2 Contents of manuscript and reports.

ings and finishing within not less than two spaces of the page numbers). Leaders should be aligned; that is, all are typed on even spaces or all are typed on odd spaces.

Other Tables. A table of illustrations, list of charts, etc., are included if necessary. These tables are also leadered.

Synopsis. A *synopsis* is a brief summary of the actual report and may be included if desired.

Report or Manuscript. The report consists of an introduction, the findings and analyses, and the conclusions and recommendations. The contents of the manuscript depend entirely on what is to be published. If technical information is presented, the contents would be similar to that of a formal report.

Appendix. An appendix is used when additional material is desired to supplement the report.

Bibliography. The bibliography contains all material used as references whether it has been cited in the report or not. If various types of references are listed, they are classified in the following order: books, encyclopedia articles, public documents, articles of magazines, reports, and unpublished materials. Items in each classification are then alphabetized by the author's name. The first line of the reference begins at the left margin; all other lines are indented five spaces.

The surname of the author is given first. If two or more authors are listed, all names appear in this *inverse order.* If no author is listed, the item is alphabetized under the title. The title of the book or magazine is underlined, followed by the edition, the volume number, the city of publication, the publisher and the date of the publication.

Index. An index may be included to aid the reader in making quick reference to specific parts of the manuscript.

COPYRIGHTS

An unpublished manuscript is covered by a *common-law copyright* which goes into effect as soon as the material is written. To protect material under a common-law copyright, the dentist may mail a copy of the manuscript to himself in a sealed envelope by Registered Mail. The unopened envelope will provide proof of the date of the material.

If the dentist or publisher wishes to have the published manuscript copyrighted, copies of the published work, a completed application form, and a nominal fee (currently $6) can be sent to the Register of Copyrights, Library of Congress, Washington, D.C. 20559. A copyright runs for 28 years and can be renewed for an additional 28 years by completing an application for renewal during the last year of the original copyright.

When copyrighted material is quoted or cited in a manuscript, the dentist is responsible for not only giving credit to the original author but also obtaining permission for its use. Permission should be requested from the copyright owner.

MINUTES OF MEETINGS

The dentist or secretarial dental assistant who is active in professional organizations may be responsible for reporting what went on, that is, recording the minutes of such meetings. A knowledge of parliamentary procedures will help in taking notes and preparing the minutes to be read at the next meeting.

Recording the Minutes

Some preliminary notes may be made before the meeting starts (the date, time and place, and name of presiding officer). A list of the membership will simplify the recording of the roll call. It also provides a means of identifying members during the meeting.

Notes should be taken in full. Summaries of discussions are usually included in the minutes, but detailed notes should be taken so that interpretations are accurate. The secretarial dental assistant may interrupt the proceedings by signaling the president if she cannot hear or failed to record important information. If *verbatim* (word-for-word) notes are required, the secretarial dental assistant may wish to make a tape of the meeting so that she will be able to verify her notes later when preparing the minutes.

Preparing the Minutes

A draft copy of the minutes should be typed and approved before the final copy is prepared. Minutes of formal meetings should be prepared in a format which is somewhat formal, figure 24-3. Minutes of committee meetings and other informal meetings may be prepared in a less formal manner. Regardless of

the format used, the minutes should contain the same information. This information includes such items as reports, motions, resolutions and adjournment.

Some follow-up activities may be necessary as a result of motions made at the meeting. Members may need to be notified of special meetings, or letters of appreciation or sympathy may need to be sent. Resolutions and petitions also require follow-up activity.

Resolutions. Each paragraph of a resolution begins with the word WHEREAS typed in capital letters except for the last paragraph which begins with the word RESOLVED. The resolution must be typed for the signature of the presiding officer.

Petitions. Each paragraph of a petition begins with the word WHEREAS typed in capital

---

THE NAME OF THE ORGANIZATION

TIME AND PLACE OF MEETING
The first paragraph gives the type of meeting, the date, hour, and place of meeting, and the name of the presiding officer. The minutes may be single or double spaced. Paragraphs may be indented five or ten spaces.

PRESENT
The names of members present are listed in alphabetic order, or the total number attending may be given if the membership is large.

ABSENT
The names of members absent are listed in alphabetic order.

READING OF MINUTES
The reading of the minutes of the previous meeting is recorded. The approval of or the corrections made to the minutes are noted.

REPORTS
Each report given is summarized and recorded in a separate paragraph with the caption indicating the specific report; such as, TREASURER'S REPORT.

MOTIONS
Motions should be given exactly as stated – typed in all capital letters or underlined so that they can be easily seen. The caption should identify the motion in as few words as possible. Each motion requires a separate paragraph. The names of the members making the motion and seconding the motion, the motion as stated, a summary of the discussion, and the results of the voting should be included.

RESOLUTION ON FORMAT OF RESOLUTIONS
WHEREAS, All Resolutions approved by the organization should become a part of the minutes, be it

RESOLVED, That this format be used when typing all Resolutions.

ADJOURNMENT
This motion need not include the names of members making and seconding the motion. The fact that the motion was made and approved and the time of adjournment should be recorded.

SECRETARY   PRESIDENT

Fig. 24-3 A format of minutes of an organization.

letters except for the last paragraph which begins with the words, "WE, the undersigned, do hereby petition . . ." The petition should be signed only by those members who wish to be included.

Correcting Minutes

When the minutes are read at the next meeting, corrections may be necessary. If corrections must be made, they are written on the original copy in ink. The minutes are NOT retyped. If the correction is a long one, an inked notation is made on the original minutes stating that the correction is attached. The correction may then be typed and attached to the original minutes.

SUMMARY

The secretarial dental assistant may be asked to help in the preparation of reports and manuscripts. A few basic things should be remembered: the copy should always be double spaced; the title and author's name should always be included; footnotes and a bibliography should be included if references have been used. The more formal the report or manuscript, the more elaborate the format will be.

Minutes of meetings should always contain the name of the organization or committee, the time and place of the meeting, the presiding officer, the roll call, the reading of previous minutes, reports given and motions made during the meeting, and the time of adjournment.

The knowledge and self-confidence gained by becoming involved in these activities will provide valuable professional growth for the secretarial dental assistant.

SUGGESTED ACTIVITY

- The following is an excerpt of the actual minutes prepared. Retype these minutes using a formal format.

MISSISSIPPI DENTAL ASSISTANTS ASSOCIATION

The Executive Board of the Mississippi Dental Assistants Association met September 8, 1973 at 10:45 a.m. at the Holiday Inn North in Hattiesburg, Mississippi.

The President called the meeting to order and declared a quorum present. The role was called by the Secretary and nine members answered. The minutes of the Post Convention Board Meeting were read and approved. The Treasurer's report was given, stating a balance of $1,397.88, listing as disbursements $1,527.55 and $1,567.94 as deposits.

A motion was made by Bobbye King that we pay Ronelda Thornhill for the cost of printing the nomination forms. The motion was seconded and carried.

Mary Ann Douglas reported on the approximate cost of attending the ADAA Annual Session in Houston, Texas, November 1973. A motion was made by Peggy Wells that $278 be given each delegate to help with expenses. The motion was seconded and carried.

A discussion on needed State Advisors were held. It was decided to ask Dr. Robert Parkes for 1974-75 Session and Dr. Wayne Sturdivant for the 1975-76 Session. Their assistants were asked to contact them about this and report on their acceptance or rejection at the next Board Meeting.

The next Board Meeting was announced to be Saturday, February 23, 1974 at Hinds Junior College, Jackson, Mississippi at 10:00 a.m. with each person bringing a covered dish for the noon meal. All committees will meet after lunch.

The meeting was adjourned at 1:00 p.m.

Peggy Wells, Secretary-Treasurer

Members Present: Bonnie Hendrix, Mary Crow, LaVelle McMorris, Mary Ann Douglas, Peggy Wells, Bobbye King, Ronelda Thornhill, Betty Jo Wicks, Flo Phillips

REVIEW

A. The following rough draft copy is a continuation of the report shown in figure 24-1. Type the report in final form using 1-inch margins and 5-space indentations. Refer to figure 24-1, study the rough draft below and submit the typed report to your instructor for evaluation.

DRAFT

FINDINGS

A brief historical review is of interest. In 1918, Prentiss[2]

> **H.J. Prentiss; "Preliminary Report Upon the Temporomandibular Articulation," C. Cosmos, Vol. 60, (1918), pp. 505-512**

pointed out that malocclusion and loss of teeth without replacement causes damage to the temporomandibular joint. In 1920, W.H. Wright[3]

> **W.H. Wright, "Deafness is influenced by Malposition of the Jaws," J. National Dental Association, Vol. 7, (1920), pp. 979-990**

reported a case in which deafness was relieved after correction of malposition of the mandibular joint. Monson in (1921) claimed both

> **Monson, G.S., "Occlusion Supplied to Crown and bridgework," J. Nat. D.A, Vol. 8, (1921), p. 833**

overclosure of the mandible and malocclusion of the teeth can force the condyle back in the articular fossa and thereby can reduce the diameter of the auditory canal which will produce deafness. During the past 30 years the literature has been filled with "proofs" and "disproofs" all based not on the symptoms but on the etiology or treatment. The first step out of this confusion is to eliminate both etiology and treatment and consider the symptoms.

B. The items listed in the first column are associated with reports, manuscripts, or minutes. Check the appropriate column or columns (A,B,C,).

ITEM	A REPORTS	B MANUSCRIPTS	C MINUTES
1. Guide Sheet	_____	_____	_____
2. Marginal Captions	_____	_____	_____
3. Headings	_____	_____	_____
4. Synopsis	_____	_____	_____
5. Motions	_____	_____	_____
6. Bibliography	_____	_____	_____
7. Rough Draft	_____	_____	_____
8. Footnotes	_____	_____	_____
9. Copyrights	_____	_____	_____
10. Roll Call	_____	_____	_____

C.   Mark the following statements True, or False.

1. Manuscripts are usually prepared when the material is to be published.   _____

2. All reports, manuscripts, and minutes should be typed in rough draft form first.   _____

3. A guide sheet is used as an outline of the report.   _____

4. When editing a rough draft copy, proofreaders' marks are usually used.   _____

5. There is only one acceptable way to prepare a manuscript.   _____

6. Footnotes are always single spaced.   _____

7. Footnotes are always numbered anew for each chapter.   _____

8. Leaders are double spaced periods.   _____

9. A synopsis is an outline of the report.   _____

10. A bibliography should contain all material used as references.   _____

11. Permission should be obtained before using copyrighted material.   _____

12. When taking minutes of a meeting, notes should always be verbatim.   _____

13. When corrections must be made to the minutes at the next meeting, they are written on the original copy in ink.   _____

14. Each motion in the minutes is written as a new paragraph.   _____

15. A preface should always appear as a part of the manuscript.   _____

Unit 25 Preparation of an Office Manual

OBJECTIVES

After studying this unit, the student should be able to

- State the purposes of a dental office manual.
- Outline recommended sections of a manual.

An office manual is an essential tool for an efficiently run dental practice. The purpose of a manual is to acquaint all members of the dental team with the philosophy of the dentist and the various policies of the office. It guides dental team members in providing optimum dental care for the patients. The duties of each member of the dental health team should be outlined in detail. A new employee would be able to study his or her specific office duties from the manual. Dental procedures may be outlined, giving the steps and/or tray setups. Again, providing the new employee with information to study is one of the major objectives of the dental office manual. It may also serve to remind the other employees of steps or information that has been forgotten.

The dentist should write or direct the writing of the office manual. Each dentist must construct the manual to suit the needs of the individual practice. A manual that would apply to every practice cannot be written. The secretarial dental assistant may help the dentist in preparing much of the manual. If she is a good writer, she may even compose portions of the manual from an outline that the dentist has prepared.

The manual should be typed neatly by the secretarial dental assistant and placed in a durable folder. The folder must allow for pages to be removed or inserted as changes will be made throughout the years. It is suggested that several copies of the manual be made. The extra copies will make it possible for new employees to take a copy home for study during early weeks of employment. The least expensive way to make extra copies is to have the original manual duplicated. If the dental office does not have a copier, the original may be taken to a professional copying company. The dental office manual should include matters such as:

- A statement of purpose or objectives.
- A statement of the dentist's philosophy regarding patients and their dental care.
- A table of contents.
- Employment policies.
- Expected conduct of dental team.
- Duties of the dental team members.
- Oral communications.
- Written communications.
- Record keeping procedures.
- Operative procedures.
- Patient education.
- Professional organizations.

FRONT PAGES

The first page of the manual, after the cover sheet, should contain a general statement of the purpose of the office manual. A list of specific objectives (written by the dentist) follows the stated purpose. These specific objectives should outline the reasons for preparing the manual. For example, one of the objectives might be "to help the new employee to become familiar with the policies and procedures of the office."

The philosophy of the dentist is written in manuscript form. This information should include the dentist's thinking about such things as how to make appointments for new patients or how to introduce the patient to dental health education. The dentist, more than likely, may want to prepare a statement on his personal philosophy of dentistry. He may include his feelings concerning the treatment of patients in the office.

A table of contents must be included for easy reference by the dental team. Each page should be numbered at the bottom for ease in locating specific items or topics. Each time a page is added or deleted, the table of contents should be corrected.

TEXT

The front pages serve as a guide to the purpose and contents. The text refers to matters which the dentist expects his staff to learn about the operation and policies of the dental practice.

Employment Policies

All employees are interested in employment policies. Salary information may or may not be stated. It is suggested that only general information relating to salaries be presented in this section. Salary schedules vary between the dental team members; it is usually not advisable to even state the beginning salaries. This matter should be privately discussed between the dentist and the employee. A clearly defined policy about salary increases is recommended. The statement should reflect that raises are given according to the performance of the employee. This type of statement is preferable to automatic raise increases.

Office hours and working days of the week should be listed. A further statement

THINGS TO DO WHILE THE DENTIST IS AWAY

Call delinquent accounts.
Prepare any packages or letters for mailing.
Straighten bookcase in the dentist's office.
Pull the cards for the next day.
Call the patients for the next day.
Organize and consolidate closets and laboratory.
Check to make sure that all recalls are up-to-date.
Catch up on all back correspondence and thank-you cards.
Inventory all printed material in the office.
Inventory and order dental and office supplies.
Clean and polish cabinets and equipment.
Clean and oil the dental handpieces.
Perform routine service on all dental equipment in the office.
Process and mount radiographs.
Clean x-ray tanks and change the solutions.
Clean all inaccessible areas.
Straighten the drug cabinet.
Autoclave paper or cloth supplies. e.g. 2 x 2 gauze.
Change cold sterilizing solutions.
Clean and sharpen the laboratory instruments.
Clean and polish the impression trays. Organize the trays neatly.

Fig. 25-1 Suggested office duties to be done in dentist's absence.

regarding overtime should be prepared. It should be emphasized that a professional health practice may require the office team to occasionally work beyond the usual office hours. It should be further stated that health occupation workers should not expect to work by a time clock.

Vacation time and sick leave should be clearly defined. If the employee is expected to schedule all vacations when the dentist is on vacation, the approximate month should be mentioned. A sick-leave policy is necessary for the welfare of the employee. However, it should be strongly emphasized that sick leave in the dental office should be kept to the absolute minimum. Stress is placed on the fact that the dental team may not function as easily or efficiently when any member is away. Paid holidays should be listed.

APPEARANCE AND GROOMING GUIDELINES

UNIFORM	Spotlessly clean at all times.
HOSE	Coordinated with uniform.
SHOES	Coordinated with uniform; clean and comfortable.
JEWELRY	Watch, and/or wedding band. The chair assistant should not wear rings, as mercury may disintegrate the jewelry.
HAIR	Neat, short, above the collar, and easily kept. Extreme hair styles have no place in the dental office. Should receive careful attention.
MAKEUP	Yes, but with the utmost discretion.
DAILY BATH OR SHOWER	Use of deodorant, a little cologne is indicated. Depilatory as needed.
CARE OF TEETH	Brush and floss each time after eating and before going to bed at night. Time out of the office will be allowed for personal appointments.
BREATH	Use of mouthwash is indicated. Never eat garlic or onions during the lunch break.
SMOKING	Is not permitted while a patient or a parent is in the office.

Fig. 25-2 A typical page in an office manual.

The dentist should also prepare a statement concerning days when he is away from the office attending professional meetings. The employees should know exactly what is expected of them while the dentist is away. It is even suggested that a list be made of "Things To Do While The Dentist Is Away," figure 25-1. The list may include items such as cleaning out the files, waxing the dental units, etc. A list such as this avoids waste of time in the office. A policy statement regarding the attendance of the employees' professional meetings should be included.

Dental care for dental team members or their families should be mentioned in the employment policies. If free dental care or a family discount is provided for the employee, the manual should include a statement and cite limitations. The employee may have a large family and expect too much dental care

DUTIES OF THE SECRETARIAL
DENTAL ASSISTANT

Call all patients the day before to remind them of their appointment with the office.

Greet and announce all incoming patients.

Type a list of scheduled appointments for the day. Call the dentist's attention to any special appointments.

Maintain the recall system in the absence of the hygienist.

Sort and screen all incoming mail.

Receive and assist all visitors calling at the office.

See that patients and parents are comfortable in the reception room.

Give Information Sheet and Medical History form to patients on arrival.

Originate and maintain records of all patients entering or now in the practice.

Send out thank-you letters to people who have referred patients to the office.

Balance charges, payments and deposits at beginning of each working day.

Maintain office payroll account.

Maintain and order all business office supplies.

Prepare tax and accounting reports.

Justify all invoices with bills payable and prepare checks for payment of these and all fixed monthly obligations. (This is to be done preferably by the 10th of the month.)

Remind the doctor of his appointments – place a note on his desk before he leaves in the afternoon.

Call patients from the day before who have had extractions or dental replacements to see how they are getting along.

Discuss and set up payment plan for patients whose balances are expected to be rather large.

Discuss overdue balances with patients and set up a plan for payment.

Fig. 25-3 Duties of the secretarial dental assistant.

from the dentist; the employee should know about these policies and limitations before beginning employment.

Conduct

Although most people working in a professional office know how to conduct themselves properly, some may need some guidance and direction. The new person may not have had the proper training relating to dress, appearance, or conduct in a professional office. The expected dress code relating to uniform shoes, etc. should be outlined, figure 25-2. Proper decorum for the dental team members was discussed in a previous unit. It is suggested unit 2 be reviewed.

TRY SAYING	INSTEAD OF . . . . .
Discomfort	Pain or hurt
Prepare	Grind
Areas of Decay	Cavities
Amalgams or Restorations	Fillings
Local Anesthesia	Shot
Primary Teeth	Baby Teeth
Investment	Cost
Protective Restoration	Temporary Filling
Reminder Due	Balance
Treating the patient	Working on the patient
Whom may I say is calling?	Who is calling?
Dentistry	Work
Reception Room	Waiting Room
Extraction	Tooth pulled
Take care of	Pay for
Necessary X-rays	Some X-rays
Cavity detecting X-rays	Bitewing X-rays
Complete mouth picture	Full mouth X-rays
Dr. Doe is with a patient	Dr. Doe is all tied up or busy
Examination	Checkup
Dr. Doe is ready to see you.	Would you like to come in?

Fig. 25-4 Guidelines for effective communication.

Duties of the Dental Team Members

Each person employed in the dental office should be able to refer to a list of duties describing expected performance skills. A list should be made for the hygienist, the secretarial dental assistant, the chairside dental assistant, and the dental laboratory technician. There may be other job classifications present in individual offices. Even though the list may be lengthy, each list should be complete according to expected duties. The duties should be subdivided into daily, weekly, and monthly duties. The secretarial dental assistant's list should also include a listing of quarterly and yearly duties, figure 25-3, page 231. She may be the only member of the dental team with specific quarterly or yearly duties; these duties involve bookkeeping procedures required by the state and federal government.

If the office manual is being prepared in an established practice, the dental team may assist. The dentist may ask the dental team members to prepare a list of their duties performed each day. From this list, the team members and the dentist work together. The input of both will make the list of duties more complete.

Oral Communications

Every dentist has his own ideas about oral communications in the dental office. Words or phrases that lessen the suggestion of pain or unpleasantness are preferred by the dentist. A list containing words to be avoided and the proper words to use should be made available for the dental team, figure 25-4. It should be stressed that successful communication depends on using words or phrases that the patient understands. Not only is the correct word or phrase a key to better understanding but it also makes a better impression on the patient.

STERILIZATION METHODS			
METHOD	TEMPERATURE	TIME	TYPE OF INSTRUMENTS
Autoclave	121° - 124°C (250° - 254°F) (15 pounds pressure)	20 to 30 minutes	Surgical Instruments Extraction forceps Elevators Syringes and needles Hemostats Rongeurs
Dry Heat	160°C (320°F)	30 minutes	Tray setups Nonstainless instruments Cotton or cloth products
Hot Oils	150°C (320°F)	15 minutes	Only hinged or geared instruments
Molten Metal	193°C (380°F)	10 seconds	Endodontic Instruments
Glass Beads	232°C (450°F)	15–30 seconds	Endodontic Instruments
Cold Sterilizing Solutions		Follow Manufacturers' Directions	Mouth Mirror Cotton Pliers (Instruments must not pierce tissue.)
Sodium Hypochlorite		15 minutes	Plastic Instruments

Fig. 25-5   A chart showing sterilization methods, temperature, times, and types of instruments.

Most of the section on oral communications should deal with telephone techniques. The importance of a favorable telephone image should be stressed. The new employee may not realize how important telephone conversations are to the dental practice. Suggested telephone messages may even be included in the manual as examples. However, it must be emphasized that messages are not to be read over the telephone. They are intended only as aids in delivering the proper message to the caller. If an automatic answering service is available in the office, a detailed explanation should be given on how to operate it; the need for a courteous recorded message should be emphasized.

Since most appointments are made by telephone, the office policy regarding appointments may be outlined in this section of the manual. The various dental procedures together with a suggested length of time for the appointment may be listed. To simplify this listing, appointment time may be divided into units. Each 15-minute segment would equal one unit; one hour would equal four units.

This is suggested because most appointment books are divided into 15 minute intervals.

Written Communications

The subject of written communications may comprise a large portion of the manual. A sample letter should be written by the dentist for all occasions which might occur that require a letter. These sample letters enable the secretarial dental assistant to prepare other letters for the dentist without his having to dictate every word. For example, letters to referring dentists may be similar except for the factual information concerning the patient. The sample letter may also show the secretarial dental assistant the preferred style for an outgoing letter.

Record Keeping

The record-keeping system should be outlined in detail. The method used to record the daily financial matters should be explained. All of the business forms used in the office should be shown in the manual with a detailed explanation. If the daily log is used, an example of each form should be shown. If the pegboard system is used, a detailed explanation of how the system works should be given. Although many forms may appear to be easy to complete, there may be certain items which the dentist desires to emphasize and expand upon. Abbreviations that the dentist prefers to use on treatment slips and record cards should be noted.

The filing system should be explained. A list of all categories of filing should be included; an explanation of each category should follow the list. Explanation of the filing system must include record keeping and the system used to file radiographs and study models.

The dentist should outline the method of recall system used and the method he prefers for collecting past-due accounts. This information should be stated so there will be no misunderstanding on the secretarial dental assistant's part as to how collections are to be handled. The last portion of the section on record keeping should deal with county, city, state, and federal tax requirements. Ideally, each form necessary for reporting financial status and other requirements of the dental practice should be explained. A list of dates should be prepared to remind the secretarial dental assistant when *all* forms are due. This list enables the secretarial dental assistant to go through the appointment book at the beginning of the year marking the specific dates. Doing this may avoid costly income tax errors.

Operative Procedures

The section of the manual which deals with operative procedures may shorten the training period of a new employee and improve the performance of all dental auxiliaries. First, a listing of duties to complete daily, weekly, or monthly in the treatment area should be outlined. Each operative procedure must be explained in steps. After each explanation, the tray setup for the procedure

should be shown. Not only does this information and format assist the new employee, but it also serves as a refresher source for the other employees (some procedures are performed only occasionally in the office). Any instructions that are to be given to the patient after certain operative procedures have been done should be stated clearly and included in the manual.

Several sterilization methods may be used in the dental office. A chart listing the types of sterilizing methods should be included. The time, temperature, or pressure should be indicated on the chart, figure 25-5. Also, the type of instruments or items to be sterilized by the particular method should be shown.

Each type of material used in the treatment area should be explained. For example, there are several classifications of cement. Various manufacturers make similar cements but with different directions for mixing. What will work for one kind of cement may not work for another. It is suggested that all the cements be classified according to certain categories. Mixing directions may then be included for each cement. Items needed to mix or pass the cement should be listed.

Patient Education

Ideally, a separate folder should be prepared as the Patient Education Packet for the dental office. This folder includes patient education procedures as well as literature suitable for distribution to the patients. If a separate folder is not available, a section in the manual should be devoted to patient education. The dentist may want to state his philosophy on preventive dentistry. How to teach the patient good oral hygiene may require an outline by the dentist.

Professional Organizations

A section in the latter part of the manual should include a listing of the dental professional organizations.   Another listing includes the various professional organizations for dental auxiliaries. Under the name and address of the organization or society, membership information is included, such as the objective, amount of the annual dues, the due date, and the address where the membership dues should be mailed.   It is desirable for the dentist to write a statement to the employee about the advantages of belonging to a professional organization.   For example, the secretarial dental assistant is eligible to become a member of the American Dental Assistants Association.   The objective of the association may be obtained from a textbook, journal, or brochure issued by the ADAA. This may encourage a new employee to seek membership. It is suggested that the name, address, and phone number of the current secretary of the local dental assistant's society be listed.   This section of the manual may be only one page in length but can be very beneficial to an enthusiastic new employee. Belonging to one's professional organization provides opportunities for growth.   By supporting their professional organizations the dental auxiliaries improve economic security and maintain high standards of performance.

SUMMARY

An office manual is desirable for every dental office.   The purpose is to acquaint all members of the dental team with the philosophy of the dentist and the various policies of the office.   The new employee may obtain valuable information by studying the manual; other employees may be reminded of steps or information that was forgotten.   The duties of each member of the dental health team may be stated in detail. Operative procedures and tray setups may be explained and listed for easy reference.

If prepared thoroughly, the dental office manual may be a very comprehensive reference guide for the efficient dental practice.

SUGGESTED ACTIVITIES

- Study in detail at least two manuals prepared for different dental offices. Write a brief summary of each manual. Compare the comprehensiveness of the two manuals.

- Invite a practice management consultant to speak to the group on "The Effectiveness of a Dental Office Manual."

- Read a dental practice management textbook. Write a two-page report on the selected textbook.

REVIEW

A.   Select the best answer.

1. The purpose of an office manual is to

   a. acquaint all members of the dental team with the philosophy of the dentist and the various policies of the office.

   b. acquaint the patients with office policy.

   c. list the beginning salaries for each position in the dental office.

   d. record the number of hours worked by each employee.

2. The office manual is

   a. purchased from a dental supply company as all manuals are the same.

   b. borrowed from a library whenever the dental team needs to refer to it.

   c. typed by the secretarial dental assistant as it must be constructed to suit the needs of the individual practice.

   d. the dentist's responsibility and does not concern the secretarial dental assistant.

3. Successful communication with the patient depends on using

   a. only written communications.

   b. only verbal communications.

   c. modern, up-to-date equipment.

   d. words and phrases that the patient understands.

4. Two reasons why membership in a professional organization is desirable for the secretarial dental assistant are

   a. the opportunity for growth it provides.

   b. it is required by the ADAA.

   c. the high standard of performance it helps to maintain.

   d. it will make her more important than the other auxiliary team members.

B. List 12 subjects that should be included in a dental office manual.

C. Match the items in Column I with their definitions in Column II.

Column I	Column II
____ 1. Dry heat (160° C.)	a. statements outlining the reasons for preparing the office manual.
____ 2. Objectives	
____ 3. A professional organization	b. guides dental team members in providing optimum dental care for the patient.
____ 4. Office manual	c. literature on good oral hygiene and preventive dentistry.
____ 5. Patient education	d. sterilization method
	e. ADAA

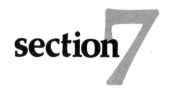

section 7

Filing Procedures

Unit 26 Basic Rules for Record Control

OBJECTIVES

After studying this unit, the student should be able to

- Define the four methods of filing.

- Explain the basic indexing rules for alphabetical files.

- List the five steps to follow when processing records to be filed.

- State five factors that must be considered when setting up a filing system.

- State the purpose of record management.

Wise organization and accurate management of records is essential for the success of any dental office. There is so much important information on paper today that one cannot possibly remember everything. A well-organized filing system serves as a memory for the office.

Filing, or records management, is the organization, protection and control of information. It is a service that is carried out to facilitate future work.

RECORD CONTROL

The organization of files is arranging items in logical, meaningful classifications. It is the first step toward control. All records are organized under headings, which are in the form of names, letters, or numbers. Filing requires personnel, space and equipment – all of which amount to a great expense. It is advisable to select a simple and quick filing system and to file only necessary items. Dental offices often file many more papers than are needed. These extra papers take up time, space and equipment unnecessarily. Papers that could be discarded are a main source of inefficiency. Organizing the files not only means deciding how to collect and put records in order, but also means establishing rules for eliminating unnecessary ones. Once items are filed, it is necessary to have a system for eliminating them when they become useless.

Protection of records from becoming damaged, lost, or burned is accomplished by proper storing facilities. Vital records should be kept in fire-proof cabinets or filed in vaults when not in use. Vital records include contracts, stockholder records, official financial records, tax records and any other records that cannot be easily replaced, yet are necessary for the operation of the dental office. *Microfilming,* a process of photographing records on rolls, strips or individual clips, is recommended for providing copies of permanent records as a way to protect against possible loss of the originals. A survey of 100 businesses whose records had been destroyed showed that only 57 of them were able to resume operation.

Frequently used records must be convenient for the office worker to retrieve quickly. Accuracy in filing is a must if a business is to operate at maximum efficiency. The telephone is being used more and more to obtain information. If the information requested is not readily accessible and easily retrievable, the time of both the caller and the receiver of the call is inefficiently used. If the call is long distance, it is even more expensive to waste time looking for requested material that has not been filed or has been incorrectly filed.

Control of records means knowing where the records are at all times, using sound methods of charge and transfer, and destroying the records when they become old and of little or no value. When material becomes inactive, it should be placed in an inactive file. Two methods used for transferring inactive files are the perpetual and the periodic. *Perpetual transfer* is removing inactive material from the active files as soon as it becomes inactive. The *periodic transfer* is made at stated intervals, determined by the needs of the office.

Experience is a good guide to determine what records to retain and for how long. The records retention system should be designed to fit the needs of the particular dental office. After observing for a few months how often records are used, a decision can be made about the selection of procedures for the type of records to be retained. The location and the space required must also be considered. A dental office is required by law to keep certain information such as wage-hour data and income tax figures. State and federal income tax returns and the records which verify the figures on the tax returns should be kept at least six years.

Different methods of filing are needed to meet the needs of different dental offices. These methods are alphabetic, numeric, geographic and subject. However, all systems of filing are based on the alphabet. This use of the alphabet in filing is explained in the following brief descriptions of the methods.

In *alphabetic filing,* records are filed according to the sequence of the alphabet. The secretarial dental assistant should be very familiar with the alphabet so she can begin at any point without hesitation and know what letters come before and after a given letter.

In *numeric filing,* records are filed by number. For example, in a dental office each patient may be assigned a number. The patient's folders are then filed in numerical order. Because one cannot remember a series of numbers easily, an alphabetic card file is needed as an index to the number files. Each patient would have a card with his index number on it.

The *geographic method,* which is filing by location, and the *subject method,* which is filing according to the main topic of the record or document, are actually alphabetic filing systems as all materials are filed in alphabetical order. These methods will be discussed in more detail in the next unit.

NEED FOR BASIC RULES

In filing, rules are necessary for consistency. Basic or standardized rules have been established yet every dental office must agree on specific rules for its particular needs. For example, should John McNair be filed in straight alphabetic sequence? Or should the "Mcs" and "Macs" be put together as if all were spelled "Mac?" To avoid inconsistency, these specific rules should be understood by everyone who has the authority to work with the files. The rules should be recorded in writing for easy reference by the secretarial dental assistant. They will be particularly helpful for the new employees who are responsible for filing. To avoid errors in filing, it is generally better to have as few people as possible do the storing and retrieving.

BASIC INDEXING RULES FOR ALPHABETIC FILING

Alphabetic filing is the basis for all methods of filing. If the basic rules for arranging names in alphabetic sequence are followed, mistakes in filing can be eliminated.

For filing purposes, names are separated in parts called *units*. For example, "Norma Jill Morris" consists of three units. Determining the order of the units is called *indexing*.

The following indexing rules should be studied and applied to insure consistency in filing. The examples give names and their indexing arrangement by units.

Rule 1.   SURNAMES

1-a.   The surname of an individual is considered the first unit; the given name is the second unit, the middle name is the third unit.

Units

	1	2	3
Bertha Lee Brown	Brown	Bertha	Lee
Mary Ann Milner	Milner	Mary	Ann

1-b.   Prefixes of a surname such as *La, Del, Mac, O',* and *Van* are considered as part of the surname and not as separate indexing units regardless of whether the surname is written as one word or two.

	1	2	3
John Del Monica	Del Monica	John	
Melvin Leo La Vail	La Vail	Melvin	Leo

1-c.   Hyphenated surnames are considered as one unit.

	1	2
Mary Lansing	Lansing	Mary
Helen Lans-Worth	Lans-Worth	Helen
Louise Miller-Jones	Miller-Jones	Louise

1-d.   Names are arranged in alphabetical order. Only the first units are considered if they are different. If the first units are the same, the second units are considered. The third units are considered if the first and second units are the same.

	1	2	3
Martha Ann Martin	Martin	Martha	Ann
Martha Jane Martin	Martin	Martha	Jane
Peggy Martin	Martin	Peggy	

1-e.   When the surname only is used, it is filed before a surname used with an initial or a given name. This rule may be remembered as "Nothing comes before something."

	1	2
Brown	Brown	
W. Brown	Brown	W.
Wood Brown	Brown	Wood

Rule 2. BUSINESS FIRMS AND ASSOCIATIONS

2-a.   Firm names and organizations are filed as written, unless they contain the full name of an individual. They are indexed in the same way as the name of an individual.

	1	2	3	4
Hays Gift Shop	Hays	Gift	Shop	
Taylor Hays Gift Shop	Hays	Taylor	Gift	Shop
National Secretaries Association	National	Secretaries	Association	

2-b.   Unimportant words such as articles, conjunctions and prepositions are not indexing units. When one comes at the beginning of a name, it is placed in parentheses at the end of the last unit. If one comes in the middle of a name, it is placed in parentheses beside the word after which it occurs.

	1	2	3
The Handy Shop	Handy	Shop (The)	
Carl Sills & Associates	Sills (&)	Carl	Associates

2-c.   Hyphenated words in a firm name are considered as separate units. Hyphenated surnames, as stated previously, are considered as one unit even when used as part of a firm name.

	1	2	3	4
Lee-Witt Dental Office	Lee-	Witt	Dental	Office
Robert Lee-Witt Dental Office	Lee-Witt	Robert	Dental	Office
Philco-Ford Corp.	Philco-	Ford	Corporation	

2-d.   Names that may be written as one or two words are considered as one unit.

	1	2	3
Airport Motel	Airport	Motel	
Municipal Air Port	Municipal	Air Port	
South West High School	South West	High	School
Southwest Lumber Co.	Southwest	Lumber	Company

Rule 3. ABBREVIATIONS

Abbreviations are indexed as if the words represented were spelled out. Single letters that are not abbreviations are considered as separate units.

	1	2	3	4
Chas. M. Mosley	Mosley	Charles	M.	
St. Paul Motel	Saint	Paul	Motel	
XYZ Company	X	Y	Z	Company

Rule 4. COMPOUND GEOGRAPHIC NAMES

Each word in a compound geographic name is a separate indexing unit except foreign prefixes such as *San* in *San Francisco.*

	1	2	3	4
Los Angeles Mobile Homes	Los Angeles	Mobile	Homes	
New Jersey Truck Lines	New	Jersey	Truck	Lines
New York News	New	York	News	

Rule 5. TITLES OR DEGREES

5-a. Titles and degrees are not indexing units unless the title is followed by only one name. The name is then filed as written.

5-b. Terms such as *Jr., Sr., IV,* are filing units and when placed on filing cards or folders, they are written in parentheses at the end of the name.

5-c. College and university degrees may be considered as the last filing unit when needed for identification.

	1	2	3	4
Mrs. Beverly Morris	Morris	Beverly (Mrs.)		
Dr. Fred Norman	Norman	Fred (Dr.)		
Princess Ann	Princess	Ann		
John Hill, Jr.	Hill	John	(Jr.)	
John Hill, Sr.	Hill	John	(Sr.)	
R.M. Jones	Jones	R.	M.	
R.M. Jones, D.D.S	Jones	R.	M.	(D.D.S.)

Rule 6. MARRIED WOMEN

The legal name of a married woman is used for filing. Her husband's surname is the first unit, her given name the second unit, and either her middle name or her maiden surname is the third unit. "Mrs." is put in parentheses at the end of the name. Her husband's name is placed in parentheses below.

	1	2	3
Mrs. Thomas A. Grant (Sue Elaine)	Grant (Thomas A.)	Sue	Elaine (Mrs.)
Mrs. John Johnson (Mary Jones)	Johnson (John)	Mary	Jones (Mrs.)

Rule 7.   POSSESSIVES

Disregard the apostrophe in possessives.

	1	2	3
May's Dress Shop	May ('s)	Dress	Shop
Mays Brothers	Mays	Brothers	
Mays' Dress Shop	Mays(')	Dress	Shop

Rule 8.   GOVERNMENT NAMES

8-a.   Federal Government names are indexed under United States Government as the first three units, followed by the name of the department, and then by the bureau, division, board, or commission. In governmental names *Department of, Division of, Kingdom of* are not indexing units and are placed in parentheses at the end of the name. Foreign government names are indexed first under the names of countries.

	1	2	3	4
Ministry of Defense Kingdom of Denmark	Denmark (Kingdom of)	Defense (Ministry of)		
U.S. Dept. of Agriculture	United	States	Government	Agriculture (Dept. of)
Internal Revenue Service	United	States	Government	Internal Revenue

8-b.   Names of other government divisions are indexed under the name of the political division followed by its classification, such as state, county, or city and then by the department, bureau, division, commission, or board.

	1	2	3
Fire Dept . of the City of Clinton	Clinton	City	Fire (Department of)
Parks Dept. of the State of Kentucky	Kentucky	State	Parks (Department of)

Rule 9.   NUMBERS

Index a number in a name as if it were spelled in letters. Numbers over 1,000, such as 2,615, should be filed as twenty-six hundred fifteen, not as two thousand, six hundred fifteen.

	1	2	3	4
The 5th Street Warehouse	Fifth	Street	Warehouse (The)	
12th Avenue Townhouse	Twelfth	Avenue	Townhouse	
22nd St. Supply House	Twenty-second	Street	Supply	House

Rule 10. ADDRESSES

The name of the firm is indexed first, followed by the city or town, then the state. If the same name is located at different addresses in the same city, the street name is considered. The street number is considered if the same name is located at different addresses on the same street, in which case the arrangement is from the lowest to the highest street number.

	1	2	3	4	5	6
Howard Bros., Cleveland, MS	Howard	Brothers	Cleveland	MS		
Howard Bros., Cleveland, OH	Howard	Brothers	Cleveland	OH		
Howard Bros., 60 Ellis Ave., Jackson TN	Howard	Brothers	Jackson	TN	Ellis Ave.	60
Howard Bros. 960 Ellis Ave., Jackson, TN	Howard	Brothers	Jackson	TN	Ellis Ave.	960

Rule 11. BANK NAMES

General bank names are indexed first by the city, then by the name of the bank. When the city and bank names are the same, the state name is considered.

	1	2	3	4	5
First National Bank Durham, N.C.	Durham	First	National	Bank	(N.C.)
First National Bank Greenville, S.C.	Greenville	First	National	Bank	(S.C.)
People's Bank & Trust Co. Hartford, Conn.	Hartford	People's	Bank (and)	Trust	Company

FILING PROCEDURES

The secretarial dental assistant may be responsible for processing all of the incoming correspondence. If so, she will find it beneficial to follow certain preliminary procedures to filing. Incoming correspondence should be sorted according to whom the mail is addressed. At the time the mail is opened, it should be time stamped with the current date and then delivered to the proper person. When the correspondence has been answered or has received the necessary attention, the person who received the correspondence will release it for filing by putting his initials and usually the current date on it.

There are five steps to follow when processing records to be filed. These steps are:

- *Inspect* the record to be filed. The paper should have a release mark to indicate that the paper is ready to be filed.

- *Index* the record. Decide under what name, subject or number the item should be filed. The caption should be the name according to the filing rules used by the dental office.

- *Code* the record by underlining the name under which it is to be filed; or if the name is not on the paper, record it in the upper right-hand corner. If the material may be asked for by a name other than the one coded, underline or write the cross-referencing caption and place an "X" in the margin beside the caption.

- *Sort* the papers to be filed. For example, sort in several stacks on a counter or desk, such as A-E, F-J, K-O, P-T, U-Z. Then sort by putting each letter in a separate stack. Arrange each stack in alphabetical order and place the stack together keeping the alphabetical arrangement.

- *Store* the record in a file container. The material is usually put in a folder with the heading to the left; then it is placed behind the proper guide in a cabinet or on an open shelf. This step is called *storing*.

Records should be filed as soon as possible after they have been released. Items should never be allowed to accumulate on the desk. It is less time-consuming to file daily than to have to look for the materials in the files (where they should be) and then look through the papers on the desk before they are found.

The use of copying machines allows the secretarial dental assistant to give a copy of requested material to be taken from the office rather than the original. This keeps materials from being lost as copies do not have to be returned. If the same material is needed by someone else, the original document will be available. If copies cannot be made, an OUT guide should be placed in the files. This guide contains a requisition form showing who has the material, when it will be returned and any other necessary information. Confidential records should be protected in files which are only used by those who have the authority.

SETTING UP A FILE SYSTEM

A few important considerations that should be reviewed when setting up a new filing system or changing the old filing system are:

- The type of records to be filed, and, thus, the method or methods to be used.

- The space available for filing equipment. The width of the aisle for four-drawer files should be 54-60 inches.

- What type of files (drawer, lateral, open-shelf, rotary, visible card, electrofile) are most suitable for the office.

- How frequently records will be needed.

- The amount of money available for filing purposes.

The filing method to use is determined by the type of records to be filed. Most dental offices use vertical filing (filing papers on edge) rather than horizontal filing (filing papers flat) to save space; it also saves time in storing and retrieving.

A small dental office may use only the alphabetic file for the patients' folders and a subject file for special papers such as tax records, current invoices, bank records, continuing education material, and correspondence. The larger dental office may use the numeric system and perhaps the open-shelf file for patients' records. In this case, an alphabetic card file is needed for recalling patients' numbers.

The revolving, circular open-shelf file in which the patients' records are filed numerically, using a color code, is popular in today's dental office. Some dental offices use the

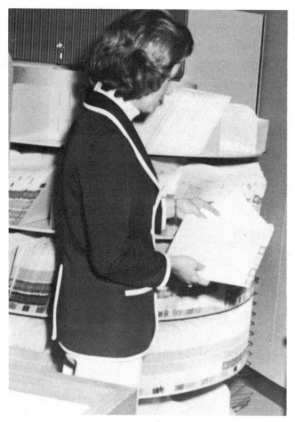

Fig. 26-1 Revolving circular open-shelf file in which records are filed numerically, using a color code.

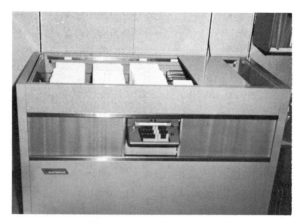

Fig. 26-2 An electrofile.

electrofile for financial records. Each patient is given a code number; when this code number is punched on the electrofile keys, the card needed is pushed up through the unit.

Filing supplies can be purchased from office supply stores. Dental supply houses have special folders designed for the dental office. The most commonly used filing supplies includes guides (primary and secondary), regular folders, hanging folders, cards, out guides, tickler files, cross-reference sheets, gummed labels, transparent gummed tape, thumbers (rubber fingerguards), colored pencils and fasteners.

SUMMARY

Filing is the organization, protection and control of records. A systematic organization of files, the proper filing equipment, and well-trained personnel will help a business to run smoothly and efficiently and will save the dental office hundreds of dollars.

The types of records to be filed determine the methods of filing to be used. The four methods of filing are alphabetic, numeric, geographic and subject. In alphabetic filing, basic rules have been established to insure consistency. For accuracy in storing and retrieving, it is necessary to follow the proper preliminary procedures to filing: opening the mail, time stamping it, delivering it to the receiver, giving it the necessary attention and releasing it for filing. When the correspondence has been released for filing, the secretarial dental assistant will follow five steps in processing it: inspecting, indexing, coding, sorting, and storing. Before purchasing filing equipment and supplies, consideration should be given to the type of records to be filed, the space available, and the budget for filing purposes.

SUGGESTED ACTIVITIES

- Make arrangements to visit a modern dental office; ask the person responsible for filing to explain the office filing system. Discuss the system with the class.

- Ask the manager of a dental supply house or an office equipment company to show and demonstrate some of the latest equipment and aids being used in filing. Prepare a report for class discussion.

REVIEW

A. Select the correct answer and place the letter before the item.

_____ 1. All systems of filing are based on (a) subjects, (b) the alphabet, (c) numbers, (d) names.

_____ 2. To store and find records effectively, it is necessary to follow indexing rules that are (a) standardized, (b) inconsistent, (c) made by the file clerk, (d) generalized.

_____ 3. Deciding the order in which the units in a name are to be considered for filing is (a) coding, (b) inspecting, (c) indexing, (d) alphabetizing.

_____ 4. Underlining the name or recording it in the upper right-hand corner is called (a) indexing, (b) coding, (c) releasing, (d) inspecting.

_____ 5. The first step to follow when processing materials to be filed is (a) coding, (b) indexing, (c) inspecting, (d) sorting.

_____ 6. Filing records on edge is called (a) lateral filing, (b) alphabetic filing, (c) horizontal filing, (d) vertical filing.

_____ 7. Incoming correspondence should be opened and stamped with (a) the employer's initials, (b) the date on the correspondence, (c) the current date, (d) the file clerk's initials.

_____ 8. Before a record is considered for filing the clerk should check it for (a) release marks, (b) the code name, (c) cross references, (d) the time stamp.

_____ 9. When you are placing records in folders, the headings should (a) face you and to the left, (b) face you and to the right, (c) be upright, (d) be at the crease of the folder.

_____ 10. The symbol "X" is used to indicate (a) the correspondence has been inspected, (b) the correspondence is released for filing, (c) a cross reference, (d) the correspondence has not been answered.

_____ 11. File guides are used (a) for faster and more efficient reference, (b) to speed the proper distribution of papers, (c) for support, (d) all of the above.

_____ 12. Transferring material from active files to inactive as soon as they become inactive is called (a) periodic transfer, (b) one-period transfer, (c) two-period transfer, (d) perpetual transfer.

B.   Matching

Read each item in Column I; select the term in Column II that best fits the description. Place the letter before the item.

Column I

_____ 1. The organization, protection and control of information.

_____ 2. Removing inactive materials from the active files
when they become inactive.

_____ 3. Transferring materials at
stated intervals as determined by the needs of
the office.

_____ 4. Filing according to the
main topic of the record.

_____ 5. Filing by location.

_____ 6. For filing purposes, names
are separated into these
parts.

_____ 7. Placed in the files when a
record or folder is removed.

_____ 8. Moving records from the
active to the inactive files.

_____ 9. Placing papers in their
proper folders.

_____ 10. A form showing the name
of the borrower of the records and the date the records are due.

_____ 11. Placing a notation or copy
in a file to indicate where
the original record is filed.

_____ 12. A process of photographing records on rolls, strips
or individual clips.

_____ 13. Popular in today's dental
office as it helps one to
determine at a glance if a
folder has been misfiled.

Column II

a. carrier
b. coding
c. color coding
d. cross referencing
e. filing
f. geographic filing
g. indexing
h. inspecting
i. microfilming
j. out guide
k. periodic transfer
l. perpetual transfer
m. requisition
n. storing
o. subject filing
p. time stamping
q. transferring
r. units

C. Alphabetic Filing.

After each group, indicate the order in which the names given should be arranged in an alphabetic file.

Example: (a) Martha Ann Lees; (b) Roy M. Johnson; (c) Johnson's Supply House   <u>bca</u>

1. (a) Harry McDowell; (b) John A. Dowell; (c) Harry McDuff   _____

2. (a) Mrs. George Lester (Elaine); (b) Jerry C. Ladner; (c) J.C. Lester   _____

3. (a) Jessie R. Watkins; (b) Mary Watkin; (c) Watkin's Equipment Company   _____

4. (a) First National Bank, Tulsa OK; (b) Col. Robert Fitz; (c) Margaret Ann Fitz   _____

5. (a) 10th Street Warehouse; (b) 100 Steak House; (c) Steve W. Thomas   _____

6. (a) Mack's, 253 Main Street, Orlando; (b) Mack's, 1253 Main Street, Orlando; (c) Mack's, 1500 Second Street, Ormond Beach   _____

7. (a) Professor Helms; (b) Helms Dental Office; (c) B.W. Helms   _____

8. (a) Police Dept., City of Detroit; (b) Janice M. Palmer; (c) Palmer's   _____

9. (a) U.S. Dept. of Defense; (b) Dottie's Beauty Shop; (c) Donald Dixon   _____

10. (a) Mrs. Jan Martin; (b) Martin Electric Company; (c) J.J. Martin   _____

11. (a) ABC Contracting Company; (b) Mary Abbott; (c) Doctor Melvin Abbott   _____

12. (a) Lee-Witt Paper Company; (b) Austin Lee-Witt; (c) Lee County Courthouse   _____

13. (a) Airport Restaurant; (b) Air Port Limousine Service; (c) The Antique Shop   _____

14. (1) (a) The Dental Specialty Company; (b) Rocky Mountain Dental Products Company; (c) Cleveland Dental Manufacturing Co.   _____

15. (a) M.F. Nations Dental Supply Company; (b) Jones Dental Laboratories; (c) Malone Dental Specialty Company   _____

Unit 27 Comprehensive Filing

OBJECTIVES

After studying this unit, the student should be able to

- Describe the alphabetic, subject and numeric methods of filing.

- List the advantages of the terminal digit system.

- Explain what records are kept in the active, inactive, and the accounts receivable files.

- List the steps in processing slides for filing.

- State what records should be kept in a dentist's office and how long they should be retained.

The secretarial dental assistant who gives careful attention to records at the patient's first visit will save much time, work and expense.   The correct spelling of a new patient's name and his accurate mailing address and telephone number in legible writing is essential to avoid errors in filing. Although errors may be discovered later, it is difficult and time-consuming to amend mistakes that have been recorded in several different places, such as the patient treatment and account records, the recall files, the birthday files, the radiograph files and even visible index files.   A patient wants his name spelled and pronounced correctly. The secretarial dental assistant should not hesitate to ask the patient to spell his name or to repeat his address and telephone number.   If the name has an unusual pronunciation, the name should be written phonetically beside the correctly spelled name. The majority of errors in filing records   are caused by failure to obtain the correct spelling of names (Catherine, Katherine), illegible handwriting (C, G), and transposing first name and surname (Allen Douglas, Douglas Allen).

FILING METHODS

Although there are four methods of filing, a dental office may use the alphabetic, the subject and the numeric filing methods.

The alphabetic method is generally used in the small dental office for patients' treatment records and financial records. An aid in filing is the *Variadex* in which color is used to speed up the location of materials and to prevent misfiling. The primary guide and the tabs on the corresponding folders have the same color.

The subject file is used for withholding and FICA tax records, invoices, bank records, dental supplies, and continuing education ma-

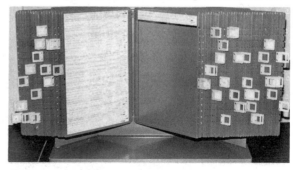

Fig. 27-1 A visible index file to the patient's assigned treatment number. Notice space is available to add names.

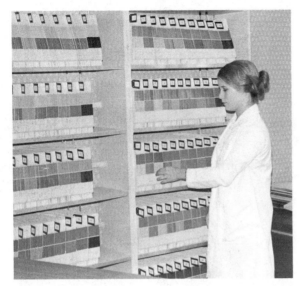

Fig. 27-2 A stationary open-shelf file may be effectively used.

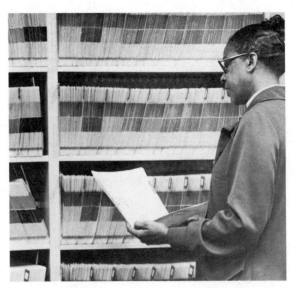

Fig. 27-3 Patient records being placed in folders prior to being filed in the stationary open-shelf file.

terial. The subjects are arranged in alphabetical order, and the materials within each subject are in alphabetical order. Records with the same code are filed by date, with the latest date forward.

There are different kinds of numeric systems used for handling patients' folders. The small dental office may use the *serial numeric system,* in which items are consecutively numbered. A more popular form for the large dental office is the *terminal digit system* in which the numbers are broken into groups. The last digits are read first. As an example of this system, the number 331255 would be shown as 33 12 55. The record would be stored in drawer or shelf 55, folder 12; 33 would determine where it would be filed in the folder. This method for use in large dental offices has several advantages:

- It eliminates the difficulty of filing almost identical names.

- It expedites locating and storing a patient's folder.

- It is convenient to use with shelf files which are less expensive than cabinet files.

- It makes for a uniform distribution of records.

As previously stated, the rotating, circular open-shelf files in which the records are color-coded and filed numerically are popular in many modern dental offices.

KINDS OF FILES

Most dental offices have active, inactive, and accounts receivable files. There may also be separate files for patient treatment records and patient account records. The treatment records are located in either the active or inactive files. The active files contain the folders of all patients who are expected to return as patients in the future. The patient's account records are placed in a card file as long as the patient's treatment folder is active. As mentioned previously, the electrofile may be used for patients' financial records. When the folder becomes inactive, the account record is placed in the patient's envelope for storage in the inactive files.

If space permits, it is good business to keep inactive records as long as possible. Some people return to their former dentists after many years for special work. These inactive folders can be placed in inexpensive corrugated files and stored outside the business office.

When a folder is filed in an inactive file, the radiographic mounts are removed. The radiographs are placed in a coin envelope which is labeled with the date the X rays were taken. All paper clips are removed. Any other records concerning the patient, such as recall control cards and birthday recall cards, should be placed in the patient's envelope. The reason for removing the records to the inactive files should be written on the patient's record card. The secretarial dental assistant must be familiar with the statute of limitations in her state regarding the number of years that a patient's records must be retained and the length of time the records of a deceased patient should be retained. The state attorney can furnish this information.

If the dental office uses a separate accounts receivable file, it contains those records of patients whose work has been completed but whose bill has not been paid in full.

FILING COLOR SLIDES

The modern dental office will probably have color slides. It is helpful to use color slides of certain dental conditions to show to patients who may have these same conditions. Slides may also be used for lectures. The slides should be properly filed so they are easily available at any time.

Roy R. Kracke, DMD, has suggested the following steps for filing slides:[1]

- As pictures are taken, the film roll number, patient's name, subject of slide and the date are recorded on an index card.

- A serial number is assigned to each slide and written on the mount.

---

[1] Roy R. Kracke, DMD, "A System of Filing and Classifying Clinical Slides," from *The Dental Assistant*, Nov. 1970. Copyright American Dental Assistants Association, reprinted by permission.

- The slides are filed numerically in a slide storage cabinet.

Another index card is made for each patient. On it are recorded the serial number of all slides made of that patient's mouth, the dates they were taken and the subject of each slide. Slides can be found in the numerical filing cabinet for any patient by taking the serial numbers from the patient's index card, which is filed alphabetically by the patient's name.

The slides should also be classified by subject, such as stomatitis, fractured incisors, dental anomalies, etc. A notebook is used to record the patient's name and serial numbers of his slides under the appropriate subject. This enables the secretarial dental assistant to find a series of slides showing a treatment of a similar condition to a patient. It also provides material for lectures or speeches. Radiographs provide a necessary addition to regular color slides. Mounts for original radiographs or their duplicates can be obtained from a local dental supply company. The name of the patient whose dental condition is shown on the slides is not given to any other patient. Patient's records are confidential!

RETENTION OF RECORDS

What records should a dentist keep in order to operate his practice successfully? What records need special protection from disasters, such as fires and storms? Deciding what ordinary records to keep depends upon the needs of the individual dental office. Experience is a guide for determining what records to retain and the length of time to retain them. Records that may be essential to recover losses and to get the business back into operation should be able to survive a disaster.

Businesses are required by law to keep certain information such as income tax records and payroll data. The Fair Labor Standards Act requires that information on employees wages and hours be kept for three years. Time cards and piecework tickets need to be kept only two years. Personnel records, such as applications and attendance records, should be retained according to the needs of the office. For example, personnel folders are usually kept for one year after the employee leaves. As a rule, all accounting records should be retained at least until the annual audit of the books is completed. The general ledger is the account summary and should be retained indefinitely. Tax returns for state and federal income tax and records which verify the figures on the returns are very important records and should be kept at least six years. One should check with the local authorities to determine how long to keep payroll records which include deductions for federal income taxes and social security taxes as state requirements vary.

SUMMARY

The secretarial dental assistant must give careful attention to recording information accurately, especially on the patients' first visit.

The three methods of filing that may be used in a dental office are alphabetic, numeric and subject. Most dental offices keep active, inactive and accounts receivable files.

Slides can be used to explain dental conditions to patients and as material for lectures given by the dentist.

It is important for the secretarial dental assistant to know what records the law requires a dental office to keep, what records the business needs to keep in order to operate efficiently and how long the different records should be retained.

SUGGESTED ACTIVITIES

- Submit a report on the management of dental records. Use current periodicals and dental texts as resource reading.

- Contact a local dentist who uses a successful method of filing color slides. Make arrangements for him, or a member of his dental team, to explain the method to the class.

- Visit a dental office and ask the secretarial dental assistant to explain the kinds of files used for the patients' folders. Report your findings to the class.

REVIEW

A.   Multiple Choice.

Review and select the correct answer.

1.   The best way to avoid misspelling a patient's name is to

a. ask the patient to spell his name.

b. spell the name the way it sounds.

c. let the patient write his name.

d. ask the dentist how to spell the patient's name.

2. The method most commonly used for filing withholding and FICA records is the

   a. alphabetic.

   b. numeric.

   c. geographic.

   d. subject.

3. The method most popular for filing patients' folders in a large dental office is the

   a. alphabetic.

   b. serial numeric.

   c. terminal digit numeric.

   d. geographic

   e. subject.

4. The open shelf files for patients' treatment records are

   a. more expensive than the cabinet files.

   b. not as popular today as the cabinet files.

   c. not used in large dental offices.

   d. frequently used because of their convenience in locating and retrieving patients' folders.

5. For patients' folders, most dental offices have

   a. only active files.

   b. active and inactive files.

   c. active, inactive and accounts receivable files.

6. The patient treatment records are found in the

   a. active files.

   b. inactive files.

   c. active or inactive files.

   d. accounts receivable files.

7. When a patient's folder is filed in an inactive file

   a. the radiographic mounts are removed and the radiograph placed in a coin envelope.

   b. paper clips are removed.

   c. records concerning the patient, such as recall cards, are placed in the patient's envelope.

   d. all of the above.

   e. none of the above.

8. The accounts receivable file contains

   a. records of patients whose work has been completed but not paid in full.

   b. records of patients who have paid in full.

   c. invoices of purchases made by the dental office.

9. Color slides of dental conditions are

   a. generally filed numerically and also classified by subject.

   b. used to educate patients who may have a similar condition.

   c. used with lectures given by the dentist.

   d. all of the above.

10. The Fair Labor Standards Act requires information on employees' wages and hours to be kept for

    a. one year.

    b. three years.

    c. five years.

    d. ten years.

B. Answer the following questions

   1. Name three causes for errors in spelling which affect filing.

   2. List three advantages of the terminal digit system.

   3. Name the three types of files where patients' folders are kept.

   4. What two factors determine the retention of records?

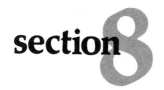
Office Supplies and Equipment

Unit 28 Office Machines

OBJECTIVES

After studying this unit, the student should be able to

- State the reasons why a typewriter is an essential office machine.
- Demonstrate the correct use of an adding machine.
- List the advantages of dictation equipment.
- State the purpose of a check writer and an imprint device.

There are several office machines that are used in the modern dental office. The secretarial dental assistant should be proficient in operating all of the machines present in the office. A special file should be kept in the dental office on the operation and maintenance of the office machines. All of the operating manuals should be included and the sections on caring for the various machines should be earmarked in each manual for easy reference. The manufacturer's directions must always be followed in using and caring for the office machines.

The office machines most commonly found in the modern dental office are:

- Typewriter
- Adding machine or calculator
- Duplicating equipment
- Dictation equipment
- Check writer
- Postage meter

There are numerous companies that manufacture these machines. The various machines illustrated in this unit are only examples of the many makes and models of machines that may be found in dental offices. Regardless of the make of the machine, operating instructions are similar in nature.

THE TYPEWRITER

Most dental offices regard the typewriter as an essential office machine. Correspondence from the dental office appears much more professional and legible when typed. Many offices prefer to type patient ledger cards or treatment records. Insurance forms that are typed are much more legible than the hand-written forms.

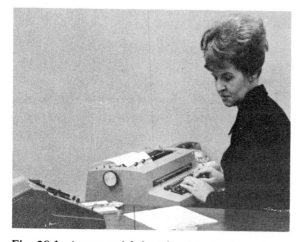

Fig. 28-1 A secretarial dental assistant using a typewriter.

256

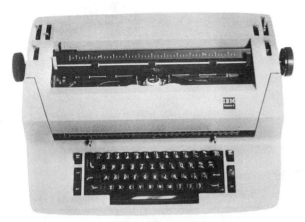

Fig. 28-2 An IBM Selectric II Typewriter.

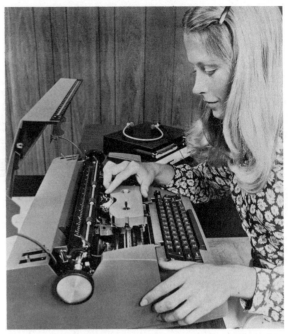

Fig. 28-3 A secretarial dental assistant installing the new IBM Tech II Ribbon in the IBM Selectric II Typewriter.

The typewriter which is selected for the dental office should be one that meets all the typing needs of the office. A manual or electric typewriter may be selected. An electric typewriter is suggested for the dental office with a heavy typing load. An IBM "Selectric" model is a machine that may be found in some dental offices, figure 28-2. The special feature of this typewriter is a small globe-shaped element. The element contains all of the type characters. Several different styles of typing elements may be selected. It is even possible to purchase several different elements at a nominal cost; the elements may be changed on the typewriter to fit the needs of the correspondence. This would permit the dental office to have different sizes and types of print for the one machine — a very useful feature for the busy office that requires typing a variety of forms. The elements may be changed in just a few seconds. One element is lifted off and quickly replaced with the second element. Since type bars are eliminated, type clash is also eliminated. The carriage does not move on this machine; this eliminates a lot of vibration and provides more work area around the machine.

An *impression control* feature allows the secretarial dental assistant to set the force with which the element strikes the paper. The higher the number on the control is set, the harder the element strikes. This feature is very useful when typing forms with several carbon copies. For example, the W-2 federal form must be typed so that all six copies are legible. The impression control feature is very helpful in preparing this type of form. The secretarial dental assistant may type for long periods of time without becoming tired. The keys are constructed so that only a very light touch is necessary to type accurately.

Ribbons, whether film or fabric, are very easily changed on this typewriter. Since the ribbons are contained in a cartridge, ribbon changing is quick, easy, and clean. A different ribbon color or a fresh ribbon may be put on within a few seconds.

The typewriter should be cared for according to the operating instructions provided by the manufacturer. When using the electric typewriter, be sure to turn the machine off when not in use. At the end of the day the electrical cord should be unplugged before leaving the office. The typewriter should always

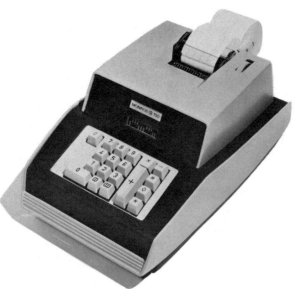

Fig. 28-4 Monroe 150 ten key adding machine.

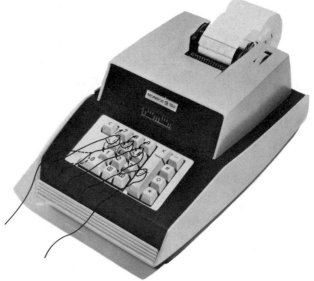

Fig. 28-5 A diagram of the proper use of a ten key keyboard.

be covered when not in use for indefinite periods of time. The cover should always be in position before leaving the office at the end of the day. Erasing should be kept to a minimum. Again, follow the operating instructions provided by the manufacturer. A special maintenance agreement may be contracted with the local representative of the typewriter company. A maintenance agreement provides preventive maintenance and emergency service during business hours. It may be less expensive in the long run for the dental office to contract such an agreement.

ADDING MACHINE OR CALCULATOR

An adding machine or calculator is an essential office machine in any dental office. All calculations — adding, subtracting, multiplying, or dividing — must be absolutely correct. The daily, monthly, and yearly financial totals must be correct. The auditor may use these totals for figuring income tax. Also, the dentist wants to know, on a daily basis, the financial status of the working day. The accounting on the patient's financial (ledger) cards must be correct to insure that both the office and the patient are receiving and remit-

ting the proper fees. Bank deposits must be added accurately to insure correct totals.

Making mistakes may result in costly errors for the dental office: Mistakes on patient records may result in unhappy patients. Patients may even leave the dental practice because of a simple error in addition. Because of the importance placed on the adding machine or calculator, care should be exercised in the selection of the machine; it should be one that will suit the needs of the individual dental office. The Monroe 150 and the Monroe 1305 are examples of machines that may be found in the modern dental office. The model 150 is an example of a modern compact ten key adding machine. A ten key machine such as this is simple to use. The number keys and the plus bar are concave in shape for easy touch. The keys in the middle which are known as the home keys are even more concave for easy location. The zero key is extended to the left.

One may learn to operate this type of machine in a few minutes. Assuming that the right hand is to be used in operating the machine, place the fingers over the keys, figure 28-5. The thumb should be positioned over

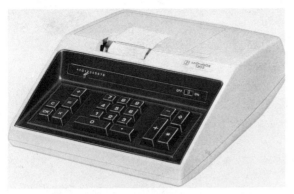

Fig. 28-6 A Monroe 1305 Printing Calculator.

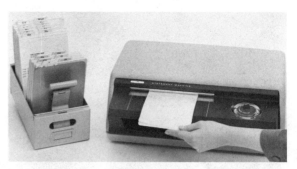

Fig. 28-7   Using ledger cards with a 3-M Statement Machine.

the zero key. The first finger is placed over the 4 key. The second finger over the 5 key, and the third finger over the 6 key. The fourth finger or little finger is then free to operate the mathematical symbol keys. Since three fingers are placed over the middle keys or home keys, it is very simple to depress any of the remaining keys. Subtraction or multiplication may also be done rapidly with this machine.

If the dental practice is a group practice a more functional machine such as an electronic printing calculator may be desired. A Monroe Model 1305 is an example of an electronic printing calculator; although more modern and functional in styling, it is also more expensive. A model such as this automatically responds to any operating pace. The open type keyboard accepts, calculates, and prints all operations as entered. A printing mechanism automatically shuts off when not in use. Any previous data remains undisturbed. The printing mechanism will automatically reactivate when work is resumed. This type of machine adds, subtracts, multiplies and divides. Operating instructions are not given for this type of model since instructions are similar to the model previously discussed.

COPYING EQUIPMENT

The most single reason for the dental office to acquire a copy machine is to aid in statement preparation. The average dental office does not have a large volume of straight copying to do other than statements. A copying machine should be selected that will copy both statement and business originals. A 3-M Statement Machine is one example of such a copier. This copier is compact enough

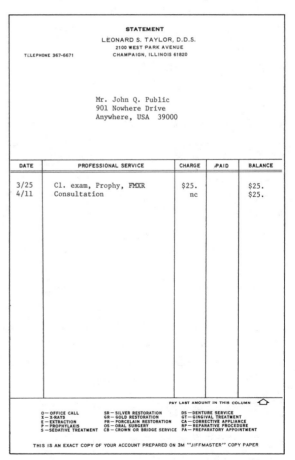

Fig. 28-8 A statement prepared on a 3-M Statement Machine.

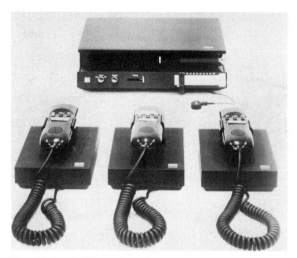

Fig. 28-9   A Microphone Input System which offers the convenience of remote dictation.

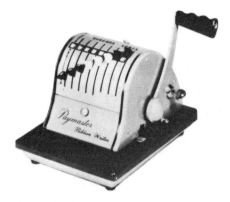

Fig. 28-10   Paymaster 8000 check writer.

to be placed on a desk top and plugged into any electrical outlet. No chemicals or powders are needed to operate it. This type of machine may be used in preparing statements from a pegboard (write-it-once) system. If ledger cards are used, these cards may simply be placed in the machine for an itemized statement to send to the patient. If a window envelope is used, the statement may be folded so that envelope addressing is eliminated.

White copies of business originals may be copied. The 3-M statement machine is even more versatile than just statement preparation and copying business originals. It is capable of laminating important documents with a plastic film, preparing transparencies from diagrams or hand-written notes, and addressing adhesive-backed mailing labels in seconds.

Learning how to operate duplicating equipment is usually simple if the operating instructions are followed. When equipment of this nature is delivered, a sales representative usually visits the office and demonstrates how to operate the equipment.

DICTATION EQUIPMENT

Many dentists desire to purchase dictation equipment to save time. It may be more

convenient for the dentist to dictate letters on a machine after hours rather than during working hours. The dentist may even prefer to take the unit home for days when heavy dictation is necessary. Dictation equipment allows the dentist to dictate whenever time permits; the secretarial dental assistant can then type the dictation at her convenience.

As with all office machines, numerous companies manufacture dictation equipment. The IBM Microphone Input System features remote indexing, built-in erase magnet, and telephone recording capability, figure 28-9; It is convenient to use because the dentist may originate, review what was said, give instructions, and indicate the end of the correspondence. Changes can be made by dictating over the unwanted material. If interrupted, the dentist can replay what was said previously in six-second increments. If the secretarial dental assistant has not had instruction in shorthand, dictation equipment can be very helpful.

CHECK WRITER

A check writer is a small machine that imprints the amount on checks, thus decreasing the possibility of the amount being changed. The check is inserted in the machine, keys of the check writer are raised to the desired amount, and a handle is pulled to inscribe the amount on the check. A visual window on the machine shows the amount selected; this eliminates errors as the secretarial dental assistant can see the amount before the handle is pulled. A signature prefix on the machine makes it impossible to add a digit to the amount of the check after the check has been imprinted. Most check writers are equipped with locks; the lock protects the office by preventing unauthorized and illegal use of the check writer. The Paymaster Series 8000 is an example of a check writer, figure 28-10.

MISCELLANEOUS

There may be other miscellaneous office machines used in the dental practice, such as an imprint machine or postage meter. An imprint machine is used for transferring informa-

tion from plastic credit cards. Postage machines were discussed in unit 20.

SUMMARY

Several office machines are used in the modern dental office. There are numerous companies that manufacture and sell many different styles and models of office machines. This allows the dentist to select the machine that best suits his dental practice. The adding machine/calculator and the typewriter are the most essential office machines for the dental office. The secretarial dental assistant should be proficient in operating all office machines. Regardless of the type of machine, the manufacturer's operating instructions should always be read and followed before operating the machine. Also, the machines should be cared for according to these instructions

SUGGESTED ACTIVITIES

- Secure and study brochures from several different companies which advertise dental office machines. Circulate them among your classmates.

- Make arrangements for a representative from a business machine company to speak to the class about available office machines for a dental office.

- Invite a secretarial science instructor to speak to the class about the care of office machines. Ask the instructor to demonstrate the use of at least two of the machines.

- If the machines are available, practice using all the machines described in this unit.

REVIEW

A. Select the best answer for the first six questions. The remaining questions require more than one answer.

    1. An electric typewriter is suggested for the dental office

        a. with a heavy patient load.

        b. with a heavy typing load.

        c. when it is a one-girl office.

        d. when delinquent accounts are difficult to collect.

2. Having several typing elements permits the dental office to

   a. have different sizes and types of print for one typewriter.
   b. type letters more professional looking.
   c. show patients how efficient the secretarial dental assistant is.
   d. set the force with which the element strikes.

3. Three home keys of a ten key adding machine or calculator are

   a. 1, 2, 3.   c. 7, 8, 9.
   b. 3, 4, 5.   d. 4, 5, 6.

4. Copying equipment is usually purchased for the purpose of

   a. aiding with statement preparation.
   b. making transparencies for the dentist to use in patient education presentations.
   c. making extra copies of business letters.
   d. typing names and addresses on patient folders.

5. An imprint machine is used in the dental office for

   a. printing collection notations on statements.
   b. making film mounts for the hygienist.
   c. transferring information from plastic credit cards.
   d. protecting the dentist against the misuse of checks.

6. Using a check writer in the dental office eliminates

   a. check writing at the end of the month.
   b. the need for the office to purchase personalized checks.
   c. the patients charging dental services.
   d. the possibility of the amount on checks being changed.

7. A typewriter is an essential office machine in the dental office because

   a. it impresses the patient to see office equipment.
   b. typed correspondence appears much more professional looking.
   c. the secretarial dental assistant may desire to type appointment cards.
   d. typed correspondence is neater and more legible than handwritten correspondence.
   e. it establishes good rapport with children by letting them type while waiting for the dentist.

8. An impression control feature on a typewriter allows the secretarial dental assistant to

   a. automatically program the copies.
   b. adequately type multiple copies.
   c. easily change the ribbon in the cartridge.
   d. set the force with which the element strikes the paper.
   e. eliminate the type bars, thus avoiding type clash.

9. An adding machine or calculator is essential to the dental office because

   a. the daily, monthly, and yearly financial totals must be correct.
   b. the auditor may use the totals for figuring income tax.
   c. the dentist desires to know the correct daily financial status of the office.
   d. financial accounting on the ledger cards must be accurate.
   e. bank deposits must be added correctly.

10. Dictation equipment is helpful to the busy dentist because

    a. office correspondence is neater and more legible.
    b. letters may be dictated after office hours.
    c. statements are easier to prepare.
    d. business originals may be copied for future use.
    e. it allows the dentist to dictate at his convenience.
    f. it allows the secretarial dental assistant to type at her convenience.

B. Using an adding machine or calculator, perform the following ten calculations. After completing all problems, have someone check your answers for accuracy.

1.	2.	3.
25.50	803.87	1,018.25
506.30	1.73	44.96
418.95	302.18	1,530.57
585.99	52.03	699.14
177.40	791.95	5,806.28
21.53	43.90	3.92
.09	9.49	34.07
3.90	405.08	35.80
125.00	8.03	6,435.20
489.07	50.18	21.60
19.90	7.01	664.81
566.33	785.33	48.30
23.98	.68	4,893.78
10.02	2.03	10.00

4. 566.40
  - 147.28

5. 251.05
  - 89.01

6. 403.20
  - 97.50

7. 325 x 2.25 = _____

8. 628 x 246 = _____

9. 458 x 152 = _____

10. 2347 x 35 = _____

Unit 29 Supplies and Inventory

OBJECTIVES

After studying this unit, the student should be able to

- List four categories of dental supplies and describe what each category includes.
- Identify items classified as dental equipment.
- State guidelines helpful in ordering and storing dental supplies.

Every member of the dental health team has a responsibility to aid in the maintenance of dental supplies. Everyone must work together to insure that the proper supplies are ordered and received before they are needed.

Most operative procedures cannot be completed without certain supplies. The absence of a necessary item results in discomfort to the patient and loss of operative time by the dental team.

The dentist delegates the ordering, receiving, and storing of supplies to members of the dental health team. Usually one person is responsible for ordering supplies. However, every member must cooperate by informing the delegated person of supplies needed. Dental supply representatives usually furnish pads of "want lists" for the dental office to use. Sheets of the pad should be securely placed in each treatment area, the laboratory, and the darkroom. The sheets should always be placed in the same place each time so the delegated person may check the sheets daily or weekly. The delegated person may very likely be the secretarial dental assistant. Many times the chairside assistant is requested to remain in the treatment area at all times with the dentist. This request may not allow enough time to properly take care of the supplies. It may be that the secretarial dental assistant will have more time to adequately perform this task.

SUPPLY CATEGORIES

Supplies needed by the dental office can be divided into four categories:

- Expendable dental supplies

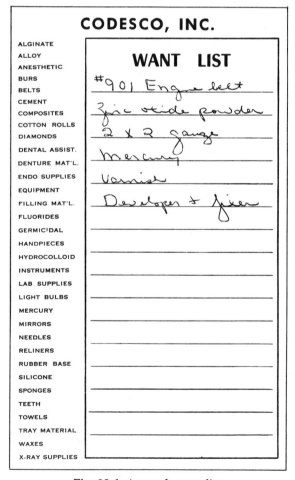

Fig. 29-1 A sample want list.

- Nonexpendable dental supplies
- Business office supplies
- Miscellaneous supplies

These four categories may include everything in the dental office with the exception of equipment.

Expendable dental supplies are those supplies which are used up periodically and must be reordered.   Examples of this category may be as follows:

- Mixing pads
- Cements
- Waxes
- Dental floss
- Radiographic film
- Disposable items such as saliva ejectors and needles
- Plaster and Stone
- Drugs
- Cotton rolls and pellets
- Discs
- Impression materials

Nonexpendable supplies include those dental supplies that are not used up periodically. However, they may have to be replaced if excessive wear is evident or if broken. These supplies include hand instruments, burs, handpieces, impression trays, glass slabs, rubber bowls, etc. Nonexpendable supplies may last a very long time if properly cared for.

Business office supplies are essential for the front desk and the dentist's private office. The following items are included in this category.

- Patient treatment records
- Stationery
- Statements
- Appointment cards
- Checkbooks

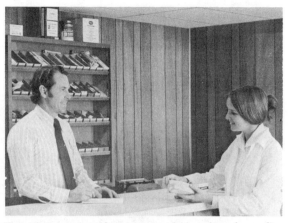

Fig. 29-2   A dental assistant ordering dental supplies from a local dental supply company.

- Pens
- Patient health forms
- Envelopes
- Receipts
- Typing paper
- Pencils
- Paper clips

Miscellaneous supplies are those supplies that are expendable but not considered dental supplies.   Furniture polish, room deodorants, hand cream, hand brushes, paper towels, cleaning supplies and, possibly, coffee are examples of miscellaneous supplies

SUPPLY AND INVENTORY CONTROL

Control of the four categories of supplies is made easier if a specific plan is adopted for the office. The dentist may have initiated a plan when the dental practice was first begun. If not, he may suggest that the secretarial dental assistant help in planning a supply control system. Practice management consultants may be contacted for suggestions and guidelines. Dental supply dealers are usually more than willing to help set up a system.

A good relationship should exist between the dental team and the dental supply companies.   A dental supply dealer represents

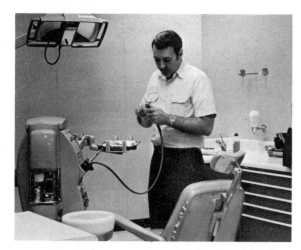

Fig. 29-3 A dental service technician making repairs on the equipment in a dental treatment area.

Item Room				Maximum Minimum			
Order Date	Rec'd Date	Quantity	Manuf.	Supply House	Unit Cost	Total Cost	Quantity On Hand

Fig. 29-4 A sample supply control and inventory card.

many manufacturing firms that make, sell, and service dental equipment and supplies. The dentist usually chooses two or three dental supply companies with whom he wishes to do business. The secretarial dental assistant should learn the names of these companies and the names of the men and women who represent the companies. If mail-order catalogs are used to purchase supplies from mail-order companies, the respective state tax commission should be consulted as some states require that dentists pay sales tax on supplies ordered from mail-order houses from another state. Failure to comply with this type of state regulation may result in tax penalties for the dentist.

A supply control system may be initiated by purchasing a file box to contain 5 x 8 index cards. Preferably the dentist and the secretarial dental assistant will design the supply and inventory control card according to the informational columns desired on the card, figure 29-4. It will be much easier and less time-consuming if a printing company is contacted to print the forms. Otherwise, a great deal of time may be spent in writing. A hand-designed card may be harder to read due to the lack of consistency in recording the supply and inventory information. Notice that the suggested printed card shows the name of the item in the upper left corner. The upper right corner may show the maximum or minimum quantity that the dentist wishes to order at one time. Any quantity ordered above the maximum listing must be approved by the dentist. For example, approval for more items than necessary may be given by the dentist if a special sales promotion is being offered by a dental supply company. Remember that usually money can be saved by buying in quantity. The larger the quantity, the less expensive each individual item may be; however, one must be aware of the shelf life of products. *Shelf life* is the length of time a product may be safely stored without deterioration of the product. The remaining columns on the card indicate the order date, when received, quantity, manufacturer, supply house, unit cost, total cost. and quantity on hand. An asterisk should be placed by the total cost if the items have a sales price.

Ideally, the index cards should be arranged alphabetically in four groups. The four groups should correspond with the four categories of supplies. Although this may require a large file box, the secretarial dental assistant should be able to quickly locate the specific item card.

This method will, at a glance, show the best price available. Local dealer prices should be compared; the secretarial dental assistant should always be interested in the best price for the dentist. Previously filed information about the last order may be very helpful. The secretarial dental assistant may look at this information and know exactly how long it will take for the item to be received as well as compare the price with the current one.

Again, the entire dental health team must cooperate by placing items on the want list in ample time for ordering. Once a week the secretarial dental assistant should use the want lists and the index file to order supplies.

EQUIPMENT CONTROL AND INVENTORY

A section on equipment may be included in the card index file. However, it may be more desirable to use a small loose-leaf notebook for equipment control and inventory. Equipment may include items essential in any area of the dental practice. The following items are a few examples of dental equipment.

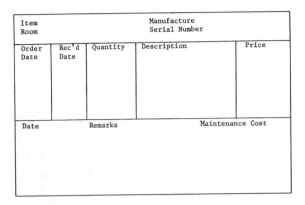

Fig. 29-5 A sample equipment control and inventory card.

- Dental chairs
- Sterilizer
- Lathe
- Typewriter
- Adding machine
- Dental units

CODESCO SUPPLY DIVISION	INVOICE							

CODESCO

Dr. John M. Doe
300 Dental Drive
Anywhere, USA 39206

ACCOUNT NAME	ACCT. TYPE	DATE
Dr. John M. Doe	A	1 / 11 /75

MFG.	DESCRIPTION	CLASS. CODE	ORDERED QUAN.	UNIT	SHIP	SHIP LATER	TAX	TOTAL	SYM CD
Greater	Engine belt # 19		1	ea.	1			1 20	mr
"	Airotor cleaner @ 1.40		2	can	2			2 80	mr
"	Airoter Lubricant @ 2.00		3	bot.	3			6 00	mr

GOLD	MDSE.	TEETH	N/EQ.	SOURCE	SLSM	FILLED	CHECKED	G. P. CODE SUMMARY		
11	⑫	13	14	PHONE ☐		✓		mr $ 10 50	SUB TOTAL	10 00
U/EQ.	PARTS	UE/PUR.		MAIL ☐					DEL.	
15	21	38		S. REP. ☒	INVOICE NUMBER			$	TAX	50
OTHER SPECIFY		SERVICE CODE		O.S. ☐	575365			$	TOTAL	10 50

FA-S-001-22   CHECK INVOICE AGAINST MONTHLY STATEMENT - INVOICE MUST ACCOMPANY RETURN MERCHANDISE

CUSTOMER

Fig. 29-6 Sample invoice for dental supplies.

- Instrument cabinets
- Radiographic machine
- Air compressor
- Vibrator

The equipment information card or sheet should be larger than the supply control card. Additional information is desired on the equipment card or sheet, figure 29-5, page 267. Space should be provided for the order date, received date, quantity, description, price, remarks, and maintenance cost. Information contained in this inventory control may be used by the auditor when computing depreciation of office equipment.

If a supply and equipment control system is being set up in an office after years of practice, one must start gradually and build up the system. Decide on a date to start and purchase the necessary supplies. Complete cards on each item ordered; as additional items are ordered, the system will grow. This is a good project to work on when the dentist is away from the office attending a meeting or convention. If a supply and equipment control system has not been in effect, it is likely that the dentist will appreciate an efficient secretarial dental assistant taking the initiative to start such a system.

RECEIVING AND STORING SUPPLIES

When items are received, the secretarial dental assistant checks the items with the packing slip or the invoice, figure 29-6, page 267. The index card should be pulled and the necessary information recorded.

Each item should be stored properly and according to the manufacturer's instructions. For example, radiographic films are placed in a cool, dark, dry area away from the radiographic equipment. Cements, impression materials, drugs, etc. should not be placed near a radiator or heating vent. Some items should not be placed near certain other items; for example disinfectants or cleaning fluids should

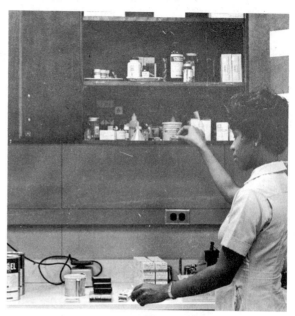

Fig. 29-7 A secretarial dental assistant storing supplies.

not be placed near gauze sponges. Consult the manufacturer's instructions for storage guidelines on each product.

Items already on hand should be moved to the front of the storage shelf or cabinet. The new items should be placed to the rear of the existing items. The older items could be marked with a dark magic marker to insure that the older items will be used first.

An additional inventory method is usually not necessary if an efficient supply and equipment control method is used. The supply and equipment control method explained, actually aids the dental office in ordering, maintaining, and taking inventory of all supplies and equipment.

SUMMARY

The entire dental health team should work together in the maintenance of dental supplies. Supplies should be ordered to allow ample time for shipment before the present supply is depleted. The absence of a necessary item may create embarrassment to the dental office. Every member of the dental team has a responsibility to check current supplies; each should inform the proper person of any needed supplies. Once a week, the secretarial dental assistant should use the want lists and the index file to order supplies.

A supply and inventory control method should be utilized by the dental office. Supply and inventory cards may be printed and filed in a small file box for this control. The dental office may consult with practice management consultants or dental supply representatives for help with this control. When the supplies arrive at the office, the control card should be completed properly. The supplies should be checked by using the invoice or packing slip. The supplies should be stored properly according to the manufacturer's instructions.

SUGGESTED ACTIVITIES

- Make arrangements for a dental supply representative to speak to the class on supply and inventory control.
- Ask permission to tour a dental supply firm. Take notes on remarks made that would be helpful in ordering and receiving dental supplies. Report your findings to the class.
- Make a list of supplies with a short shelf life, using package instructions from dental supplies.
- Write a one-page report on the proper method of storing dental supplies.

REVIEW

A. Define the following terms.

1. Expendable dental supplies.

2. Nonexpendable dental supplies.

3. Business office supplies.

4. Miscellaneous supplies.

5. Shelf life.

B.   Match each of the items listed below with the number of its proper category: (1) expendable dental supplies, (2) nonexpendable dental supplies, (3) business office supplies, (4) miscellaneous supplies, or (5) equipment.

____	dental units	____	alloy
____	typewriter	____	burs
____	radiographic film	____	lathe
____	typing paper	____	plaster and stone
____	glass slabs	____	patient treatment records
____	room deodorants	____	hand instruments
____	air compressors	____	staples
____	impression materials	____	autoclave
____	handpieces	____	drugs

C.   Select the best answer for the first five questions.   The remaining questions require more than one answer.

1. State tax commission offices should be contacted if supplies are purchased from mail-order catalogs because

a. some states require that sales tax be paid on supplies ordered from another state.

b. 10% tax may be added to mail-order sales.

c. state income tax may have to be paid to mail-order companies.

d. a special state income tax return may have to be filed at the end of the business year.

2. Usually, the larger the quantity purchased

a. the more expensive each item may be.

b. the more superior the product may be.

c. the less expensive each item may be.

d. the quicker the shipment may be.

3. The auditor may use the inventory control system to aid in computing depreciation for

a. expendable dental supplies.

b. nonexpendable dental supplies.

c. business office supplies.

d. equipment.

4. Radiographic films should be stored

   a. in a cool, dark, dry area away from the dental radiographic equipment.

   b. inside the dental radiographic unit.

   c. in the radiographic treatment area.

   d. in a warm, moist quiet area.

5. Items already on hand should be placed

   a. at the rear of the storage area.

   b. near the front of the storage shelf or cabinet.

   c. directly behind the newer items.

   d. in the treatment area to insure quick use.

6. Failure to reorder supplies at the proper time may result in

   a. discomfort to the dental patient.

   b. embarrassment to the dental office.

   c. the inability to complete an operative procedure.

   d. loss of operative time by the dental team.

7. Professionally printed supply and inventory control cards are recommended because

   a. they are easier and quicker to use.

   b. dental supply companies require that their customers use a printed supply and inventory control card.

   c. they are easier to read since they are consistent in form.

   d. the auditor may use the cards in determining depreciation of dental supplies.

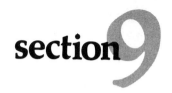

section **9**

A Career as a Secretarial Dental Assistant

Unit 30 Preparing for the Job Interview

OBJECTIVES

After studying this unit, the student should be able to

- Name and define eight specialty areas of dental practice.
- List sources of employment.
- Identify items to include in a job resume.
- Prepare a personal resume.

Employment in a dental office is one of the most challenging positions available in the health field. It is challenging because of the opportunity to work with people and to serve mankind. The main objective of the profession of dentistry is to provide dental health care to the public. The different types of positions available in a dental practice were defined in the first unit of this text. The purpose of this unit is to establish some objectives and guidelines to use when applying for a position in a dental office.

Much thought and preparation should be given to applying for a dental office position. The positions should provide an opportunity for one to grow in poise, personality, professional responsibility, and salary. A prospective secretarial dental assistant must be interested in the profession of dentistry and enjoy working with people. The dental practice should be one that the dental health team member can be proud to be associated with. Never should a person remain in a position if he or she cannot support the employer or the office. For that reason, it is reemphasized that much thought should be given to the possibility of new employment.

JOB OPPORTUNITIES

There are many job opportunities available in the dental profession. The demand for trained dental office personnel usually exceeds the availability of such persons. The secretarial dental assistant with training has a wide variety of job opportunities. All of the units in this text may be adapted for a general dentistry practice or one of the eight specialties of dentistry.

The eight specialities of dentistry are:
- Pedodontics (dentistry for children)
- Prosthodontics (deals with artificial fabrications)
- Periodontics (areas around the teeth; gingiva, periodontal membrane and the alveolar bone)
- Oral Surgery (surgical procedures of the oral cavity)
- Oral Pathology (diseases of the oral cavity)
- Endodontics (treatment of the pulp and surrounding tissues)
- Orthodontics (correction of malocclusion and irregularities of the teeth and arches.)

• Public Health Dentistry (dental health of the people)

Positions are also available in county, state, or federal facilities. The Civil Service Commission frequently has openings for which a secretarial dental assistant may qualify by successful completion of the Civil Service Examination. These positions may also be found in dental clinics of the Veterans Administration or in a branch of the Armed Forces. A secretarial dental assistant might also apply for a position in an educational institution such as a community college dental assisting program or a university dental school.

In a 1973 survey of 13 graduates of an accredited dental assisting program, it was found that 12 graduates were employed in private dental offices either as chairside assistants, roving assistants, patient education assistants, or as secretarial dental assistants. One was employed as a receptionist and secretary to the executive secretary of a state dental association. This survey is mentioned to show that there are opportunities available for varied employment in the dental assisting field.

SEEKING EMPLOYMENT

There are several ways of finding out about job openings in dental offices. If the student is enrolled in a dental assisting program, the director or instructor may have leads concerning job opportunities. Perhaps the clinical phase of the curriculum includes a term in a private dental office. This is an excellent opportunity for a student to learn about job openings. Many times the school or college may have a graduate placement office. This type of office helps students find employment after graduation. Some college libraries periodically receive microfilm of state or national job openings which can be viewed by prospective graduates.

The newspaper is an excellent source to consult when looking for a new position.

SECRETARIAL DENTAL ASSISTANT

General dentist desires to employ a Certified Dental Assistant to manage the dental office. Salary open. Apply by sending a resume to Daily News, P. O. Box 155, Albany, N.Y.

Fig. 30-1 A typical newspaper advertisement.

Check the help wanted section for any dental office listings. The advertisement may list a telephone number to call. Others may request that the interested party reply by sending a resume to a particular box number. If the latter is requested, it is suggested that the applicant follow the resume guidelines in this unit.

Employment agencies may be found by consulting the yellow pages of the local telephone directory. Most states provide a non-profit employment office to provide employment services to the residents of the state. All of the fifty state offices are a part of the United States Employment Service (USES); these offices employ persons who counsel prospective applicants in an effort to match applicants to jobs for which they are best qualified.

Private employment agencies charge a specified percent of the salary for the first few months as a job placement fee. However, the fee may seem small when compared to the need for finding gainful employment. Most employment agencies require a visit to their office in order for the applicant to complete an application. Also, one or more aptitude type tests may be required. The agency may then arrange interviews for the applicant with prospective employers.

It is a good idea to tell friends, acquaintances, or relatives that you are looking for a new position. Tell them your qualifications and the type of job you are looking for. Many times, people who are interested in you may hear of interesting job opportunities.

One of the best methods of finding out about available jobs is to attend local meetings

RESUME

Mary Jane Smith
200 State Street
Callahan, N.Y. 12300
Telephone: 459-3993
Position Applied for: Secretarial Dental Assistant

PERSONAL DATA

Birthdate:	November 30, 1954
Weight:	123 pounds
Height:	5' 6"
Marital Status:	Single
Health:	Excellent

EDUCATION

Central Community College, 398 Jay Street, Troy, N.Y. Sept. 1973 – June 1975
Certificate in Dental Assisting. ADAA Certification examination taken on May 18, 1975
Subjects relating to this position:
    Typing, Dental Practice Management, Bookkeeping, Filing.
Central High School, May 1969
    General Education Courses

EXPERIENCE

Clinical Training Internship
Dr. Jack Simpson   (160 clock hours)
General Dentistry, 350 Jackson Drive, Callahan, N.Y. 12300

AWARDS AND ACTIVITIES

Student Dental Assistant of the year, 1973
Central Community College
DAR Good Citizenship Award, 1968

SPECIAL INTERESTS

Volunteer dental assistant, Good Samaritan Center (two Saturdays per month)

REFERENCES

Dr. Jack Simpson, 350 Jackson Drive, Callahan, N.Y. 12300

Dr. John P. Walker, 487 Dover Drive, Hawthorne, N.Y. 12408

Mrs. Linda J. Jones,
Dental Assisting Instructor, Central Community College
398 Jay Street,
Troy, N.Y. 12401

Fig. 30-2 Example of a resume.

of the Dental Assistants Association. During the announcement segment of the meeting, members often announce openings in their offices. If you are seeking a new position, tell the members present during the social period just before or after the meeting.

HOW TO APPLY

A prospective dental health team member may apply by telephone, in writing, or in person. The method used may depend on the requirements of the prospective dental office. If telephoning, dial the office, state your name and the purpose of the call. Wait for the other person to tell you what steps should be taken. The dentist may have instructed the receptionist to request a resume (rez-ou-may) or to set up an interview.

The Summary of Qualification

A *resume* is a summary of one's qualifications. It should be brief but comprehensive. This written summary might also be called a personal data sheet, a qualifications summary, a dossier, or possibly just background information. The prospective employer usually prefers to read a resume rather than a long wordy letter of application, figure 30-2.

The summary should be typed in a consistent form. If at all possible, all the information should be typed on *one* sheet of white bond unlined paper. No errors or erasures should appear on the page. If necessary, type the resume over until a perfect copy is complete. It is suggested that a recent black and white photograph be attached. The following information should be included.

A Heading should appear at the top of the page. It should include complete name, address, and telephone number. The position applied for should be stated in the heading.

Personal Data should follow the heading. Information should include birth date, height, weight, marital status and condition of health.

Education. An applicant's educational background should be listed; the most recent is listed first. For example, any college training should be listed first followed by high school information. It is not necessary to list junior high or elementary schools. The school or college should be listed by name and address. The years of attendance should follow. The areas of specialization should be stated. The degree or certificate earned and the date awarded should also appear. If the certification examination given by the Certifying Board of the American Dental Assistants Association has been taken, be sure to list the date of the examination. It is quite possible that the results may not be known at the time of writing. Any significant courses that would apply to the job sought should be written. The number of courses may vary greatly from one applicant to another. Be sure to list all courses directly related to the type of office.

Experience. The name and address of all previous employers is recorded. The most recent place of employment is listed first. The duties performed in each place of employment are briefly described. If this is to be the first full time job, it is permissible to list vacation type jobs or part-time employment. If a dental assisting school has been attended, be certain to list the clinical experience received during the program. Clinical experience may include private dental offices or experience in clinical facilities of dental schools. It is usually not necessary to list previous salaries. There will be a time during the interview to discuss salaries.

Awards and Activities. Do not be too modest when listing awards. However, be very concise and do not elaborate on awards received. Activities should include clubs and associations in which the applicant participates. Be certain to list the professional organizations; for example, Student Member of the American Dental Assistants Association.

200 State Street
Callahan, N.Y. 12300
March 29, 1975

Dr. John Melvin Doe
300 Thompson St.
Hawthorne, N.Y. 12408

Dear Doctor:

Please consider this letter an application for the position of Secretarial Dental Assistant
advertised in today's edition of the Daily News.

My graduation date from Central Community College will be June 1, 1975. I am completing a twelve-month course in Dental Assisting. My training has included all phases of dental
assisting. However, I prefer to find employment as a Secretarial Dental Assistant rather than
a chairside assistant. The enclosed resume will give you detailed information about my
background.

May I make an appointment for an interview? I am free on Wednesday afternoons and any-
time Saturday. If these times are not convenient for you, possibly, I could arrange with my
instructor for an early dismissal from class on another day.

Sincerely,

Mary Jane Smith

Fig. 30-3 An example of a cover letter to attach to a resume.

Special Interests. It is suggested that special interests be listed that might have a bearing on the chances for employment. This might include any voluntary work engaged in which might relate to dentistry or medicine. The dentist may be able to estimate an appli-cant's initiative or personality by reviewing both the awards and activities sections and the special interest section.

References. Three references should be re-corded. Do not list a reference without first obtaining permission. Write or telephone the person and request permission to use his name as a reference. Record the name, address, and telephone number of each reference. It is strongly suggested that at least two of the ref-erences be able to recommend the applicant on the basis of work and school accomplish-ments. One of the references should be able to recommend the applicant on the basis of ethical or moral values. An applicant may wish to list one of the following:

- Director of a Dental Assisting Program
- High School Counselor
- Clergyman

The resume is now complete and may be mailed to the prospective employer. A short cover letter should be written to accompany it. The times when the applicant will be avail-able for interviews may be stated in the cover letter. It is also suggested that a prospective graduate of a dental assisting program state

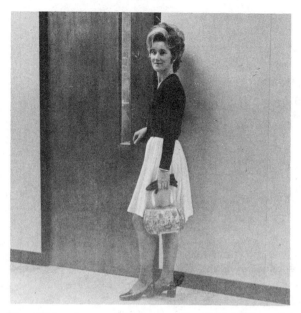

Fig. 30-4   An applicant properly dressed for a job interview.

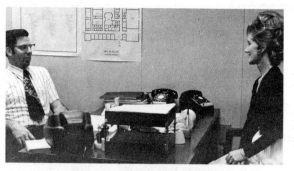

Fig. 30-5   The job interview.

the day of graduation and the date available for employment.

The Interview

The personal interview is usually the final phase of applying for a new position. Much thought and preparation should be given to personal appearance on the day of the interview. Unfortunately, many people do not realize what their appearance or actions tell the prospective employer. The following paragraphs may be helpful to applicants in preparing for an interview.

Personal appearance of an applicant is most important when preparing for an interview. The applicant should not be over or under dressed. A conservative outfit with tasteful accessories should be worn. It is strongly suggested that a dress or two-piece outfit be worn rather than pantsuits. Pantsuits are appropriate for many occasions including working in the dental office but not for the personal interview. Hose should match the outfit and be free of snags or runs. Shoes and bag should be exceptionally clean and in good repair. The same is true for the arrangement

of the handbag. It may be necessary to open the bag during the interview. One overflowing with a variety of items such as paper and cosmetics may be embarrassing. Jewelry should be kept to a minimum. Hair should be arranged neatly in a style suitable for employment in the professional office. Avoid heavy perfume; strong fragrances are offensive to many people. General appearance should be checked in a full-length mirror before leaving for the interview.

Being punctual for a job interview is important. Plenty of time should be allowed for heavy traffic or unexpected obstacles. Time should be allowed for calling a taxi in the event of car trouble. Do not appear too anxious by arriving too early. The trip should be timed so that you are at the office five minutes before scheduled time.

Upon arrival, courteously give the receptionist your name, the name of the interviewer, and the time of the appointment. Converse with the receptionist while waiting only if she includes you in a conversation. When you are called to meet the interviewer, thank the receptionist if possible.

The dentist will usually interview the applicants in his private office. Do not offer to shake hands with the dentist unless he or she offers the hand first. Do not sit down until the dentist indicates where you should sit. Place handbag or gloves on your lap or on the floor near your chair. Never place anything on the dentist's desk. If you are a smoker, do

200 State Street
Callahan, N.Y. 12300
April 6, 1975

Dr. John Melvin Doe
300 Thompson Street
Hawthorne, N.Y. 12408

Dear Doctor Doe:

Thank you for talking with me today about the job opportunity in your dental office.

I have studied the job description sheet you gave me from your office manual. Reviewing my experience and interest, I feel that I could perform the work to your satisfaction.

It would please me very much to become a part of your dental team.

Sincerely,

Mary Jane Smith

Fig. 30-6 A thank-you letter following an interview.

not ask the dentist if he minds if you smoke; neither should a cigarette be accepted during an interview. Many dentists do not allow smoking in their office. Since very little time is available for smoking during working hours, smoking during the interview may cancel one's chance of employment.

The dentist should begin the interview as well as end it. The applicant should listen very carefully and answer all questions as adequately as possible. When the dentist has indicated the interview is over, thank him courteously for taking his time to talk with you.

A thank-you letter should be written to the dentist after the interview. This may improve chances for employment.

SUMMARY

A position in a dental office is one of the most challenging positions in the health field. It provides an opportunity to work with and to serve people. There are many job opportunities available in the dental profession since the demand for trained personnel exceeds the availability. These job opportunities may become known by consulting with instructors or directors of dental assisting programs, newspapers, employment agencies, and friends or relatives.

A prospective dental team member may apply by telephone, in writing, or in person. A resume is a written summary of one's qualifications. It should be comprehensive but brief. A personal interview means applying for a position in person. Much thought and preparation should be given to personal appearance and punctuality on the day of the interview. The applicant should listen carefully during the interview and answer all questions as adequately as possible. A thank-you letter should be written after the interview.

SUGGESTED ACTIVITIES

- Read "Job Preparation" sections of at least two practice management reference textbooks.
- Look in the local newspapers in the classified section for advertisements of job openings in the dental assisting field. Compare the advertisements for job descriptions and salary, if listed.
- Interview three employed dental assistants and inquire how they obtained their current employment.

REVIEW

A.   List and define the eight specialties of dentistry.

1.

2.

3.

4.

5.

6.

7.

8.

B.   List six ways of seeking employment in the dental field.

1.

2.

3.

4.

5.

6.

C. List the information categories to include in a resume.

D. Select the best answer.

1. There are usually many job opportunities available for the trained dental assistant because

a. any type of person may work as a dental assistant.

b. the demand is usually far greater than the availability of such persons.

c. everyone likes to work with people.

d. dental assisting salaries are far better than other health occupation fields.

2. Pedodontics is the branch of dentistry dealing with

a. the gingiva, periodontal membrane, and the alveolar bone.

b. the dental care of children.

c. treatment of the pulp and the surrounding tissue.

d. correction of malocclusion and irregularities of the teeth.

3. State employment offices are a part of the

a. Department of Health, Education and Welfare.

b. Civil Service Commission.

c. Veterans Administration area office.

d. United States Employment Service (USES).

4. A resume may also be called

a. a personal data sheet.

b. a bibliography.

c. an interview.

d. an application form.

5. Educational background information is listed

a. beginning with elementary school.

b. beginning with junior high school.

c. only if college has been attended.

d. beginning with the most recently attended school.

6. The awards, activities, and special interest section of a resume may

    a. enable the dentist to estimate the applicant's initiative or personality.

    b. Help the dentist to determine the starting salary.

    c. enable the dentist to figure out references to contact.

    d. indicate the applicant's experience in dental assisting.

7. On the day of the interview, the applicant should

    a. wear a conservative outfit with tasteful accessories.

    b. go to a beauty salon and try a new fashionable hair style.

    c. arrive a couple of minutes late so as not to appear anxious.

    d. ask as many questions as possible to show interest in the position.

E. Prepare a personal resume to a prospective employer.

RESUME

HEADING

PERSONAL DATA

EDUCATION

EXPERIENCE

AWARDS AND ACTIVITIES

SPECIAL INTERESTS

REFERENCES

Unit 31 The Value of Medical Terminology

OBJECTIVES

After studying this unit, the student should be able to

- Define prefix and suffix.
- Associate the prefixes in this unit with the correct meanings.
- Associate the suffixes in this unit with the correct meanings.

The person who selects the career of a secretarial dental assistant must continue to grow professionally. Skill in office management includes knowledge of business and office procedures, but the value of understanding medical terms and being able to speak with confidence cannot be overemphasized. Therefore, this unit on prefixes and suffixes will provide the student with an educational tool which can be used regardless of what specialty she wishes to pursue.

Following the unit is a glossary of dental terms which may be used as a quick reference; however, if one masters the basics of medical terminology, the glossary will provide a smooth transition from this unit into the specialized area of dental terminology. The glossary also includes business terms used in dental office management.

MEDICAL TERMINOLOGY

Medical and dental words will not be difficult to pronounce or understand if the prefixes and suffixes are known. Particular prefixes and suffixes listed in this unit should be helpful to the person employed as a secretarial dental assistant. It is suggested that five terms be selected and memorized daily until all the terms are learned.

Prefixes

A *prefix* is a letter or sequence of letters attached to the beginning of a word. It is the most frequently used element in forming medical words. A prefix may also tell something about the root word such as: how many, where located, or what color.

Some of the prefixes that follow may also be seen in medical terms as a root word. For example, *ortho* is a prefix meaning *straighten* or *correct; odont* pertains to *tooth* or *teeth*. Therefore, the word *orthodontics* is defined as the branch of dentistry that deals with straightening or correcting teeth.

Prefixes	Meanings
a, an	without, not
ab	away from
ad	to, near, toward
adeno	gland
album	white
ante	before
ant, anti	against
bi, bin	two
bio	life
blast	a formative cell; bud
cardio	heart
cata, kata	down, lower, under
cephal	head
cheil	lip
co, com, con	with, together
counter	against
crani	skull
cyano	blue
cyst	sac, bladder, bag
cyt	cell
deci, deca	ten
dermato, dermo	skin
dextro	to the right of

Prefixes	*Meanings*	*Prefixes*	*Meanings*
di	two	octo, octi	eight
dis	free of, separation, reversal	ortho	straight, correct
dys	difficult, painful, faulty	osteo	bone
e, ex	out, away from, without outside	oti	ear
		para	beside, alongside of
ecto, exo, extra	without, on the outside	path	disease
encephal	brain	penta	five
endo, ento	within	per	between, through, across
entero	intestine	peri	around
erythro	red	pharm	drugs
galact	milk	phlebo	vein
gastro	stomach	phreno	diaphragm or mind
glosso	tongue	pneum	air
gynec	woman	polio	gray
hemato, hemo, hema	blood	poly	many
hepato, hepatico	liver	post	after
histo	tissue, web-like	proto	first
homo	common, same	pseudo	false
hydro	water	psycho	soul or mind
hypo	below, under	ptery	wing
ilio	ilium	ptya	saliva
ileo	ileum	pyo	accumulation of pus
infra	under	re, retro	behind, backward, again
inter	between	rhino	nose
intro	into	rube	red
kerato	horn or corn	sarco	flesh
kin	movement	scirrho, sclero	hard
labia	lip	semi	half
latero	to the side of	septa	seven
lipo	fat	septic	poison
lith	stone	sexa	six
macro	great	sial	saliva
mast	breast	sphygmo	pulse
media, medial	middle	steno	narrowness, constriction
meta	change	sub	less, deficient
micro	small	super, supra	above, over, excess
milli	thousand	tachy	fast or swift
mono	one	ter, tri	three
morpho	form	tetra	four
myelo	bone marrow, spinal cord	thermo	heat
myo	muscle	thoraco	chest
myx	mucus	thrombo	clot
narco	numbness	toxi, toxo	poison
naso	nose	tracheo	windpipe or air passage
necro	dead	troph	nourishment
nephro	kidney	trans	across or through
neo	new	uni	mono or one
neuro	nerve	ultra	beyond or excess
nona	nine	vaso	vessel
odonto	tooth or teeth	xero	dry

Suffixes

A *suffix* is a letter or sequence of letters attached to the end of a word; it describes the prefix or the root word. For example, since *naso* means *nose,* the word *paranasal* would re- fer to the area *alongside* of the nose (*para* is the prefix for *beside* or *alongside of*). Therefore, upon hearing "paranasal sinuses," the secretarial dental assistant knows that the sinuses alongside of the nose are being discussed.

Suffixes	*Meanings*	*Suffixes*	*Meanings*
-able, ible	capacity	-malacia	softening
-ac, al	pertaining to, resembling	-mania	madness
-agra	seizure, acute pain	-oma	tumor
-ago, igo	disease	-orexia	appetite
-algesia, algia	pain	-osis	condition of
-cele	hernia, tumor, swelling	-oscopy	inspection, looking into
-centesis	perforation or aspiration	-ostomy	making a permanent opening (surgical passageway)
-clasis	breaking		
-clysis	injection, washing out	-otomy	incision, cutting into
-cide	a destroyer, killer	-penia	decrease, lack of
-desis	binding, fusing	-plasty	repair, reconstruction by surgery
-dynia	pain	-plegia	paralysis
-eal, eous	of the nature of	-plexy	stroke
-ectasia, estasis	stretching, dilation, expansion	-phagy, phagia	eating, swallowing
-ectomy	excision, removal	-phonia	voice or sound
-emesis	vomiting	-phylaxis	protection against
-emia	condition of the blood	-pnea	breathing
-fuge	something that drives away or expels	-ptosis	downward displacement
-genia	origin, producing	-rrhage	excessive flow
-gnosis	knowledge, recognition	-rrhaphy	suture
-ia, iasis, id, ism	abnormal or diseased condition	-rrhexis	rupture
-ites	dropsy of a part	-stasis	stopping the flow
-itis	inflammation	-staxis	dripping, oozing
-ize	action or treatment	-therapy	treatment, heal
-lith, lithiasis	stone	-trophy	nutrition, nourishment
-logy	study of	-uria	condition of the urine
-lysis	loosening, freeing		

REVIEW

A. Define the following.

   1. Prefix

   2. Suffix

B. Given a list of <u>meanings</u>, indicate the correct prefix or suffix to which each meaning applies. The instructor (or student in self-study situations) will make the selection from those listed in this unit.

Dental Glossary

abrasion — Mechanical wearing down of teeth.

abutment — The supporting natural teeth of a removable or nonremovable bridge.

account — A record of the patient's financial business with the dental office.

acrylic — A synthetic substance that is used in commercial restorative materials such as an acrylic filling, crown, or bridge.

ADA — American Dental Association.

ADAA — American Dental Assistants Association.

ADHA — American Dental Hygienists Association.

alginate — An extraction of marine kelp used in making certain impression materials.

allergy — Hypersensitivity of man to a foreign protein.

alloy — Two or more metals fused together.

alveolar bone — The process of bone of the maxilla and mandible that supports the teeth.

amalgam — The combination of a silver alloy and mercury.

amalgamate — The process of combining silver alloy and mercury.

ameloblast — A cell that aids in forming the enamel of the teeth.

analgesia — Loss of feeling without the loss of consciousness.

analgesic — An agent that relieves pain.

anesthesia — Loss of feeling.

    local — Loss of feeling in a localized area.

    general — Loss of feeling with a loss of consciousness.

anesthetic — A drug that produces either local or general anesthesia.

anodontia — Without teeth.

anterior — Located in the front or forward area.

antibiotic — A drug used to destroy pathogenic microorganisms.

antiseptic — An agent that stops or inhibits the growth of bacteria.

apex — The tip-end of the root of a tooth.

armamentarium — (1) All items needed to practice dentistry. (2) All items needed to perform a certain procedure. e.g. Amalgam Armamentarium.

articulator — A device used to articulate or bring together the teeth.

attrition — Normal wearing down of teeth.

autoclave — A piece of equipment used to render dental instruments and materials sterile.

back order — A written notice from a supply company showing items ordered but not delivered.

base — A type of cement used between the tooth preparation and the restorative material for protection of the pulp of the tooth.

bicuspid — Teeth with two cusps; a premolar tooth.

bite — An impression that shows the relationship between the maxillary and mandibular teeth.

bridge — An artificial replacement for missing teeth in an arch.

buccal — Pertaining to the cheek side.

buffer time — Time reserved each day to take care of problems and emergencies that arise during the regularly scheduled appointments.

business summary sheet — Page in the daily log to compute the total business and total cash for the month.

bur — A small rotary cutting instrument used in dental handpieces for the purpose of preparing (cutting) teeth for restorations and/or crowns and bridges.

calculus — A hard deposit that may accumulate on the crowns and roots of teeth; tartar.

cancellation list — A written list of patients who desire to come for an appointment sooner than they are appointed.

caries — A disease characterized by the molecular death of teeth.

case history — Past medical and/or dental information on a patient.

cavity — The lesion that is produced by the disease of caries.

CDA — Certified Dental Assistant.

CDT — Certified Dental Technician.

cementum — That part of the tooth that surrounds the root.

cephalometric radiograph — X ray of bones and teeth of the head and profile.

Certified Mail — First class mail with a return receipt but not insured.

cervical — Pertaining to the neck of a tooth.

contract — An agreement in writing between two or more people.

coronal — Pertaining to the crowns of teeth.

crown — (1) The part of the tooth that is covered with enamel. (2) An artificial replacement of a portion of a tooth.

cusp — A point on the grinding surface of a tooth.

cuspid — Having one cusp; a canine tooth.

daily log — A ledger for maintaining all financial records of the dental office.

daily page — A lined page to record name of the patients, services rendered, and amounts that are charged or paid.

darkroom — A room where dental radiographs are developed, fixed, and washed.

D.D.S. — Doctor of Dental Surgery.

deciduous — The primary teeth; teeth that fall out at the end of a development stage which are then replaced by the secondary teeth.

dental floss — A string like mechanical aid used in cleaning between the teeth.

dental laboratory technician — A person responsible for the laboratory procedures requested by the dentist. These responsibilities include making dental appliances, casting crowns and bridges, and fabricating artificial dentures.

dental unit — A piece of equipment that provides gas, water, and electricity for the dentist's use in treating dental patients.

dentifrice — An agent used in cleaning the teeth such as toothpaste or tooth-powder.

dentin — The tissue that forms the bulk of the tooth and is covered by enamel and cementum.

dentistry — The profession that deals in the prevention, diagnosis, and treatment of dental disorders.

denture — Artificial replacement of all the teeth in a given arch.

distal — Pertaining to areas.

D.M.D. — Doctor of Dental Medicine.

edentulous — Without teeth.

emergency period — Buffer time; time reserved to take care of problems and emergencies that arise during the regularly scheduled appointments.

employee's earning record — A form in the daily log for recording payroll records on each employee.

enamel — The tissue that forms the outer covering of the crown of a tooth.

endodontics — Branch of dentistry that deals with diseases of the dental pulp and surrounding tissues.

equilibrate — To balance.

ethical — Pertaining to values of right and wrong.

etiology — Study of the cause of diseases.

expendable supplies — Supplies that are used up and reordered regularly.

expense sheet — A page in the daily log to record all expenses incurred during the month.

exodontics — Area of dentistry that deals with the extraction of teeth.

extraction — Removing a tooth from the alveolar bone.

FICA — Federal Insurance Contribution Act (Social Security).

filling — Material used to restore carious lesions; restoration.

First class mail — Sealed letters or a type of postcard.

fissure — A faulty groove in the enamel of teeth.

forceps — Surgical instruments used in the extraction of teeth.

Fourth class mail — Parcel post, includes packages or printed materials that weigh more than 16 ounces.

generalist — In dentistry, a laboratory technician who performs all laboratory procedures the dentist requires.

gingiva — The tissue that surrounds the teeth, commonly referred to as gum.

gingivitis — Inflammation of the gingiva.

gross pay — Amount of an employee's salary before any deductions are made.

gypsum — Calcium sulfate minus the water; plaster of paris, used to pour into impressions to obtain a positive reproduction of a structure.

hemorrhage — Excessive flow of blood.

hemostat — Instrument or agent that stops the flow of blood.

hygienist — In dentistry, a licensed person employed to perform prophylaxis, take radiographs, take impressions for study models, and teach dental health education to the patient.

I.M. — Intramuscular (into the muscle).

impression — A mold of an area of the mouth, usually of an entire arch.

imprint device — A small piece of equipment used for transferring information from plastic credit cards to patient records.

incisal — Pertaining to the cutting edges of teeth.

inferior — Lower.

inlay — A restoration shapted like the form of a cavity and inserted with a cement.

Insured mail — Third and Fourth class mail that is insured.

interdental — Between the teeth.

interproximal — Pertains to the area between surfaces of two adjacent teeth.

IRS — Internal Revenue Service.

I.V. — Intravenous (into the vein).

jurisprudence — The understanding and application of the science of law.

kvp — Kilovoltage peak of an X-ray machine.

labial – Pertaining to the lips or the area near the lips.

lingual – Pertaining to the tongue or the area near the tongue.

luting – A substance for sealing (cement).

malocclusion – Abnormal occlusion of the maxillary and mandibular arches.

malpractice – Improper or careless treatment of a patient; injurious or negligent practice.

mandible – Lower jaw.

mandibular – Pertaining to the lower jaw.

masticate – To chew.

mastication – Act of chewing.

materia alba – Soft white deposit found on the exposed surfaces of improperly cleaned teeth.

maxilla – Upper jaw.

maxillary – Pertaining to the upper jaw.

median – Pertaining to the middle.

Medicaid – A federal and state program providing medical assistance to needy persons.

Medicare – A federal program that helps provide medical care for people over age 65.

mesial – Pertaining to the area nearest to the mid-line.

model – A reproduction of a tooth, quadrant, or arch.

molar – The posterior teeth that are used for grinding food.

morphology – The study of form or structure. Dental morphology includes the study of the form of the individual teeth.

nasal – Pertaining to the nose.

necrotic – Pertaining to death of a cell or group of cells.

net pay – Amount of a payroll check after deductions have been made.

nitrous oxide – A gas used in dentistry as an analgesia to relieve hypertension and raise the pain threshold during dental procedures, sometimes called "laughing gas."

occlude – To close the teeth.

occlusal – Pertaining to closing the teeth; the biting surfaces of the posterior teeth.

occlusion – The act of bringing opposing surfaces of the teeth of the two jaws into contact.

odontalgia – Toothache. Pain in the tooth area.

odontoblast – A cell that aids in the formation of dentin.

office manual – A manual prepared to acquaint all members of the dental team with the philosophy of the dentist and the various problems of the office.

operatory – A room where dental patients are treated; treatment room.

oral – Pertaining to the mouth.

orthodontics – Branch of dentistry that deals with preventing and correcting malocclusion.

outstanding check – A written check that has not cleared the bank.

overhead expense – The total expense involved in maintaining an office.

palatal – Pertaining to the palate (roof) of the mouth.

panoramic survey – An extra-oral radiograph exposure showing the maxillary and mandibular areas in one film.

parotid – Pertaining to an area near the ear.

parulis – A gingival abscess.

pathology – Branch of medicine or dentistry that deals with the study of the causes and effects of disease.

pedodontics – Branch of dentistry that deals with the treatment of children's teeth and oral cavity.

periapical – Pertaining to the area around the apex or tip end of the tooth.

pericoronal – Pertaining to the area around the crown of a tooth.

periodontal – Pertaining to the area around the entire tooth such as the gingiva, periodontal ligaments, and the alveolar bone.

periodontics – The branch of dentistry that deals with the prevention and treatment of the gingiva, periodontal ligaments, and alveolar bone.

periodontium – The gingiva, periodontal ligaments, and alveolar bone.

permanent – Lasting; The second dentition sometimes referred to as secondary teeth.

petty cash – A small office fund maintained for the purpose of purchasing miscellaneous inexpensive items.

pharmacology – The study of drugs, their properties and actions.

pit – A depression.

plaque – A bacterial patch that forms on the exposed surfaces of teeth.

plastic – Something that is capable of being molded.

pontic – The artificial tooth or teeth that replaces missing teeth on a bridge or partial.

posterior – Pertaining to the area toward the rear of an object.

postoperative – Occurs after the operation.

premolar – The two teeth that appear before the molars in normal dentition.

prescription – A written order from a doctor to a pharmacist describing the drugs to be dispensed to a patient.

private practice – A practice without public or government control.

prophylaxis — The prevention of disease.

prothesis — An artificial substitute that is used whn a part is missing.

prosthodontics — The branch of dentistry that deals with replacing missing structures (such as teeth and tissues) by artificial substitutes.

proximal — Pertaining to the eara nearest to the midline of a structure.

psychology — The study and functions of the mind.

public health dentistry — The branch of dentistry that deals with the dental health of the general public.

pulp — The interior portion of the tooth.

pulpectomy — the removal of the pulp of a tooth.

pulpitis — Inflammation of the pulp.

pulpotomy — A dental procedure that removes the crown portion of the dental pulp.

purulent — Containing, consisting of, or being pus.

pyorrhea — A discharge that is purulent. Periodontitis is a more scientific term.

radiation — A transfer of energy through space or matter.

radiograph — An X-ray photograph.

radiology — In dentistry, the branch that deals with methods and techniques of obtaining X-ray photographs and the reading of the photographs for diagnostic purposes.

RDH — Registered Dental Hygienist.

recall — A systematic method of reminding a patient it is time for a visit to the dental office.

receptionist — A person employed to greet the patient and perform the daily business procedures of the front office.

record — An official method of retaining information about a patient; treatment charts, financial records, X rays, and study models are all classified as patient records.

registration form — A form for the new patient to record information such as address, telephone number, place of employment, etc.

restoration — The method of replacing a missing portion of a tooth or replacing teeth by artificial substitutes.

resume — A thorough, brief summary of one's education and experience.

root — The unexposed portion of a tooth.

roving assistant — Dental team member who moves among treatment area, front desk, laboratory, supply area, and dark room.

rubber dam procedure — A method of isolating teeth with thin sheets of latex to keep the area dry during dental procedures.

Second class mail — Newspapers and periodical publications.

shelf life — Length of time a product may be safely stored without deterioration of the product.

sigmoid — An area or structure that is shaped like an S.

sodium fluoride — Chemical effective in reducing dental decay when applied topically to children's teeth.

Special Delivery mail — Mail that requires delivery as soon as it reaches the post office; available only in towns and cities.

Special Handling mail — Third and fourth class mail that requires quick handling.

specialist — A qualified person who limits professional practice to a specific branch of health care.

SS-4 — A federal form used to obtain employer identification numbers.

statement — An office form showing the balance of one's account.

sterilization — In dentistry, the destruction of microorganisms present on dental instruments.

stomatitis — Inflammation of the soft tissues of the mouth.

study model — In dentistry, a reproduction usually in plaster or stone of the teeth for the purpose of studying and planning a treatment plan.

subgingival — Below the gingiva.

sublingual — Below the tongue.

submaxillary — Below the jaw, especially the upper portion.

succedaneous — Something that follows after, such as a permanent tooth that replaces a deciduous tooth.

superior — Pertaining to the uppermost parts.

syncope — Fainting.

tartar — A layman's term for calculus.

temporomandibular — Pertaining to the bones of the temporal and mandible.

Third class mail — Bulk type mail weighing less than 16 ounces such as circulars and catalogs.

TMJ — Temporomandibular Joint.

treatment plan — An explanation to the patient of exactly what the dentist recommends as treatment and the approximate cost.

trituration — Mixing of alloy and mercury for an amalgam restoration.

W-2 — Wage and Tax Statement; A federal form that employers prepare yearly for each employee that was on the payroll during the year.

W-3 — A federal form which is a reconciliation of income tax withheld and a transmittal of tax statements.

W-4 — Employee's Withholding Exemption Certificate. A federal form for employees to record their exemption status at the beginning of employment.

withholding tax — Holding back a portion of a salary for income tax purposes.

zinc oxide — In dentistry, a fine white powder that is combined with liquid to be used in treatment fillings, temporary lutings, and impression materials.

No attempt has been made to provide a complete dental glossary. Only those terms that a secretarial dental assistant may need to use frequently in the processing of dental records and conversing with the dental patient, are listed.

Acknowledgments

The author is grateful to all who helped in the writing and final preparation of this text. Special thanks are extended to the following persons.

Technical Consultant: Claire Williamson, Medical University of South Carolina and past president of ADAA.

Photographers: Cecil Landrum, Robert Mullins and Barbara Schultz

Contributors: Donna Meeler for Units 19 and 24; Dell Broadway for Units 26, 27, Wanda C. Dell for Unit 21.

Others whose contributions are appreciated:

American Dental Assistants Association's Journal, *The Dental Assistant* for figure 2-1.

American Telephone and Telegraph Co. for figures 5-1, 5-2, 5-3 and 5-4.

Codesco Davidson Dental Supply Co. for figures 2-8, 8-6, 29-1, 29-2 and 29-6.

Colwell Company for figures 6-4, 6-5, 6-6, 7-1, 8-2, 8-3, 8-4, 8-8, 8-9, 9-2, 9-3, 9-7, 9-8, 9-9, 10-1, 10-3, 10-6, 10-7, 10-8, 10-9, 12-1, 13-1, 13-2, 13-3, 13-4, 13-5, 15-5, 22-3, 22-4, 22-5, 23-1, 23-2.

Deposit Guaranty National Bank for figures 14-1, 14-4, 14-6 and 14-7.

Dr. Charles Davis, Jackson, MS, for figure 24-1.

Dr. Heber Simmons, Jackson, MS, for figures 1-1, 1-4, 2-5, 2-7, 3-1, 3-5, 6-1, 6-2, 8-7, 9-1, 11-8, 12-4, 14-2, 14-5, 15-6, 20-1, 20-2, 20-3, 25-1, 25-2, 27-1, 27-2.

Dr. Wayne McLaughlin, Auburn, AL for help with unit 25.

Dr. Peter Mills, Atlanta GA, for figure 21-4.

Dr. Robert Parkes, Jackson, MS, for figures 1-5, 1-6, 2-4, 13-6, 17-3, 26-1, 26-2.

Hinds Junior College, Jackson Branch, for figures 1-2, 1-3, 2-2, 2-3, 2-6, 2-9, 3-3, 5-6, 6-3, 6-7, 7-5, 8-1, 8-5, 11-4, 11-5, 11-6, 16-4, 16-5, 18-4, 22-1, 27-4, 28-1, 29-7, 30-4, 30-5.

Histacount Corporation for figures 7-3, 9-4, 9-5.

IBM Corporation for figures 28-2, 28-3, 28-9.

Monroe Calculator Co. for figures 28-4, 28-5 and 28-6.

3-M Company for figures 28-7 and 28-8.

Paymaster for figure 28-10.

Pitney Bowes for figures 20-6 and 20-8.

Professional Equipment Service Co. for figure 29-3.

Record-O-Fone for figure 5-5.

Social Security Administration for figure 16-6.

State of Mississippi, Medicaid Commission, for figure 12-2.

Summit Orthodontic Laboratory for figure 21-7.

Veterans Administration for figure 12-3

Contributions by Delmar Staff:

Director of Publications — Alan N. Knofla

Source Editor — Angela Emmi

Copy Editor — Ruth Saur

Director of Manufacturing and Production — Frederick Sharer

Illustrators — Anthony Canabush, George Dowse, Michael Kokernak

Production Specialists — Sharon Lynch, Patti Manuli, Jean LeMorta, Betty Michelfelder, Lee St. Onge, Debbie Monty and Alice Schielke

Index

Various blank forms have been reproduced for student use, and begin on the next page. For guidance in completing each one, refer to the list and text page indicated below:

Forms are reproduced through courtesy of the Colwell Co., Veterans Administration, and Codesco Davidson Dental Supply Co. Some are duplications of those illustrated in the text; others are updated or alternate forms which are used for the same purpose.

DAILY SCHEDULE

8:00	
15	
30	
45	
9:00	
15	
30	
45	
10:00	
15	
30	
45	
11:00	
15	
30	
45	
12:00	
15	
30	
45	
1:00	
15	
30	
45	
2:00	
15	
30	
45	
3:00	
15	
30	
45	
4:00	
15	
30	
45	
5:00	

Daily Schedule

```
┌─────────────────────────────────────────────────────────────┐
│  Mr.                        REGISTRATION                      │
│  Mrs.                                                         │
│  Miss                              S M W D        DATE ____   │
│  _____         │
│  HOME ADDRESS                   HOME TEL.                     │
│  _____         │
│  DATE OF BIRTH                  SOC. SEC. NO.                 │
│  _____         │
│  EMPLOYER                    ADDRESS                          │
│  _____         │
│  OCCUPATION                  BUS. TEL.                        │
│  _____         │
│  PREVIOUS                                                     │
│  ADDRESS            CITY              STATE                   │
│  _____         │
│  PERSON RESPONSIBLE                                           │
│  FOR ACCOUNT                                                  │
│  _____         │
│  ADDRESS                                                      │
│  _____         │
│  REFERRED BY                 PHYSICIAN                        │
│  _____         │
│  DENTAL INSURANCE PROGRAM            LOCAL NO.                │
│  _____         │
│  PURPOSE OF CALL                                             │
│  _____         │
│  PREFERRED DAY FOR APPTS.    TIME          AM  PM            │
│  _____         │
│  REMARKS                                                     │
│  _____         │
│  _____         │
│  _____         │
│                                                              │
│        Form 1063 Colwell Co., Champaign, Illinois            │
└─────────────────────────────────────────────────────────────┘
```

Registration Form

PATIENT MEDICAL-DENTAL HISTORY

Date _____

Name _____   Residence _____
       Last   First   M. In.   Date of Birth _____

PATIENT MEDICAL HISTORY

Physician _____ Office Phone _____ Home Phone _____

Approximate date of last physical examination _____

	Yes	No
1. Are you under any medical treatment now?	☐	☐
2. Have you had any major operations? If so what?	☐	☐
3. Have you ever had a serious accident involving head injuries?	☐	☐
4. Have you had any adverse response to any drugs including penicillin?	☐	☐
5. Has a physician ever informed you that you had: A Heart Ailment?	☐	☐
6. High blood pressure?	☐	☐
7. Respiratory disease?	☐	☐
8. Diabetes?	☐	☐
9. Rheumatic fever?	☐	☐
10. Rheumatism or arthritis?	☐	☐
11. Tumors or growths?	☐	☐
12. Any blood disease?	☐	☐
13. Any liver disease?	☐	☐
14. Any kidney disease?	☐	☐
15. Any stomach or intestinal disease?	☐	☐
16. Any venereal disease?	☐	☐
17. Yellow jaundice or hepatitis?	☐	☐
18. Do you have night sweats accompanied by weight loss or cough?	☐	☐
19. Are you on a diet at this time?	☐	☐
20. Are you now taking drugs or medications?	☐	☐
21. Are you allergic to any known materials resulting—in hives, asthma, eczema, etc.?	☐	☐
22. Are you in general good health at this time?	☐	☐
23. Have any wounds healed slowly or presented other complications?	☐	☐
24. Are you pregnant?	☐	☐
25. Do you have a history of fainting?	☐	☐
26. Have you ever had any X-RAY TREATMENTS (other than diagnostic)?	☐	☐

PATIENT DENTAL HISTORY

	Yes	No
27. Do you have pain in or near your ears?	☐	☐
28. Do you have any unhealed injuries or inflamed areas in or around your mouth?	☐	☐
29. Have you experienced any growth or sore spots in your mouth?	☐	☐
30. Does any part of your mouth hurt when clenched?	☐	☐
31. Have you ever had Novocaine anesthetic?	☐	☐
32. Any reactions or allergic symptoms to novocaine?	☐	☐
33. Any difficult extractions in the past?	☐	☐
34. Prolonged bleeding following extractions in the past?	☐	☐
35. Trench Mouth?	☐	☐
36. Do your gums bleed?	☐	☐
37. Have you ever had instruction on the correct method of brushing your teeth?	☐	☐
38. Have you ever had instructions on the care of your gums?	☐	☐
39. Do you chew on only one side of your mouth? If so why?	☐	☐
40. Do you at the present time have any dental complaints?	☐	☐
41. Do you habitually clench your teeth during the night or day?	☐	☐
42. When was your last full mouth X-RAY taken? _____ Where? _____		
43. Any part of your mouth sore to pressures or irritants (cold, sweets, etc.)	☐	☐
If so locate _____		

Signature _____

FORM 9879 COLWELL CO., CHAMPAIGN, ILL.

Medical-Dental History Form

LAST NAME FIRST NAME CITY STATE

OCCUPATION

RESIDENCE TEL. RESIDENCE ADDRESS CITY DATE OF EXAM

BUSINESS TEL. BUSINESS ADDRESS

NAME OF PHYSICIAN

RECOMMENDED BY

S M D W C

LEFT

RIGHT

MISSING TEETH, EXISTING RESTORATIONS, CAVITIES, ABNORMALITIES

DENTAL RESTORATIONS AND TREATMENTS

LEFT

RIGHT

1 2 3 4 5 6 7 8 9 10 11 12 13 14 15 16 17
32 31 30 29 28 27 26 25 24 23 22 21 20 19 18

PROSTHETICS & SURGERY

L. R. L. R.

STUDY MODELS

PHOTOGRAPHS – BEFORE

AFTER

RADIOGRAPHIC HISTORY DATE TYPE

TOOTH	MOULD		SHADE	
	UPPER	LOWER	UPPER	LOWER
CENT.				
LAT.				
CUSP.				
POST.				

REMARKS

BIRTHDAY SCHOOL GRADE

PETS NICKNAME

OUTSIDE INTERESTS

HABITS: THUMB OR FINGER SUCKING

MOUTH BREATHER

LIP OR CHEEK BITE

OTHER

PAST ILLNESSES: TONSILS AND OR ADENOIDS

MEASLES MUMPS

CHICKEN POX DIPHTHERIA

WHOOPING COUGH RHEUMATIC FEVER

SCARLET FEVER ALLERGIES

HEALTH HISTORY

CHIEF COMPLAINT

ORAL FINDINGS

HYGIENE 1 2 3 4

DEPOSITS 1 2 3 4

PERIODONT 1 2 3 4

OCCLUSION

ABNORMALITIES

WHEN WAS LAST DENTAL VISIT

PROPHYLAXIS RESTORATIONS EXTRACTIONS

OTHER TREATMENT

GENERAL PHYSICAL CONDITION

LAST COMPLETE PHYSICAL EXAM

UNDER PHYSICIAN'S CARE NOW?

WHOM NATURE OF TREATMENT

RECEIVING ANY MEDICATION

PREVIOUS HISTORY OF BLEEDING

REACTION TO ANESTHETICS

ALLERGIES

CHRONIC AILMENTS: HEART RHEUMATIC FEVER

BLOOD PRESSURE ARTHRITIS

ANEMIA NERVOUSNESS

HEADACHES SINUS

PAIN IN REGION OF EAR SMOKE

PREGNANT

OTHER

DENTURES:

UPPER TYPE HOW LONG

LOWER TYPE HOW LONG

PARTIALS: TYPE HOW LONG

TYPE HOW LONG

FORM 9766 COLWELL CO., CHAMPAIGN, ILL.

A Comprehensive Dental Chart.

297

NAME		DATE		AGE
ADDRESS			TELEPHONE	
BUSINESS ADDRESS		TELEPHONE		
CHARGE TO		ADDRESS		
ESTIMATE		REFERRED BY		
REMARKS				

FORM 2420   COLWELL CO. CHAMPAIGN, ILL.

NAME			ADDRESS				
DATE	TOOTH		SERVICE RENDERED	CHARGE		PAID	BALANCE

An Adult Dental Chart

298

NOTE – ALL ENTRIES SHOULD BE TYPEWRITTEN. IF BALLPOINT PEN MUST BE USED, APPLY HEAVY PRESSURE.

1. ISSUING OFFICE: Veterans Administration

MEDICAL ADJUNCT CERTIFICATION	2. DENTAL TREATMENT IS ☐ IS NOT ☐ NECESSARY AS ADJUNCT TO MEDICAL DISABILITY OF:	3. SIGNATURE AND DATE

4. FOR VA FISCAL USE ONLY			5. FISCAL SYMBOL	6. OB. NO. AND D.S.	9. EXAMINATION AUTHORIZATION (Authorizing Signature and Date – for services and fees listed in Items 17 and 22)
APPROVED	VOUCHER AUDIT	DATE	36__0160.001		
$			7. VA REGULATION	8. AUTH. EXP. DATE	

FEE DENTIST

EXAMINATION AUTHORIZATION does *NOT* allow for proceeding with definitive dental care. Complete all applicable Items 10 thru 21 and return (with X-rays) for *TREATMENT AUTHORIZATION.* After all treatment is completed return remaining packet as invoice for payment.

10. NAME AND ADDRESS OF FEE DENTIST	11. SOC. SEC. OR GROUP IRS NO.	12. LICENSE NO.
	13. SIGNATURE OF FEE DENTIST	
ZIP		
TELEPHONE NO.		

14. "X" OUT MISSING TEETH

ENTER ONLY ONE TOOTH NO., ONE PROCEDURE, ONE DATE OF SERVICE AND ONE FEE PER LINE.

15. TOOTH #	16. SUR-FACES (MO, DO, MOD, etc.)	17. DESCRIPTION OF SERVICE (List treatment recommendations)	18. DATE SERVICES PERFORMED			19. CODE NO.	20. FEE	22. FOR VA USE ONLY
			MO.	DAY	YR.			
		X-RAYS (Type and No.)						
		EXAMINATION (Indicate date) ⟶						
							23. TOTAL ▶	

21. REMARKS (Include significant periodontal disease, soft tissue lesions, presence and serviceability of existing prostheses, pathogenicity of impacted teeth and statement concerning teeth extracted while in service. (Attach additional sheet if necessary.)

24. SERVICES NOT LINED OUT IN ITEM 17 ARE APPROVED (Signature of Chief, Dental Service or Designee and Date)	25. FISCAL SYMBOL	26. OB. NO. AND D.S.	29. TREATMENT AUTHORIZATION (Authorizing Signature and Date)
	36__0160.001		
	27. VA REGULATION	28. AUTH. EXP. DATE	

30. PRINT BENEFICIARY'S NAME, IDENTIFICATION NO., CURRENT ADDRESS, ZIP CODE, AND TELEPHONE NO.	31. THE SERVICES AND FEES LISTED ARE APPROVED EXCEPT –
	32. SIGNATURE OF APPROVING OFFICIAL AND DATE

VA FORM MAR 1973 **10-2570d**

DENTAL RECORD, AUTHORIZATION AND INVOICE FOR OUTPATIENT SERVICES – COPY 1

Veterans Administration Form for Participating Dentist

ATTENDING DENTIST'S STATEMENT   ADS (71)

CHECK ONE:
☐ DENTIST'S PRE-TREATMENT ESTIMATE
☐ DENTIST'S STATEMENT OF ACTUAL SERVICES
Spaced for Typewriter - Marks for Tabulator Appear on this Line

1. EMPLOYEE NAME			2. SOCIAL SECURITY NUMBER

3. ADDRESS	CITY	STATE OR PROVINCE	ZIP

4. PATIENT NAME (IF A DEPENDENT)	5. RELATIONSHIP TO EMPLOYEE	6. BIRTH DATE MO. DA. YR.	7. DATE FIRST VISIT (CURRENT SERIES)

8. EMPLOYER NAME	9. DOES PATIENT HAVE OTHER HEALTH COVERAGE? YES ☐ NO ☐ IF "YES" PLEASE IDENTIFY.

10. GROUP DENTAL PLAN NAME	11. POLICY NUMBER	12. UNION LOCAL NO.

13. DENTIST'S NAME (PRINT)	14. LICENSE NO.	15. INDIVIDUAL PRACTITIONERS - SS# ALL OTHERS - EMPLOYER I.D.#

16. ADDRESS CITY STATE OR PROVINCE ZIP	MUST BE FURNISHED UNDER AUTHORITY OF LAW

17. IS ANY OF THE TREATMENT FOR:
(A) ORTHODONTIC PURPOSES? YES ☐ NO ☐   (B) ACCIDENTAL INJURY? YES ☐ NO ☐   (C) OCCUPATIONAL INJURY? YES ☐ NO ☐

18. IF PROSTHESIS, IS THIS INITIAL PLACEMENT? YES ☐ NO ☐ IF NO, REASON FOR REPLACEMENT:
19. DATE OF PRIOR PLACEMENT? MO. DA. YR.
20. ARE X-RAYS ENCLOSED? YES ☐ NO ☐ IF YES, HOW MANY?

EXAMINATION AND TREATMENT RECORD - USE CHARTING SYSTEM SHOWN

TOOTH # OR LETTER	SURFACES	DESCRIPTION OF SERVICE (INCLUDING X-RAYS, PROPHYLAXIS MATERIALS USED, ETC.)	DATE SERVICE PERFORMED MO. DA. YR.	ADA PROCEDURE NUMBER	FEE	FOR CARRIER USE ONLY

LABIAL
LINGUAL
RIGHT   LEFT
UPPER   PERMANENT
LOWER   PRIMARY
LINGUAL
LABIAL

INDICATE MISSING TEETH WITH AN "X"

REMARKS FOR UNUSUAL SERVICES

ORTHODONTICS: *(give diagnosis, class of malocclusion and describe appliance(s) in above treatment section)*

DATE FIRST APPLIANCE INSERTED _____
DATE LAST APPLIANCE REMOVED _____
TREATMENT PERIOD (NUMBER MONTHS) _____
TOTAL FEE $ _____

TOTAL FEE ACTUALLY CHARGED	
PATIENT PAYS	
BALANCE	
CARRIER %	
CARRIER PAYS	

I HAVE REVIEWED THE FOREGOING TREATMENT PLAN. I AUTHORIZE RELEASE OF ANY INFORMATION RELATING TO THIS CLAIM.

_____ DATE _____
SIGNED (PATIENT, OR PARENT IF MINOR)

I HEREBY CERTIFY THAT THE SERVICES LISTED ABOVE   WILL BE ☐   HAVE BEEN ☐ PERFORMED

_____ DATE _____
SIGNED (DENTIST)

I HEREBY AUTHORIZE PAYMENT DIRECTLY TO THE ABOVE-NAMED DENTIST OF THE GROUP INSURANCE BENEFITS OTHERWISE PAYABLE TO ME, BUT NOT TO EXCEED THE CHARGES SHOWN. I UNDERSTAND THAT I AM FINANCIALLY RESPONSIBLE FOR ANY CHARGES NOT COVERED BY THIS AUTHORIZATION.

_____ DATE _____
SIGNED (INSURED PERSON)

SEE INSTRUCTIONS ON REVERSE SIDE   *Form Approved by the Council on Dental Care Programs of the A.D.A. 1971*

Attending Dentist's Statement

			Friday	July 9			

HOUR	NAME OF PATIENT	SERVICE RENDERED	CHARGE	CASH	REC'D ON ACCOUNT	√
1						
2						
3						
4						
5						
6						
7						
8						
9						
10						
11						
12						
13						
14						
15						
16						
17						
18						
19						
20						
21						
22						
23						
24						
25						
26						
27						
28						
29						
30						
31						
32						
33						
34						
35						
36						
37						
38						
39						
40						
CARRY TOTALS FORWARD TO BUSINESS SUMMARY		TOTALS				

FORM 4201   COLWELL CO. CHAMPAIGN. ILL.

Page from a Daily Log

January   Expense Sheet One

JAN

	DRUGS AND SUPPLIES				SALARIES				DUES, MEETINGS		
DAY	ITEM	AMOUNT		DAY	ITEM	AMOUNT		DAY	ITEM	AMOUNT	
									TOTAL		
								OFFICE SUPPLIES, STAMPS ETC.			
					TOTAL						
				OFFICE RENT, UPKEEP							
	TOTAL										
AUTOMOBILE UPKEEP											
					TOTAL						
				LAUNDRY SERVICE							
								TOTAL		
								PROFESSIONAL INSURANCE			
					TOTAL				TOTAL		
				ELECTRICITY, GAS, WATER				BUSINESS TAXES			
								DO NOT INCLUDE WITHHOLDING TAX. INCLUDE ONLY ½ SOCIAL SECURITY TAX			
					TOTAL						
				TELEPHONES, TOLLS				TOTAL		
								INTEREST PAID			
	TOTAL				TOTAL				TOTAL		

FORM 42028 COLWELL CO., CHAMPAIGN, ILL.

First Page of Expense Sheet

Expense Sheet Two   January

ENTERTAINMENT						MISCELLANEOUS		
DAY	ITEM	AMOUNT	DAY	ITEM	AMOUNT	DAY	ITEM	AMOUNT
	TOTAL			TOTAL				
	TOTAL			TOTAL			TOTAL	

CARRY TOTALS FORWARD TO **SUMMARY** OF **EXPENSE**

SUMMARY OF EXPENSE		
	AMOUNT	
DRUGS AND SUPPLIES		
AUTOMOBILE UPKEEP		
SALARIES		
OFFICE RENT UPKEEP		
LAUNDRY SERVICE		
ELECTRICITY, GAS, WATER		
TELEPHONES TOLLS		
DUES MEETINGS		
OFFICE SUPPLIES, STAMPS, ETC.		
PROFESSIONAL INSURANCE		
BUSINESS TAXES		
INTEREST PAID		
ENTERTAINMENT		
MISCELLANEOUS		
TOTAL FOR PRESENT MONTH		
FORWARDED FROM PREVIOUS MONTH		
GRAND TOTAL		

MONTHLY BALANCES		
FOR THE PRESENT MONTH		
TOTAL CASH RECEIVED		
TOTAL EXPENSE		
NET EARNINGS		
FOR THE YEAR TO DATE		
GRAND TOTAL CASH		
GRAND TOTAL EXPENSE		
NET EARNINGS		
EQUIPMENT (NONDEDUCTIBLE)		
DAY	ITEM	AMOUNT
	* TOTAL	

* ENTER THIS TOTAL DIRECT IN **ANNUAL SUMMARY**

FORM 4203A COLWELL CO., CHAMPAIGN, ILL.

Second Page of Expense Sheet

Business Summary   September

DAY OF MONTH	CHARGE BUSINESS		CASH BUSINESS		RECEIVED ON ACCOUNTS		TOTAL BUSINESS		TOTAL CASH RECEIVED	
1										
2										
3										
4										
5										
6										
7										
8										
9										
10										
11										
12										
13										
14										
15										
16										
17										
18										
19										
20										
21										
22										
23										
24										
25										
26										
27										
28										
29										
30										
31										
TOTAL FOR THE MONTH										
BROUGHT FORWARD										
GRAND TOTAL										

CARRY ALL **GRAND TOTALS** FORWARD TO **BUSINESS SUMMARY** OF FOLLOWING MONTH

FORM 4202A COLWELL CO CHAMPAIGN ILL

SEPT

Business Summary

Check No. 8110

John A. Doe, D.D.S.
3005 Anywhere St.
Great City, N.Y. 20000

No. **8110**

58-345 / 356

19____

PAY TO THE ORDER OF _____ $ _____

_____ DOLLARS

FOR _____

PROGRESSIVE BANK AND TRUST CO.
Great City, N.Y.

John A. Doe, D.D.S.

⑈035⑈0345⑈ ⑈82⑈068⑈17⑈

Check No. 8111

John A. Doe, D.D.S.
3005 Anywhere St.
Great City, N.Y. 20000

No. **8111**

58-345 / 356

19____

PAY TO THE ORDER OF _____ $ _____

_____ DOLLARS

FOR _____

PROGRESSIVE BANK AND TRUST CO.
Great City, N.Y.

John A. Doe, D.D.S.

⑈035⑈0345⑈ ⑈82⑈068⑈17⑈

Check No. 8112

John A. Doe, D.D.S.
3005 Anywhere St.
Great City, N.Y. 20000

No. **8112**

58-345 / 356

19____

PAY TO THE ORDER OF _____ $ _____

_____ DOLLARS

FOR _____

PROGRESSIVE BANK AND TRUST CO.
Great City, N.Y.

John A. Doe, D.D.S.

⑈035⑈0345⑈ ⑈82⑈068⑈17⑈

Check Stub No. 8110

No. **8110**

BAL. BRO'T FOR'D

19____

ORDER OF

FOR

DEPOSITS

TOTAL

AMOUNT THIS CHECK

BALANCE

Check Stub No. 8111

No. **8111**

19____

ORDER OF

FOR

DEPOSITS

TOTAL

AMOUNT THIS CHECK

BALANCE

Check Stub No. 8112

No. **8112**

19____

ORDER OF

FOR

DEPOSITS

TOTAL

AMOUNT THIS CHECK

BALANCE

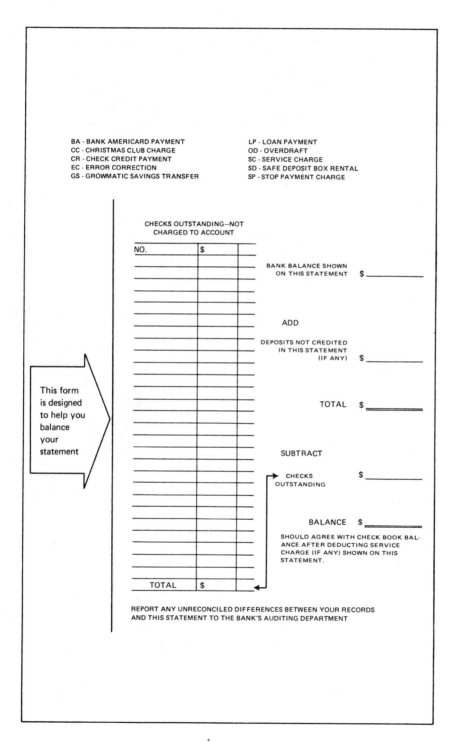

BA - BANK AMERICARD PAYMENT
CC - CHRISTMAS CLUB CHARGE
CR - CHECK CREDIT PAYMENT
EC - ERROR CORRECTION
GS - GROWMATIC SAVINGS TRANSFER

LP - LOAN PAYMENT
OD - OVERDRAFT
SC - SERVICE CHARGE
SD - SAFE DEPOSIT BOX RENTAL
SP - STOP PAYMENT CHARGE

CHECKS OUTSTANDING—NOT CHARGED TO ACCOUNT

NO.	$	

This form is designed to help you balance your statement

BANK BALANCE SHOWN ON THIS STATEMENT $ _____

ADD

DEPOSITS NOT CREDITED IN THIS STATEMENT (IF ANY) $ _____

TOTAL $ _____

SUBTRACT

CHECKS OUTSTANDING $ _____

BALANCE $ _____

SHOULD AGREE WITH CHECK BOOK BALANCE AFTER DEDUCTING SERVICE CHARGE (IF ANY) SHOWN ON THIS STATEMENT.

TOTAL	$	

REPORT ANY UNRECONCILED DIFFERENCES BETWEEN YOUR RECORDS AND THIS STATEMENT TO THE BANK'S AUDITING DEPARTMENT

Reconciliation Form

NAME:				SOC. SEC. NO.				NUMBER OF EXEMPTIONS			
DATE	HOURS	RATE	GROSS PAY	WITHHOLDING	F. I. C. A.					NET PAY	
		TOTALS									
QUARTER		BROUGHT FWD.									
		TO DATE									
YEAR		BROUGHT FWD.									
		TO DATE									

NAME:				SOC. SEC. NO.				NUMBER OF EXEMPTIONS			
DATE	HOURS	RATE	GROSS PAY	WITHHOLDING	F. I. C. A.					NET PAY	
		TOTALS									
QUARTER		BROUGHT FWD.									
		TO DATE									
YEAR		BROUGHT FWD.									
		TO DATE									

NAME:				SOC. SEC. NO.				NUMBER OF EXEMPTIONS			
DATE	HOURS	RATE	GROSS PAY	WITHHOLDING	F. I. C. A.					NET PAY	
		TOTALS									
QUARTER		BROUGHT FWD.									
		TO DATE									
YEAR		BROUGHT FWD.									
		TO DATE									

AUG

NAME:				SOC. SEC. NO.				NUMBER OF EXEMPTIONS			
DATE	HOURS	RATE	GROSS PAY	WITHHOLDING	F. I. C. A.					NET PAY	
		TOTALS									
QUARTER		BROUGHT FWD.									
		TO DATE									
YEAR		BROUGHT FWD.									
		TO DATE									

FORM 4233   COLWELL CO., CHAMPAIGN, ILL.

Employee's Earning Record

Form W–4 (Revised April 1975)
Employee's Withholding Allowance Certificate
(Use for wages paid after April 30, 1975 and before January 1, 1976)
The explanatory material below will help you determine your correct number of withholding allowances, and will assist you in completing the Form W–4 at the bottom of this page.

Avoid Overwithholding or Underwithholding

By claiming the proper number of withholding allowances you are entitled to, you can fit the amount of tax withheld from your wages to your tax liability. In addition to the allowances for personal exemptions to be claimed in items (a) through (g) below, be sure you claim any additional allowances you are entitled to in item (h) "Special withholding allowance," and item (i) "Allowance(s) for itemized deductions." While these allowances may be claimed on Form W–4 for withholding purposes, they are not to be claimed under "Exemptions" on your tax return Form 1040 or Form 1040A.

You may claim the special withholding allowance if you are single with only one employer, or married with only one employer and your spouse is not employed. If you have unusually large itemized deductions, you may claim the allowance(s) for itemized deductions to avoid having too much income tax withheld from your wages. On the other hand, if you and your spouse are both employed or you have more than one employer, you should take steps to assure that enough has been withheld. If you find that you need more withholding, claim fewer exemptions or ask for additional withholding. If you are currently claiming additional withholding allowances based on itemized deductions, check the table on the back to see that you are claiming the proper number of allowances.

How Many Withholding Allowances May You Claim?

Please use the schedule below to determine the number of allowances you may claim for tax withholding purposes. In determining the number, keep in mind these points: If you are single and hold more than one job, you may not claim the same allowances with more than one employer at the same time; or if you are married and both you and your spouse are employed, you may not claim the same allowances with your employers at the same time. A nonresident alien, other than a resident of Canada, Mexico, or Puerto Rico, may claim only one personal allowance.

Figure Your Total Withholding Allowances Below

(a) Allowance for yourself—enter 1 . . . . _____

(b) Allowance for your spouse—enter 1 . . . . _____

(c) Allowance for your age—if 65 or over—enter 1 . . . , ... _____

(d) Allowance for your spouse's age—if 65 or over—enter 1 . . . . _____

(e) Allowance for blindness (yourself)—enter 1 . . . . _____

(f) Allowance for blindness (spouse's)—enter 1 . . . . _____

(g) Allowance(s) for dependent(s)—you are entitled to claim an allowance for each dependent you will be able to claim on your Federal income tax return. Do not include yourself or your spouse * . . . . _____

(h) Special withholding allowance—if you are single with only one employer, or married with only one employer and your spouse is not employed—enter 1** . . . . _____

(i) Allowance(s) for itemized deductions—if you do plan to itemize deductions on your income tax return, enter the number from the table on back** . . . . _____

(j) Total—add lines (a) through (i) above. Enter here and on line 1, Form W–4 below . . . . _____

* If you are in doubt as to whom you may claim as a dependent, see the instructions which came with your last Federal income tax return or call your local Internal Revenue Service office.

** This allowance is used solely for purposes of figuring your withholding tax, and cannot be claimed when you file your tax return.

See Table on Back if You Plan to Itemize Your Deductions

Completing Form W–4.—If you find that you are entitled to one or more allowances in addition to those which you are now claiming, increase your number of allowances by completing the form below and filing it with your employer. If the number of allowances you previously claimed decreases, you must file a new Form W–4 within 10 days. (Should you expect to owe more tax than will be withheld, you may use the same form to increase your withholding by claiming fewer or "0" allowances on line 1, or by asking for additional withholding on line 2, or both.)

▼ Give the bottom part of this form to your employer; keep the upper part for your records and information ▼

- Cut along this line -

Form **W-4** (Rev. April 1975) Department of the Treasury Internal Revenue Service	# Employee's Withholding Allowance Certificate (This certificate is for income tax withholding purposes only; it will remain in effect until you change it.)	
Type or print your full name		Your social security number
Home address (Number and street or rural route)		Marital status ☐ Single ☐ Married
City or town, State and ZIP code		(If married but legally separated, or spouse is a nonresident alien, check the single block.)

1 Total number of allowances you are claiming . . . . _____

2 Additional amount, if any, you want deducted from each pay (if your employer agrees) . . . . $ _____

I certify that to the best of my knowledge and belief, the number of withholding allowances claimed on this certificate does not exceed the number to which I am entitled.

Signature ▶ .... Date ▶ ...., 19 ....

Employee's Withholding Allowance Certificate (Form W–4)

APPLICATION FOR A SOCIAL SECURITY NUMBER

ID   CN   DO

See Instructions on Back.   Print in Black or Dark Blue Ink or Use Typewriter.   ⌐ DO NOT WRITE IN THE ABOVE SPACE ⌐

1 *Print* FULL NAME YOU WILL USE IN WORK OR BUSINESS   (First Name)   (Middle Name or Initial – if none, draw line ___)   (Last Name)

2 *Print* FULL NAME GIVEN YOU AT BIRTH   **6** YOUR DATE OF BIRTH   (Month) (Day) (Year)

3 PLACE OF BIRTH   (City)   (County if known)   (State)   **7** YOUR PRESENT AGE (Age on *last* birthday)

4 MOTHER'S FULL NAME AT HER BIRTH (Her maiden name)   **8** YOUR SEX   MALE   FEMALE

5 FATHER'S FULL NAME (Regardless of whether living or dead)   **9** YOUR COLOR OR RACE   WHITE   NEGRO   OTHER

10 HAVE YOU EVER BEFORE APPLIED FOR OR HAD A SOCIAL SECURITY, RAILROAD, OR TAX ACCOUNT NUMBER?   NO   DON'T KNOW   YES   (If "YES" Print STATE in which you applied and DATE you applied and SOCIAL SECURITY NUMBER if known)

11 YOUR MAILING ADDRESS   (Number and Street, Apt. No., P.O. Box, or Rural Route)   (City)   (State)   (Zip Code)

12 TODAY'S DATE   NOTICE: Whoever, with intent to falsify his or someone else's true identity, willfully furnishes or causes to be furnished false information in applying for a social security number, is subject to a fine of not more than $1,000 or imprisonment for up to 1 year, or both.

13 TELEPHONE NUMBER   **14** Sign YOUR NAME HERE (Do Not Print)

TREASURY DEPARTMENT Internal Revenue Service   ☐ RESCREEN   ☐ ASSIGN   ☐ DUP ISSUED   Return completed application to nearest SOCIAL SECURITY ADMINISTRATION OFFICE
FORM **SS-5** (2-73)

An Application for a Social Security Number (Form SS-5).

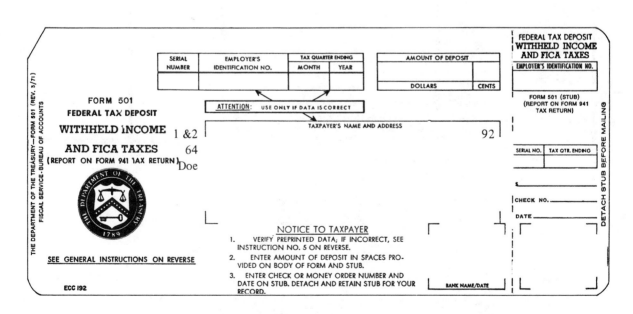

Monthly Federal Tax Deposit Form 501.

Form **941**
(Rev. Apr. 1977)
Department of the Treasury
Internal Revenue Service

Employer's Quarterly Federal Tax Return

Schedule A—Quarterly Report of Wages Taxable under the Federal Insurance Contributions Act—FOR SOCIAL SECURITY

List for each nonagricultural employee the WAGES taxable under the FICA which were paid during the quarter. If you pay an employee more than $16,500 in a calendar year, report only the first $16,500 of such wages. In the case of "Tip Income," see instructions on page 4. IF WAGES WERE NOT TAXABLE UNDER THE FICA, MAKE NO ENTRIES IN ITEMS 1 THROUGH 9 AND 14 THROUGH 18.

SSA Use Only

F ☐ 2 ☐ U ☐ E ☐
S ☐ 1 ☐ L ☐ T ☐
X ☐ 0 ☐ V ☐ A ☐

1. Total pages of this return including this page and any pages of Form 941a ▶	2. Total number of employees listed ▶	3. (First quarter only) Number of employees (except household) employed in the pay period including March 12th ▶

4. EMPLOYEE'S SOCIAL SECURITY NUMBER	5. NAME OF EMPLOYEE (Please type or print)	6. TAXABLE FICA WAGES Paid to Employee in Quarter (Before Deductions)		7. TAXABLE TIPS REPORTED (See page 4)	
000 00 0000 ▼	▼	Dollars	Cents	Dollars	Cents

If you need more space for listing employees, use Schedule A continuation sheets, Form 941a.

Totals for this page—Wage total in column 6 and tip total in column 7 ⟶

8. TOTAL WAGES TAXABLE UNDER FICA PAID DURING QUARTER. $ ◁

(Total of column 6 on this page and continuation sheets.) Enter here and in item 14 below.

9. TOTAL TAXABLE TIPS REPORTED UNDER FICA DURING QUARTER. $ ◁

(Total of column 7 on this page and continuation sheets.) Enter here and in item 15 below. (If no tips reported, write "None.")

Name (as distinguished from trade name)   Date quarter ended

Employer's name, address, employer ▶

Trade name, if any   Employer Identification No.

Address and ZIP code

Employer's Quarterly Federal Tax Return (Form 941)

STATEMENT

LEONARD S. TAYLOR, M.D.
2100 WEST PARK AVENUE
TELEPHONE 367-6671   CHAMPAIGN, ILLINOIS 61822

DATE	FAMILY MEMBER	PROFESSIONAL SERVICE	CHARGE	CREDITS		BALANCE
				PAYM'TS	ADJ	
		BALANCE FORWARD ▷				

1625   PAY LAST AMOUNT IN THIS COLUMN ⬆

OC - OFFICE CALL	INS - INSURANCE	PE - PHYSICAL EXAMINATION
HC - HOUSE CALL	OB - OBSTETRICAL CARE	EKG - ELECTROCARDIOGRAM
HOSP - HOSPITAL CARE	PAP - PAPANICOLAOU TEST	XR - X-RAY
L - LABORATORY	OS - OFFICE SURGERY	M - MEDICATION
I - INJECTION	HS - HOSPITAL SURGERY	NC - NO CHARGE

Financial Record or Ledger Card

311

CUSTOMER

CODESCO DISTRIBUTION DIVISION

SUP-01 9/75

INVOICE

ACCOUNT NAME

DATE / /

QUANTITY OR UNIT	QUANTITY SHIPPED		TAX	MANUFACTURER OR DESCRIPTION
	NOW	LATER		

ACCOUNT NUMBER

CD INVENTORY NUMBER

TYPE

SYM

TERR

TAX

TOTAL AMOUNT

SUB TOTAL

DELIVERY/POSTAGE

TAX

INVOICE TOTAL

INVOICE MUST ACCOMPANY RETURNED GOODS

SALESMAN | FILLED | CHECKED

1 — MAIL
2 — PHONE
3 — SALESMAN
4 — COUNTER
5 — BACK ORDER
6 — OTHER

SOURCE

PURCHASE ORDER NUMBER

INVOICE NUMBER

903722

CODESCO

CODESCO

Sample Invoice for Dental Supplies

312

Item Room				Maximum Minimum			
Order Date	Rec'd Date	Quantity	Manuf.	Supply House	Unit Cost	Total Cost	Quantity On Hand

A Sample Equipment Control and Inventory Card.

Item Room			Manufacture Serial Number	
Order Date	Rec'd Date	Quantity	Description	Price
Date		Remarks		Maintenance Cost

A Sample Supply Control and Inventory Card.